# Nutrition and Quality of Life for Patients with Chronic Disease

# Nutrition and Quality of Life for Patients with Chronic Disease

Guest Editors

**Evridiki Patelarou**
**Konstantinos Giakoumidakis**

MDPI

Basel • Beijing • Wuhan • Barcelona • Belgrade • Novi Sad • Cluj • Manchester

*Guest Editors*
Evridiki Patelarou
Department of Nursing
Hellenic Mediterranean University
Heraklion
Greece

Konstantinos Giakoumidakis
Department of Nursing
Hellenic Mediterranean University
Heraklion
Greece

*Editorial Office*
MDPI AG
Grosspeteranlage 5
4052 Basel, Switzerland

This is a reprint of the Special Issue, published open access by the journal *Nutrients* (ISSN 2072-6643), freely accessible at: https://www.mdpi.com/journal/nutrients/special_issues/ZN9MZ6WY61.

For citation purposes, cite each article independently as indicated on the article page online and as indicated below:

Lastname, A.A.; Lastname, B.B. Article Title. *Journal Name* **Year**, *Volume Number*, Page Range.

**ISBN 978-3-7258-4855-3 (Hbk)**
**ISBN 978-3-7258-4856-0 (PDF)**
**https://doi.org/10.3390/books978-3-7258-4856-0**

# Contents

**About the Editors** . . . . . . . . . . vii

**Preface** . . . . . . . . . . ix

**Evridiki Patelarou and Konstantinos Giakoumidakis**
Nutrition and Quality of Life for Patients with Chronic Disease
Reprinted from: *Nutrients* **2025**, *17*, 2170, https://doi.org/10.3390/nu17132170 . . . . . . . . . . 1

**Francesca Galletta, Angela Klain, Sara Manti, Francesca Mori, Carolina Grella, Leonardo Tomei, et al.**
Parental Knowledge and Preventive Strategies in Pediatric IgE-Mediated Food Allergy—Results from a Cross-Sectional Survey
Reprinted from: *Nutrients* **2025**, *17*, 2387, https://doi.org/10.3390/nu17152387 . . . . . . . . . . 5

**Konstantinos Giakoumidakis, Evridiki Patelarou, Anastasia A. Chatziefstratiou, Dimitra Aloizou, Nikolaos Vaitsis, Hero Brokalaki, et al.**
Validation of the Greek Cardiovascular Diet Questionnaire 2 (CDQ-2) and Single-Center Cross-Sectional Insights into the Dietary Habits of Cardiovascular Patients
Reprinted from: *Nutrients* **2025**, *17*, 1649, https://doi.org/10.3390/nu17101649 . . . . . . . . . . 16

**Fifi Retiaty, Nuri Andarwulan, Nurheni Sri Palupi, Fitrah Ernawati, Renata Kazimierczak and Dominika Średnicka-Tober**
Contribution of Food, Energy, Macronutrients and Fiber Consumption Patterns to Obesity and Other Non-Communicable Disease Risks in the Indonesian Population
Reprinted from: *Nutrients* **2025**, *17*, 1459, https://doi.org/10.3390/nu17091459 . . . . . . . . . . 28

**Miguel García Samuelsson, Pedro Juan Tárraga López, Ángel Arturo López-González, Hernán Paublini, Emilio Martínez-Almoyna Rifá and José Ignacio Ramírez-Manent**
Assessment of the Risk of Insulin Resistance in Workers Classified as Metabolically Healthy Obese
Reprinted from: *Nutrients* **2025**, *17*, 1345, https://doi.org/10.3390/nu17081345 . . . . . . . . . . 46

**José M. Alcaide-Leyva, Manuel Romero-Saldaña, María García-Rodríguez, Rafael Molina-Luque, María del Rocío Jiménez-Mérida and Guillermo Molina-Recio**
Metabolic Syndrome in the Amazon: Customizing Diagnostic Methods for Urban Communities
Reprinted from: *Nutrients* **2025**, *17*, 538, https://doi.org/10.3390/nu17030538 . . . . . . . . . . 62

**Nan Hu, Jingyi Sun, Yujia Cao, Hongji Zhao, Meng Sun, Guanlong Li, et al.**
Anti-Fatigue Activity of Corn Protein Hydrolysate Fermented by Lactic Acid Bacteria
Reprinted from: *Nutrients* **2025**, *17*, 199, https://doi.org/10.3390/nu17020199 . . . . . . . . . . 78

**Maria Notarnicola, Valeria Tutino, Valentina De Nunzio, Anna Maria Cisternino, Miriam Cofano, Rossella Donghia, et al.**
Daily Orange Consumption Reduces Hepatic Steatosis Prevalence in Patients with Metabolic Dysfunction-Associated Steatotic Liver Disease: Exploratory Outcomes of a Randomized Clinical Trial
Reprinted from: *Nutrients* **2024**, *16*, 3191, https://doi.org/10.3390/nu16183191 . . . . . . . . . . 94

**Shaye Ludlow, Katherine Farragher, Kelly Squires, Susan Heaney, Jessica Orman, Sarah Pullen, et al.**
A Qualitative Study Supporting Optimal Nutrition in Advanced Liver Disease—Unlocking the Potential for Improvement
Reprinted from: *Nutrients* **2024**, *16*, 2403, https://doi.org/10.3390/nu16152403 . . . . . . . . . . 108

**Jacopo Ciaffi, Luana Mancarella, Claudio Ripamonti, Andrea D'Amuri, Veronica Brusi, Federica Pignatti, et al.**
Ultra-Processed Food and Its Impact on Bone Health and Joint Diseases: A Scoping Review
Reprinted from: *Nutrients* **2025**, *17*, 1188, https://doi.org/10.3390/nu17071188 . . . . . . . . . . . **124**

**Miroslaw Perlinski and Jacek Sobocki**
The Impact of Home Parenteral Nutrition on Survival and Quality of Life in Patients with Intestinal Failure and Advanced Cancer: A Comprehensive Review
Reprinted from: *Nutrients* **2025**, *17*, 905, https://doi.org/10.3390/nu17050905 . . . . . . . . . . . . **142**

# About the Editors

**Evridiki Patelarou**

Evridiki Patelarou has an educational background in medicine (University of Crete) and nursing (National and Kapodistrian University of Athens). She holds a master's in public health and a PhD in epidemiology. Her research career began at the Department of Social Medicine, Faculty of Medicine-University of Crete, where she was a researcher in a mother–child prospective study, "The RHEA" study. Her PhD examined the effect of environmental pollutants on pregnancy outcomes. Since then, her research has mainly focused on the evaluation of environmental exposures in the prenatal period and in early childhood and how they correlate with the development of the fetus and early-life diseases. Evridiki has a demonstrated record of accomplished and productive research projects that have been of high international relevance. Evridiki is the Editor in Chief of the *Population Medicine* journal and a member of the Editorial Board of several scientific journals (including the *World Journal of Meta-Analysis*, *European Journal of Midwifery*, *Tobacco Induced Diseases*, *Journal of Respiratory Medicine and Lung Disease*, etc.). She also serves as a regular reviewer for more than 20 peer-reviewed journals, including the *International Journal of Environmental Research and Public Health*, *Journal of Asthma*, *Journal of Developmental Origins of Health and Disease*, *Journal of Pediatric Biochemistry*, and *Journal of the American College of Nutrition*.

**Konstantinos Giakoumidakis**

Konstantinos Giakoumidakis is an Associate Professor in the Department of Nursing, Faculty of Health Sciences, at the Hellenic Mediterranean University, Heraklion (Greece). He is a graduate of the Department of Nursing of the National and Kapodistrian University of Athens, Greece; he holds a master's degree in clinical nursing and a PhD in nursing. He has been working as a Clinical Registered Nurse for 20 years in intensive care units. His research includes numerous peer-reviewed international and Hellenic journal publications, with an h-index of 19 and over 1000 citations according to Google Scholar. Dr. Giakoumidakis is certified in Cardiac Surgery Unit Advanced Life Support, Immediate Life Support, and the Morisky Scale, and he is a member of the Hellenic Nurses' Association Council on Cardiovascular Nursing and Allied Professions of the European Society of Cardiology. His current research interests focus on clinical nursing, cardiovascular nursing, and chronic diseases nursing management.

# Preface

This Special Issue highlights research on nutrition's role in improving quality of life for patients with chronic diseases, including diabetes, heart and kidney disease, cancer, and digestive disorders, and aims to provide healthcare professionals with practical insights into improving patient care through nutritional therapy. We thank all authors, reviewers, and the editorial team for their contributions to this important collection.

**Evridiki Patelarou and Konstantinos Giakoumidakis**
*Guest Editors*

nutrients

MDPI

*Editorial*

# Nutrition and Quality of Life for Patients with Chronic Disease

**Evridiki Patelarou and Konstantinos Giakoumidakis ***

Department of Nursing, School of Health Sciences, Hellenic Mediterranean University, 71410 Heraklion, Greece; epatelarou@hmu.gr
* Correspondence: kongiakoumidakis@hmu.gr; Tel.: +30-2810379549

## 1. Introduction

Chronic conditions such as cancer, heart disease, metabolic syndrome, liver disease, and renal failure significantly influence patients' social, emotional, and functional well-being, in addition to their physical symptoms [1,2]. Among the many modifiable aspects of health in chronic illness, nutrition has a significant impact on both overall quality of life (QoL) and clinical outcomes [3]. It appears that targeted nutrition interventions can modify immune and inflammatory responses, which are crucial parameters in the development of chronic disease [4]. Additionally, personalized nutrition therapy enhances the clinical course of patients with a wide range of chronic diseases, enhancing muscle functionality and fostering recovery mechanisms [5,6].

This Special Issue of *Nutrients*, titled "Nutrition and Quality of Life for Patients with Chronic Disease," brings together a multidisciplinary collection of original research and thorough reviews that clarify how individualized nutritional approaches can change the course of many chronic diseases, enhance functional ability, and increase life satisfaction. The nine published articles, which span the fields of hepatology, nephrology, rheumatology, cancer, cardiovascular health, public health, and public policy, demonstrate the complexity and potential of nutrition-based interventions in improving patient care. Apart from physical health, social and emotional domains, including social isolation and behavioral compliance, are also important factors influencing patient outcomes and health-related quality of life [7]. These behavioral interventions, which can help maintain lifestyle and dietary changes, are key to long-term adherence to dietary recommendations, which emphasizes the need for interdisciplinary care when dealing with chronic disease [8,9].

## 2. Key Contributions

Perlinski and Sobocki [10] thoroughly investigated advanced malignancy in chronic intestinal failure, home parenteral nutrition (HPN), and malignant bowel obstruction. Their pooled analysis of 34 studies showed that, with appropriate management, HPN can enhance QoL and, in some cases, prolong survival. Positive outcomes were associated with higher albumin levels, better performance status, and continued treatment. In the meantime, the authors emphasized the significant psychological effects of chronic HPN and supported patient-centered care strategies that combine nutritional therapy with mental health and social support.

Ciaffi et al.'s [11] scoping review of 19 studies explained the detrimental effects of ultra-processed foods (UPFs) on bone health and joint diseases, particularly in postmenopausal women and patients with knee osteoarthritis. UPF consumption was linked to an increased risk of osteoporosis, reduced bone mineral density, and a higher incidence of gout and rheumatoid arthritis. These results call for immediate public health measures to lower UPF consumption and encourage musculoskeletally appropriate whole-food eating habits.

 https://doi.org/10.3390/nu17132170

A qualitative study of advanced liver disease identifies several intricate causes of malnutrition, including gaps in healthcare delivery, dietary and physical limitations, symptom burden, a lack of social support, and structural issues [12]. The shortcomings of the current screening tools, which fail to adequately capture psychological and systemic factors, are revealed through interviews with doctors, caregivers, and patients. This leads to recommendations for comprehensive, customized screening techniques that will more effectively detect and address nutritional risk.

Notarnicola et al. [13] present compelling evidence from a randomized controlled study showing that daily orange consumption significantly reduces liver steatosis in metabolic dysfunction-associated steatotic liver disease. Individuals consuming 400 g of oranges per day showed a 30% decrease in liver fat after just four weeks, regardless of weight loss, suggesting the direct hepatoprotective effect of phytochemicals. The study supported the inclusion of foods high in phytochemicals in therapeutic diets for liver illnesses, even though fibrosis remained unchanged.

In a mouse model, experimental data from Hu et al. [14] showed that maize protein hydrolysate fermented by lactic acid bacteria (FCH) has anti-fatigue properties. High-dose FCH improved endurance, decreased oxidative stress, restored liver and muscle glycogen, and changed the ecology of the gut by raising Lactobacillus abundance. These results point to a potential gut–muscle axis mechanism and support further research on FCH as a functional meal with the goal of reducing fatigue.

To treat metabolic syndrome in low-resource settings, Alcaide-Leyva et al. created a highly sensitive and reasonably priced diagnostic methodology specifically for an urban population in the Peruvian Amazon [15]. The model achieved over 90% sensitivity in detecting metabolic syndrome in a population with a nearly 48% prevalence using systolic blood pressure and very-low-density lipoprotein cholesterol, highlighting the need for population-specific tools to guide targeted public health interventions in rapidly urbanizing settings.

According to the Spanish researchers García Samuelsson et al. [16], even if they do not have any overt signs of metabolic syndrome, metabolically healthy obese (MHO) people are more likely to develop insulin resistance. Low levels of physical activity, poor adherence to the Mediterranean diet, and socioeconomic disparities were identified as the primary causes of metabolic deterioration in a cohort of 68,884 obese workers, underscoring the transient nature of the MHO phenotype and the urgent need for early lifestyle interventions, particularly in occupational health settings.

An eight-year Indonesian cohort study by Retiaty et al. [17] examined the relationship between rising central and body mass index-based obesity rates and changing dietary patterns, which were characterized by a high intake of fat and oil and a low intake of fiber. Interestingly, despite increasing obesity rates, the biomarkers for non-communicable diseases remained relatively stable, highlighting the intricate connection between diet, obesity, and metabolic health, and pointing to important areas for intervention.

Finally, our research team translated and validated the Greek version of the Cardiovascular Diet Questionnaire 2 (CDQ-2), providing a validated tool for assessing the dietary habits of patients with cardiovascular disease. The Greek version of the CDQ-2 demonstrated high reliability and strong agreement with the current Mediterranean Diet Adherence Screener (MEDAS) measure, particularly among smokers, younger adults, men, and those who were less physically active. This proven technique provides a useful way to evaluate and adjust dietary interventions in cardiovascular disease management [18].

## 3. Conclusions

This Special Issue underscores the central role of nutrition in the comprehensive management of chronic diseases, addressing not only physical symptoms, but also mental health and overall quality of life. The studies collectively demonstrate how targeted dietary interventions—ranging from functional food compounds and validated screening tools to lifestyle modifications and micronutrient therapies—can prevent metabolic deterioration, support organ integrity, and alleviate disease burden. These findings advocate for integrated, individualized care models that address the biological, psychological, and social dimensions of nutrition-related health, recognizing the need for both clinical precision and cultural relevance [19,20]. Future research should adopt longitudinal, interdisciplinary designs to enhance risk stratification, unravel the mechanisms of nutrition–disease interactions, and scale effective nutritional care models—from clinical practice to occupational, community, and public health settings. Building stronger teamwork among healthcare professionals is key to successfully putting these care models into practice [21]. Ultimately, advancing nutrition as a pillar of evidence-based clinical practice holds the potential to transform the lives of millions living with chronic diseases worldwide [22].

**Author Contributions:** Conceptualization, E.P. and K.G.; writing—original draft preparation, E.P. and K.G.; writing—review and editing, E.P. and K.G.; supervision, E.P. and K.G.; project administration, E.P. and K.G. All authors have read and agreed to the published version of the manuscript.

**Funding:** This research received no external funding.

**Conflicts of Interest:** The authors declare no conflicts of interest.

## References

1. Taylor, R.M.; Haslam, R.L.; Herbert, J.; Whatnall, M.C.; Trijsburg, L.; de Vries, J.H.M.; Josefsson, M.S.; Koochek, A.; Nowicka, P.; Neuman, N.; et al. Diet quality and cardiovascular outcomes: A systematic review and meta-analysis of cohort studies. *Nutr. Diet.* **2024**, *81*, 35–50. [CrossRef] [PubMed]
2. Vajdi, M.; Farhangi, M.A. A systematic review of the association between dietary patterns and health-related quality of life. *Health Qual. Life Outcomes* **2020**, *18*, 337. [CrossRef]
3. Law, L.; Heerey, J.L.; Devlin, B.L.; Brukner, P.; Kemp, J.L.; Attanayake, A.; Hulett, M.D.; De Livera, A.; Mosler, A.B.; Morris, H.G.; et al. Effectiveness of an anti-inflammatory diet versus low-fat diet for knee osteoarthritis: The FEAST randomised controlled trial protocol. *BMJ Open* **2024**, *14*, e079374. [CrossRef] [PubMed]
4. Calder, P.C. Nutrition, immunity and COVID-19. *BMJ Nutr. Prev. Health* **2020**, *3*, 74–92. [CrossRef]
5. Lambell, K.J.; Tatucu-Babet, O.A.; Chapple, L.A.; Gantner, D.; Ridley, E.J. Nutrition therapy in critical illness: A review of the literature for clinicians. *Crit. Care* **2020**, *24*, 35. [CrossRef]
6. Deutz, N.E.; Bauer, J.M.; Barazzoni, R.; Biolo, G.; Boirie, Y.; Bosy-Westphal, A.; Cederholm, T.; Cruz-Jentoft, A.; Krznariç, Z.; Nair, K.S.; et al. Protein intake and exercise for optimal muscle function with aging: Recommendations from the ESPEN Expert Group. *Clin. Nutr.* **2014**, *33*, 929–936. [CrossRef]
7. Kobayashi, L.C.; Steptoe, A. Social Isolation, Loneliness, and Health Behaviors at Older Ages: Longitudinal Cohort Study. *Ann. Behav. Med.* **2018**, *52*, 582–593. [CrossRef]
8. Greaves, C.J.; Sheppard, K.E.; Abraham, C.; Hardeman, W.; Roden, M.; Evans, P.H.; Schwarz, P.; IMAGE Study Group. Systematic review of reviews of intervention components associated with increased effectiveness in dietary and physical activity interventions. *BMC Public Health* **2011**, *11*, 119. [CrossRef]
9. Swinburn, B.A.; Kraak, V.I.; Allender, S.; Atkins, V.J.; Baker, P.I.; Bogard, J.R.; Brinsden, H.; Calvillo, A.; De Schutter, O.; Devarajan, R.; et al. The Global Syndemic of Obesity, Undernutrition, and Climate Change: The Lancet Commission Report. *Lancet* **2019**, *393*, 791–846. [CrossRef]
10. Perlinski, M.; Sobocki, J. The Impact of Home Parenteral Nutrition on Survival and Quality of Life in Patients with Intestinal Failure and Advanced Cancer: A Comprehensive Review. *Nutrients* **2025**, *17*, 905. [CrossRef]
11. Ciaffi, J.; Mancarella, L.; Ripamonti, C.; D'Amuri, A.; Brusi, V.; Pignatti, F.; Lisi, L.; Ursini, F. Ultra-Processed Food and Its Impact on Bone Health and Joint Diseases: A Scoping Review. *Nutrients* **2025**, *17*, 1188. [CrossRef] [PubMed]

12. Ludlow, S.; Farragher, K.; Squires, K.; Heaney, S.; Orman, J.; Pullen, S.; Attia, J.; Wynne, K. A Qualitative Study Supporting Optimal Nutrition in Advanced Liver Disease—Unlocking the Potential for Improvement. *Nutrients* **2024**, *16*, 2403. [CrossRef] [PubMed]
13. Notarnicola, M.; Tutino, V.; De Nunzio, V.; Cisternino, A.M.; Cofano, M.; Donghia, R.; Giannuzzi, V.; Zappimbulso, M.; Milella, R.A.; Giannelli, G.; et al. Daily Orange Consumption Reduces Hepatic Steatosis Prevalence in Patients with Metabolic Dysfunction-Associated Steatotic Liver Disease: Exploratory Outcomes of a Randomized Clinical Trial. *Nutrients* **2024**, *16*, 3191. [CrossRef]
14. Hu, N.; Sun, J.; Cao, Y.; Zhao, H.; Sun, M.; Li, G.; Liu, X.; Cong, S. Anti-Fatigue Activity of Corn Protein Hydrolysate Fermented by Lactic Acid Bacteria. *Nutrients* **2025**, *17*, 199. [CrossRef]
15. Alcaide-Leyva, J.M.; Romero-Saldaña, M.; García-Rodríguez, M.; Molina-Luque, R.; Jiménez-Mérida, M.d.R.; Molina-Recio, G. Metabolic Syndrome in the Amazon: Customizing Diagnostic Methods for Urban Communities. *Nutrients* **2025**, *17*, 538. [CrossRef]
16. García Samuelsson, M.; Tárraga López, P.J.; López-González, Á.A.; Paublini, H.; Martínez-Almoyna Rifá, E.; Ramírez-Manent, J.I. Assessment of the Risk of Insulin Resistance in Workers Classified as Metabolically Healthy Obese. *Nutrients* **2025**, *17*, 1345. [CrossRef]
17. Retiaty, F.; Andarwulan, N.; Palupi, N.S.; Ernawati, F.; Kazimierczak, R.; Średnicka-Tober, D. Contribution of Food, Energy, Macronutrients and Fiber Consumption Patterns to Obesity and Other Non-Communicable Disease Risks in the Indonesian Population. *Nutrients* **2025**, *17*, 1459. [CrossRef]
18. Giakoumidakis, K.; Patelarou, E.; Chatziefstratiou, A.A.; Aloizou, D.; Vaitsis, N.; Brokalaki, H.; Fotos, N.V.; Geniataki, E.; Patelarou, A.E. Validation of the Greek Cardiovascular Diet Questionnaire 2 (CDQ-2) and Single-Center Cross-Sectional Insights into the Dietary Habits of Cardiovascular Patients. *Nutrients* **2025**, *17*, 1649. [CrossRef]
19. Price, J.S.; Larsen, S.E.; Miller, L.A.; Smith, H.M.; Apps, J.A.; Weis, J.M. Clinical Biopsychosocial Reflection on Coping with Chronic Illness and Reliance Upon Nutrition Support: An Integrated Healthcare Approach. *Nutr. Clin. Pract.* **2019**, *34*, 220–225. [CrossRef]
20. van Dijk-de Vries, A.; Moser, A.; Mertens, V.C.; van der Linden, J.; van der Weijden, T.; van Eijk, J.T. The Ideal of Biopsychosocial Chronic Care: How to Make It Real? A Qualitative Study among Dutch Stakeholders. *BMC Fam. Pract.* **2012**, *13*, 14. [CrossRef]
21. Volkert, D.; Beck, A.M.; Cederholm, T.; Cruz-Jentoft, A.; Goisser, S.; Hooper, L.; Kiesswetter, E.; Maggio, M.; Raynaud-Simon, A.; Sieber, C.C.; et al. ESPEN Guideline on Clinical Nutrition and Hydration in Geriatrics. *Clin. Nutr.* **2019**, *38*, 10–47. [CrossRef] [PubMed]
22. Koh, L.M. Culturally Tailoring Plant-Based Nutrition Interventions for Hispanic/Latino Adults at Risk for or with Type 2 Diabetes: An Integrative Review. *Hisp. Health Care Int.* **2023**, *21*, 89–103. [CrossRef] [PubMed]

nutrients

MDPI

*Article*

# Parental Knowledge and Preventive Strategies in Pediatric IgE-Mediated Food Allergy—Results from a Cross-Sectional Survey

**Francesca Galletta [1,†], Angela Klain [2,†], Sara Manti [1,*], Francesca Mori [3], Carolina Grella [2], Leonardo Tomei [3], Antonio Andrea Senatore [4], Amelia Licari [5], Michele Miraglia del Giudice [2] and Cristiana Indolfi [2]**

1 Pediatric Unit, Department of Human Pathology in Adult and Developmental Age 'Gaetano Barresi', University of Messina, 98124 Messina, Italy; francygall.92@gmail.com
2 Department of Woman, Child and General and Specialized Surgery, University of Campania 'Luigi Vanvitelli', 80138 Naples, Italy; klainangela95@gmail.com (A.K.); caro.grella94@gmail.com (C.G.); michele.miragliadelgiudice@unicampania.it (M.M.d.G.); cristianaind@hotmail.com (C.I.)
3 Allergy Unit, Meyer Children's Hospital IRCCS, 50139 Florence, Italy; francesca.mori@meyer.it (F.M.); leonardo.tomei@unifi.it (L.T.)
4 Department of Clinical, Surgical, Diagnostic, and Pediatric Sciences, University of Pavia, 27100 Pavia, Italy; antonioandrea.senatore01@universitadipavia.it
5 Pediatric Clinic, Fondazione IRCCS Policlinico San Matteo, 27100 Pavia, Italy; amelia.licari@unipv.it
* Correspondence: sara.manti@unime.it
† These authors contributed equally to this work.

**Abstract: Background/Objectives**: Food allergy (FA) is a growing concern in pediatric care, requiring effective avoidance strategies and timely emergency responses. The role of caregivers is central to the daily management of FA. This study aimed to assess parental knowledge, preparedness, and behaviors regarding pediatric FA management, focusing on both prevention and emergency readiness. **Methods**: A cross-sectional survey was conducted from December 2024 to April 2025 through the SurveyMonkey® platform, promoted by the Italian Society of Pediatric Allergology and Immunology (SIAIP). The anonymous, structured questionnaire was distributed online and in two Italian university hospitals. A total of 129 fully completed responses from caregivers of children with FA were analyzed. The survey explored self-perceived knowledge, symptom recognition, preventive actions, emergency preparedness, and communication practices. **Results**: Only 9.3% of parents considered themselves "very informed," while 54.3% reported limited or no knowledge. Just 16.0% recognized all symptoms of an allergic reaction, and only 24.0% could distinguish mild reactions from anaphylaxis. Notably, 67.4% reported not knowing how to respond to anaphylaxis, and 83.7% did not possess an epinephrine auto-injector. Preventive measures at home were inconsistently applied, and 41.1% took no precautions when eating out. Communication with external caregivers was often informal or absent. Only 33% updated physicians regularly. **Conclusions**: The findings reveal significant gaps in parental preparedness and highlight critical areas for educational intervention. Enhanced caregiver training, standardized communication protocols, and improved clinical follow-up are essential to strengthen pediatric FA management and safety.

**Keywords:** food allergy; parental knowledge; anaphylaxis management; pediatric allergy education

## 1. Introduction

Food allergy (FA) is a growing public health concern, particularly in the pediatric population, where prevalence rates have significantly increased over the past two decades [1].

FA can lead to a broad range of clinical manifestations, from mild skin reactions to life-threatening anaphylaxis [2]. Management primarily relies on strict allergen avoidance and prompt administration of epinephrine in case of accidental exposure [2]. While emerging therapeutic options such as oral immunotherapy (OIT) and biologic agents have shown promise for selected patients, they remain accessible to a limited subset and require specialist supervision [2–4]. Consequently, the cornerstone of effective FA management in real-life settings remains the knowledge, vigilance, and preparedness of caregivers, particularly parents, who serve as primary coordinators of dietary choices, emergency preparedness, and communication with other caregivers (e.g., teachers, relatives) [5]. Therefore, parental education plays a crucial role in reducing the risk of accidental exposure and improving the outcomes of allergic reactions. However, gaps in knowledge and preventive behaviors remain a challenge [5,6]. Limited understanding of symptom severity, insufficient communication with secondary caregivers, and underuse or misuse of emergency medications such as epinephrine auto-injectors have been documented in various settings [5,6].

## 2. Materials and Methods

This study aims to assess parental knowledge and self-reported readiness in managing pediatric food allergies, using a structured and accessible questionnaire. This cross-sectional study was promoted by the "Primary and Secondary Prevention of Allergic Diseases" Committee of the Italian Society of Pediatric Allergology and Immunology (SIAIP), to assess the knowledge, attitudes, and behaviors of caregivers managing food allergies (FAs) in children and adolescents aged 0 to 18 years. The questionnaire was created and administered through the SurveyMonkey® platform (Momentive Inc., San Mateo, CA, USA) and was open from December 2024 to April 2025. Participants were enrolled at their initial allergological evaluation at the pediatric allergy outpatient services of two tertiary university hospitals: AOU "G. Martino" in Messina and AOU "Luigi Vanvitelli" in Naples, Italy. Eligible subjects included children with a previously confirmed diagnosis of IgE-mediated food-induced anaphylaxis established at another healthcare institution, as well as those presenting with a clinical history strongly suggestive of such condition. In all cases, the assessment was performed by board-certified pediatric allergists in accordance with the diagnostic criteria outlined by the European Academy of Allergy and Clinical Immunology (EAACI), which describes anaphylaxis as a serious, rapidly evolving, and potentially life-threatening allergic reaction. It is a systemic hypersensitivity response that typically involves multiple organ systems, most commonly the skin, respiratory tract, and/or cardiovascular system [7]. Importantly, not all of the patients had already been prescribed an epinephrine auto-injector at the time of the visit. Participation was entirely voluntary and anonymous. No identifying data were collected. The survey consisted of ten closed-ended, multiple-choice questions, each offering three to four fixed response options. Caregivers were instructed to select a single answer for each item. The questionnaire was specifically designed to explore multiple dimensions of FA management, including caregivers' self-perceived knowledge, their ability to recognize the main symptoms of an allergic reaction, and their understanding of the distinction between mild and severe reactions, such as anaphylaxis. Other areas of focus included strategies for allergen avoidance at home and outside the home, preventive behaviors in everyday settings, communication practices with external caregivers (such as teachers and relatives), the frequency with which medical updates are provided to healthcare professionals, knowledge of emergency procedures in the event of anaphylaxis, and the availability of an epinephrine auto-injector. Descriptive statistical analysis was carried out using Microsoft Excel® (Microsoft Corporation, Redmond, WA, USA). Prevalence data were calculated for each response option to identify trends in knowledge and behavior, and to highlight areas in which additional caregiver education may be warranted.

## 3. Results

A total of 129 fully completed responses were collected.

### *3.1. Caregiver Knowledge and Perceptions*

The first question investigated parents' self-perceived level of knowledge in managing their child's FA. Results showed that 41.1% of participants considered themselves "a little informed," 36.4% "fairly informed," while only 9.3% reported being "very informed". Notably, 13.2% admitted to feeling "not at all informed" [Figure 1]. The second question focused on symptom recognition, a critical element of timely and effective intervention. While 70.0% of respondents reported knowing "some" of the main symptoms of a FA reaction, only 16.0% said they were familiar with all of them. Alarmingly, 14.0% acknowledged not knowing the symptoms at all [Figure 1]. The third item explored whether caregivers understood the distinction between mild allergic reactions and severe ones like anaphylaxis. While 24.0% of parents reported having a solid understanding of this difference, 53.5% stated that they had some awareness but were not confident in distinguishing the two. Furthermore, 22.5% admitted they had no knowledge on this point [Figure 2]. Question four evaluated knowledge of emergency response procedures in the case of anaphylaxis. Just 19.4% of caregivers reported knowing exactly what to do, including how to use an epinephrine auto-injector and when to call emergency services. An additional 13.2% said they were unsure how to use the auto-injector, and 67.4% admitted they would not know how to respond at all [Figure 3]. Question five focused on the availability of an epinephrine auto-injector, which represents the first-line treatment for anaphylaxis. Only 11.6% of respondents reported always having an auto-injector readily available. A further 4.7% had one but did not carry it consistently. A total of 83.7% of participants stated they did not have an epinephrine auto-injector at all [Figure 4].

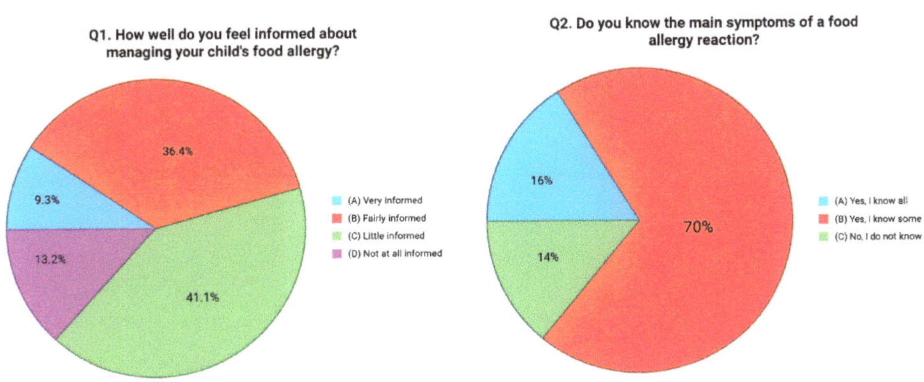


**Figure 1.** Distribution of responses to Q1 ("How well do you feel informed about managing your child's food allergy?") and Q2 ("Do you know the main symptoms of a food allergy reaction?").

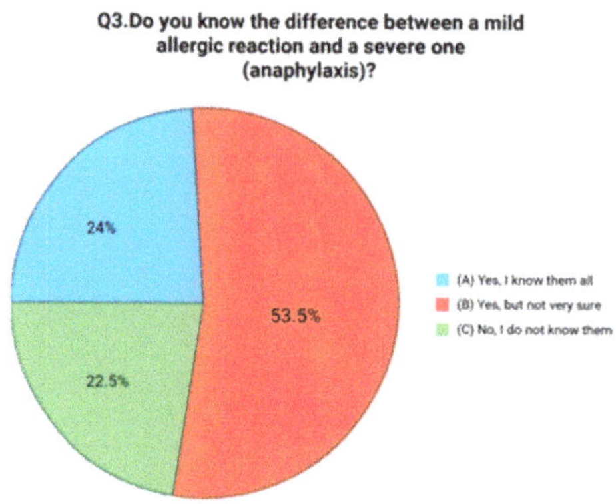


**Figure 2.** Distribution of responses to Q3 ("Do you know the difference between a mild allergic reaction and a severe one [anaphylaxis]?").

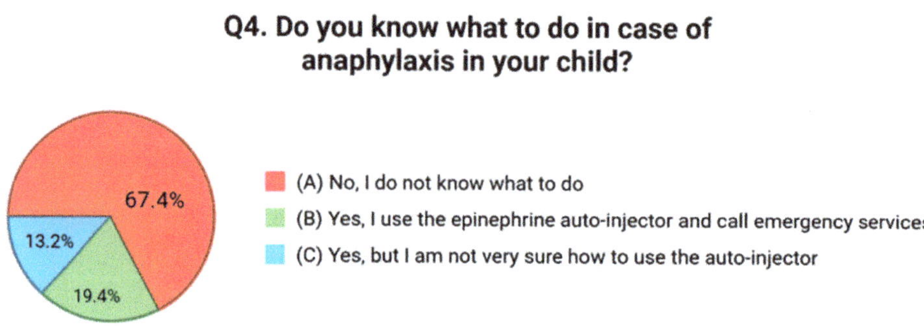


**Figure 3.** Distribution of responses to Q4 ("Do you know what to do in case of anaphylaxis in your child?").

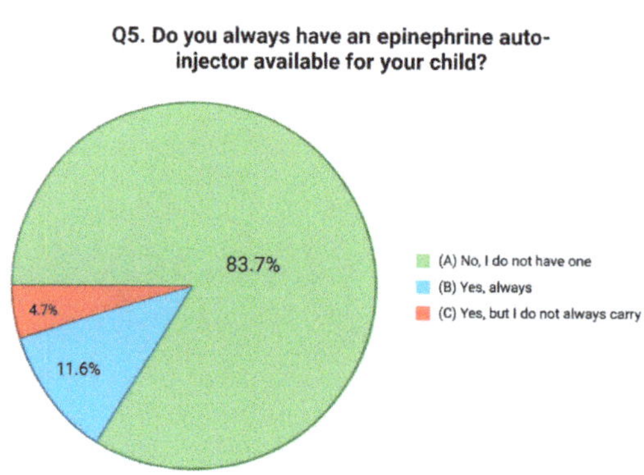


**Figure 4.** Distribution of responses to Q5 ("Do you always have an epinephrine auto-injector available for your child?").

### *3.2. Behavioral Practices and Risk Management*

Question six addressed behavioral strategies for avoiding allergenic foods. Just 30.2% of respondents reported that they always read food labels carefully, and 13.9% said they limit avoidance to known allergens. Interestingly, 27.9% reported using both approaches, but an equal proportion, 27.9%, admitted to not adopting any specific avoidance strategies at all [Figure 5]. Preventive actions taken within the home environment were assessed in question seven. A total of 40.3% of respondents reported not adopting any targeted preventive measures. Among those who did, 17.1% stated they cook separate meals and clean surfaces carefully, while 16.3% avoid keeping allergenic foods in the home. A further 26.4% indicated that they follow both strategies [Figure 6]. The eighth question examined how families manage FA risks while eating outside the home. A total of 44.9% reported informing restaurant staff about their child's allergy, while 13.9% said they avoid eating out entirely. However, a concerning 41.1% stated that they do not take any specific precautionary measures when dining in public venues [Figure 7]. Communication with external caregivers and institutions was the focus of question nine. Slightly more than half of the respondents (52.7%) reported providing written instructions to others about their child's allergy. Meanwhile, 23.3% relied only on verbal communication, and 24.0% admitted that they do not inform others at all [Figure 7]. Question ten explored the frequency with which caregivers update healthcare providers about their child's allergy status. Only 33.3% reported discussing the allergy during every medical visit. A larger group, 43.4%, stated they do so only in the event of new symptoms or allergic reactions. Notably, 23.3% reported rarely or never updating their physician unless prompted [Figure 8].

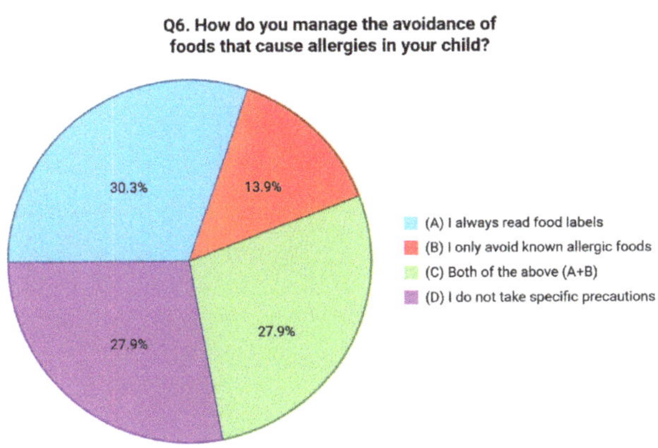


**Figure 5.** Distribution of responses to Q6 ("How do you manage the avoidance of foods that cause allergies in your child?").

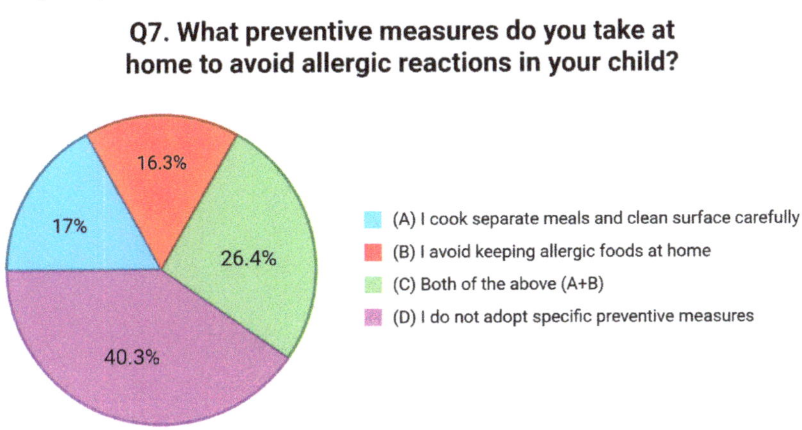


**Figure 6.** Distribution of responses to Q7 ("What preventive measures do you take at home to avoid allergic reactions in your child?").

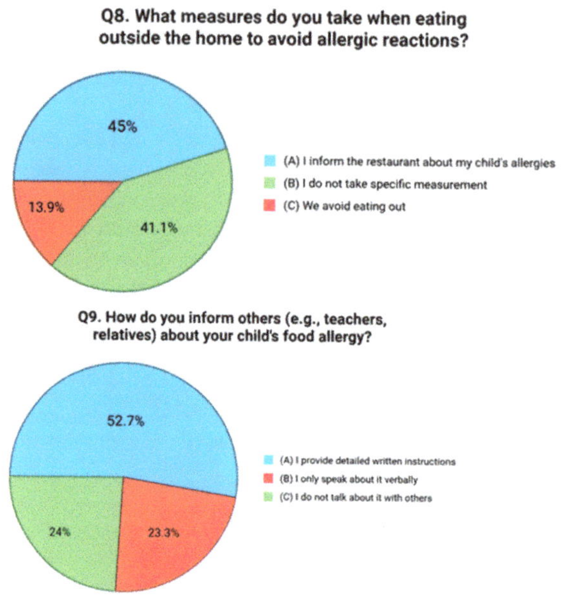


**Figure 7.** Distribution of responses to Q8 ("What measures do you take when eating outside the home to avoid allergic reactions?") and response to Q9 ("How do you inform others [e.g., teachers, relatives] about your child's food allergy?").

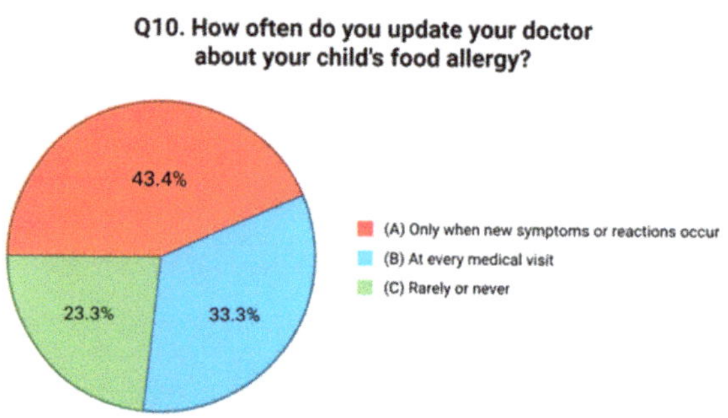


**Figure 8.** Distribution of responses to Q10 ("How often do you update your doctor about your child's food allergy?").

## 4. Discussion

Our survey findings highlight a complex picture of parental knowledge and behavior regarding pediatric food allergies. While a substantial proportion of parents reported being aware of allergic reactions and preventive measures, several areas of concern emerged, particularly in emergency preparedness and external communication. Despite growing public attention to food allergies, the results suggest that a large proportion of families still feel underinformed and underprepared, especially in emergency contexts. Self-perceived knowledge was generally limited: although 36.4% rated themselves as "fairly informed", only 9.3% of respondents considered themselves "very informed" about FA management, while a combined 54.3% rated themselves as only "a little" or "not at all" informed.

These findings are consistent with prior research, which documented substantial parental knowledge gaps. Taha et al. [8], in a cross-sectional study, reported a median knowledge score of 7 out of 15 among parents of children with food allergies, with wide variability across different sections. Knowledge was significantly influenced by factors such as educational level, income, and the number of interactions with healthcare professionals, indicating substantial informational gaps within the general population [8]. Notably, most caregivers are not adequately aware of allergy symptoms, and many are unable to distinguish between a mild allergic reaction and a life-threatening anaphylactic episode. In addition, parental knowledge regarding the correct use of an epinephrine auto-injector remains limited, compromising their ability to respond effectively in emergencies. This limit is clinically significant, as delayed or incorrect administration of epinephrine is a well-documented factor contributing to the progression and severity of allergic reactions [7].

Several studies have highlighted limited practical knowledge regarding the use of epinephrine auto-injectors among caregivers [9–12]. Polloni et al. [9] highlighted a gap between parents' self-perceived knowledge and their actual ability to manage food-induced anaphylaxis. Despite many rating their knowledge as moderate to high, only 20% had ever administered epinephrine, with widespread insecurity and fear regarding its use and side effects. These findings suggest that emotional and psychological barriers, alongside technical skills, play a critical role in emergency response [9]. Similarly, Narchi et al. [10] reported that many parents, despite having received medical training on the use of the epinephrine auto-injector, exhibited considerable hesitation when faced with real-life emergency situations. While 79% of participants were aware of the clinical indications for epinephrine use, only 36% felt competent following practical experience [9,10]. As with Polloni et al.'s findings, key barriers included fear, anxiety, and a lack of confidence in their ability to act appropriately [9,10]. To address these challenges, the authors advocate for implementing comprehensive support strategies, including structured theoretical and practical training sessions, clear and detailed written instructions, access to psychological support, and establishing peer support groups. Such multifaceted interventions may help reduce parental anxiety, enhance confidence, and ultimately improve the timely and effective use of epinephrine in anaphylactic emergencies [9,10]. This need is further confirmed by two recent cross-sectional studies, which show that parents not only continue to seek more practical guidance on when and how to administer epinephrine but also explicitly call for additional educational resources, clear step-by-step instructions, and ongoing support, including access to psychological counselling and peer groups [11,12]. In Cronin et al. [11], for example, only 26.7% of parents performed all the critical steps of the auto-injector correctly, while the Australian survey by Stockhammer et al. [12] highlighted persistent frustration and anxiety directly linked to the lack of practical training and support networks. Preventive actions within the home environment are inconsistently implemented among surveyed families. In our sample, 40.3% of respondents reported not adopting any targeted preventive measures despite the critical role of home-based strategies in minimizing allergen exposure. Among those who implemented precautions, 17.1% reported cooking separate meals and cleaning surfaces carefully, while 16.3% avoided keeping allergenic foods at home. Notably, only 26.4% of participants combined both practices, suggesting that comprehensive allergen avoidance protocols are not routinely applied.

Moen et al. [13] characterize the home as a perceived "safe zone" for families managing food allergies; however, preserving this safety requires continuous vigilance, structured routines, and careful planning. The responsibility for allergen control often falls on mothers, a role frequently associated with significant psychological burden, including anxiety and social withdrawal. In this context, a correct understanding of food labels is crucial in enabling families to identify hidden allergens and reduce the risk of accidental exposure. Strengthening parental labelling skills could significantly improve home-based food allergy management [14,15]. Another critical finding involves the management of food allergies outside the home. While many parents adopt effective avoidance strategies at home, fewer report feeling confident when dining out or leaving their child in the care of others, such as at school.

Particularly, school is where children spend most of their time. This context makes the school environment pivotal for effective food allergy management. As reported in the scoping review by Santos et al. [5], up to 20% of anaphylactic reactions occur in schools, yet preparedness remains inconsistent. Many staff members lack training in allergy and anaphylaxis management, and some are unaware of students' food allergies. The absence of standardized policies and emergency plans is common. While educational interventions have shown benefit, the review underscores the need for mandatory training, ready access to epinephrine auto-injectors, and individualized emergency protocols to ensure student safety [5]. An important insight emerges from the analysis of parental strategies at restaurants. Although 45% of respondents reported informing restaurant staff about their child's food allergies, this was a positive and proactive behavior. Over 41% declared they did not take any specific precautionary measures, and 13.9% explicitly stated that they avoided dining out altogether. These findings highlight a fragmented and inconsistent approach to risk management in restaurant settings. The high percentage of parents who do not adopt specific measures may reflect a combination of low-risk perception, lack of practical guidance, or skepticism about the effectiveness of communicating with food service staff. This is particularly concerning given the evidence in the literature showing that restaurants are frequent sites of accidental allergic reactions [16,17]. Furthermore, systematic reviews confirm that restaurant staff often lack adequate knowledge and training in allergen management, increasing the potential for cross-contamination and miscommunication [18,19]. The coexistence of proactive and avoidant behaviors highlights the need for targeted education and clear public health messaging to enhance caregiver preparedness in public settings. Equally important is effective communication with external caregivers, such as teachers, relatives, and family friends, which remains a key component of food allergy management. Survey results revealed substantial variability in how parents communicate information about their child's allergy: 53% reported providing detailed written instructions, 23% relied solely on verbal explanations, and 24% admitted not informing others at all. This inconsistency is concerning, as informal or absent communication increases the likelihood of misunderstandings or errors in allergen avoidance and emergency response. These findings suggest a gap between recommended safety practices and real-world parental behavior. Clinical guidelines emphasize the importance of written documentation, including individualized emergency plans and symptom recognition tools, as essential components of safe allergy management outside the home [2,8]. As such, greater efforts are needed to promote and facilitate the use of standardized communication tools, ideally supported by healthcare professionals and institutional frameworks, to enhance safety across all caregiving environments [2,8]. The frequency with which caregivers update healthcare providers about their child's food allergy status represents an important indicator of continuity and quality of care. In our survey, only 33% of respondents reported informing their physician at every medical visit, while a larger proportion (43%) stated they do so only when new symptoms or allergic reactions occur. Notably, 23% reported rarely or never updating their doctor unless specifically prompted.

This pattern highlights a reactive rather than proactive approach to food allergy management in the clinical setting. Regular communication with healthcare providers is essential for monitoring the child's condition and updating emergency care plans, reviewing avoidance strategies, and evaluating the continued need for epinephrine auto-injectors or diagnostic re-assessment [20,21]. The lack of consistent dialogue may hinder timely interventions and contribute to gaps in prevention and preparedness, particularly as new triggers or changes in symptom severity can emerge over time [20,21].

*Strengths and Limitations*

The main limitations of the study include the cross-sectional design and self-reported nature of the survey, which may introduce bias. However, the structured questionnaire offers a comprehensive overview of real-world behaviors and beliefs, making the findings relevant for clinical and educational policy development. Importantly, we deliberately chose not to collect individual demographic (e.g., age, sex) or clinical (e.g., specific food allergens) information about the children involved. This decision was based on multiple considerations. First, the core objective of the study was to explore parental knowledge, preparedness, and management practices at the initial clinical visit rather than to establish correlations with child-specific clinical profiles. Second, ethical and privacy concerns guided our methodology: by avoiding collecting sensitive or identifiable health data, we ensured anonymity and avoided the need for formal ethical approval or data protection procedures. Third, from a logistical perspective, maintaining a concise and non-invasive questionnaire contributed to higher completion rates and greater patient adherence, particularly in the real-life context of busy outpatient clinical settings. Lastly, as highlighted in the literature, the core principles of food allergy management, such as label reading, availability of an epinephrine auto-injector, and preparedness for emergency response, are broadly consistent across pediatric age groups and allergen types [7,9–12]. Therefore, the omission of detailed clinical variables does not compromise the relevance or validity of the study's primary findings.

## 5. Conclusions

This study highlights several gaps in parental knowledge and preparedness in managing pediatric food allergies among patients presenting with food-induced anaphylaxis at their first clinical evaluation and initial care. While some caregivers demonstrate awareness of allergic symptoms and prevention strategies, a substantial proportion report limited understanding of anaphylaxis, uncertainty in emergency response, and inconsistent use of epinephrine auto-injectors. Communication with healthcare professionals and external caregivers is also suboptimal, potentially compromising the safety of allergic children. These findings underscore the need for comprehensive, accessible educational initiatives that promote practical skills, confidence in emergency management, and consistent communication practices for families of children with food allergies and the general population. Integrating structured parental education into routine clinical care may enhance long-term outcomes and reduce the risk of severe allergic reactions.

**Author Contributions:** Conceptualization, C.I. and S.M.; methodology, C.I. and S.M.; investigation, A.K. and F.G.; data curation, F.M., C.G., L.T., A.A.S. and A.L. writing—original draft preparation, F.G. and A.K.; writing—review and editing, S.M., C.I. and M.M.d.G.; supervision, A.L., M.M.d.G. All authors have read and agreed to the published version of the manuscript.

**Funding:** This research received no external funding.

**Institutional Review Board Statement:** Ethical review and approval were waived for this study due to the anonymous collection of non-sensitive, non-identifiable data through a voluntary questionnaire administered in a non-interventional context.

**Informed Consent Statement:** Informed consent was obtained from all subjects involved in the study.

**Data Availability Statement:** Data are contained within the article.

**Acknowledgments:** We want to thank Elisabetta Frontino for her technical support as well as all the patients and caregivers who participated in the survey.

**Conflicts of Interest:** The authors declare no conflicts of interest.

## Abbreviations

The following abbreviations are used in this manuscript:

| | |
|---|---|
| FA | Food Allergy |
| OIT | Oral Immunotherapy |
| IgE | Immunoglobulin E |
| FDA | Food and Drug Administration |
| EAACI | European Academy of Allergy and clinical Immunology |
| SIAIP | Italian Society of Allergy and Immunology |
| PTSD | Post Traumatic Stress Disorder |

## References


1. Sampath, V.; Abrams, E.M.; Adlou, B.; Akdis, C.; Akdis, M.; Brough, H.A.; Chan, S.; Chatchatee, P.; Chinthrajah, R.S.; Cocco, R.R.; et al. Food allergy across the globe. *J. Allergy Clin. Immunol.* **2021**, *148*, 1347–1364. [CrossRef] [PubMed]
2. Santos, A.F.; Riggioni, C.; Du Toit, G.; Skypala, I. An algorithm for the diagnosis and management of IgE-mediated food allergy, 2024 update. *Allergy* **2025**, *80*, 629–632. [CrossRef] [PubMed]
3. Nurmatov, U.B.; Lo Scalzo, L.; Galletta, F.; Krasnenkova, M.; Arasi, S.; Ansotegui, I.J.; Tagiyeva-Milne, N.; Fiocchi, A. Biologics in IgE-mediated food allergy: A systematic review and meta-analysis of interventional studies. *World Allergy Organ. J.* **2025**, *18*, 101069. [CrossRef] [PubMed]
4. U.S. Food and Drug Administration. FDA Approves First Medication to Help Reduce Allergic Reactions to Multiple Foods After Accidental Exposure. Available online: https://www.fda.gov/news-events/press-announcements/fda-approves-first-medication-help-reduce-allergic-reactions-multiple-foods-after-accidental (accessed on 4 June 2025).
5. Santos, M.J.L.; Merrill, K.A.; Gerdts, J.D.; Ben-Shoshan, M.; Protudjer, J.L.P. Food Allergy Education and Management in Schools: A Scoping Review on Current Practices and Gaps. *Nutrients* **2022**, *14*, 732. [CrossRef] [PubMed]
6. Sugunasingha, N.; Jones, F.W.; Jones, C.J. Interventions for caregivers of children with food allergy: A systematic review. *Pediatr. Allergy Immunol.* **2020**, *31*, 805–812. [CrossRef] [PubMed]
7. Muraro, A.; Worm, M.; Alviani, C.; Cardona, V.; DunnGalvin, A.; Garvey, L.H.; Riggioni, C.; de Silva, D.; Angier, E.; Arasi, S.; et al. EAACI guidelines: Anaphylaxis (2021 update). *Allergy* **2022**, *77*, 357–377. [CrossRef] [PubMed]
8. Taha, S.; Rabaiah, R.; Dweikat, A.; Abu-Ali, L.; Yaeesh, H.; Jbour, R.; Al-Jabi, S.W.; Zyoud, S.H. Parental knowledge and attitudes toward food allergies: A cross-sectional study on determinants and educational needs. *BMC Public Health* **2024**, *24*, 2668. [CrossRef] [PubMed]
9. Polloni, L.; Baldi, I.; Amadi, M.; Tonazzo, V.; Bonaguro, R.; Lazzarotto, F.; Toniolo, A.; Gregori, D.; Muraro, A. Management of Children with Food-Induced Anaphylaxis: A Cross-Sectional Survey of Parental Knowledge, Attitude, and Practices. *Front. Pediatr.* **2022**, *10*, 886551. [CrossRef] [PubMed]
10. Narchi, H.; Elghoudi, A.; Al Dhaheri, K. Barriers and challenges affecting parents' use of adrenaline auto-injector in children with anaphylaxis. *World J. Clin. Pediatr.* **2022**, *11*, 151–159. [CrossRef] [PubMed]
11. Cronin, C.; Keohane, H.; O'Rourke, E.; O'Kelly, C.; Ramesh, Y.; Flores, L.; Gallagher, A.; Dumitrescu, A.; Velasco, R.; Trujillo, J. Assessing the Knowledge of Anaphylaxis Management and Adrenaline Auto-Injector Administration Among Parents of Children with Food Allergies: A Cross-Sectional Study. *Allergies* **2024**, *4*, 80–93. [CrossRef]
12. Stockhammer, D.; Katelaris, C.H.; Simpson, M.D.; Vanniasinkam, T. Parent perceptions in managing children with food allergy: An Australian perspective. *World Allergy Organ. J.* **2020**, *13*, 100468. [CrossRef] [PubMed]
13. Moen, Ø.L.; Opheim, E.; Trollvik, A. Parents' Experiences Raising a Child with Food Allergy: A Qualitative Review. *J. Pediatr. Nurs.* **2019**, *46*, e52–e63. [CrossRef] [PubMed]
14. Dinardo, G.; Fierro, V.; Del Giudice, M.M.; Urbani, S.; Fiocchi, A. Food-labeling issues for severe food-allergic consumers. *Curr. Opin. Allergy Clin. Immunol.* **2023**, *23*, 233–238. [CrossRef] [PubMed]
15. Fiocchi, A.; Risso, D.; DunnGalvin, A.; González Díaz, S.N.; Monaci, L.; Fierro, V.; Ansotegui, I.J. Food labeling issues for severe food allergic patients. *World Allergy Organ. J.* **2021**, *14*, 100598. [CrossRef] [PubMed]
16. Dominguez, S.; Théolier, J.; Gerdts, J.; Godefroy, S.B. Dining Out with Food Allergies: Two Decades of Evidence Calling for Enhanced Consumer Protection. *Int. J. Hosp. Manag.* **2024**, *122*, 103825. [CrossRef]
17. Konstantinou, G.N.; Pampoukidou, O.; Sergelidis, D.; Fotoulaki, M. Managing Food Allergies in Dining Establishments: Challenges and Innovative Solutions. *Nutrients* **2025**, *17*, 1737. [CrossRef] [PubMed]
18. Figueroa-Gómez, X.A.; Oliveras-López, M.J.; Poyanco-Bugueño, M.F.; Ocaña-Peinado, F.M.; López-García de la Serrana, H.; Araya Quezada, M. Knowledge, attitude, and practices of restaurant and foodservice personnel in food allergy: A systematic review and meta-analysis. *Heliyon* **2024**, *10*, e33431. [CrossRef] [PubMed]

19. Ajibade, T.; Bukutu, C.; Marinkovic, A.; Okorie, C.; Izurieta, R.; Sanyaolu, A. A Systematic Review of the Knowledge and Training of Food Service Workers on Food Allergies. *AIMS Allergy Immunol.* **2023**, *7*, 195–212. [CrossRef]
20. Berni Canani, R.; Caffarelli, C.; Calvani, M.; Martelli, A.; Carucci, L.; Cozzolino, T.; Alvisi, P.; Agostoni, C.; Lionetti, P.; Marseglia, G.L.; et al. Diagnostic therapeutic care pathway for pediatric food allergies and intolerances in Italy: A joint position paper by the Italian Society for Pediatric Gastroenterology Hepatology and Nutrition (SIGENP) and the Italian Society for Pediatric Allergy and Immunology (SIAIP). *Ital. J. Pediatr.* **2022**, *48*, 87. [CrossRef] [PubMed]
21. Muraro, A.; Mendoza Hernandez, D.A. Managing food allergy and anaphylaxis: A new model for an integrated approach. *Allergol. Int.* **2020**, *69*, 19–27. [CrossRef] [PubMed]

nutrients

Article

# Validation of the Greek Cardiovascular Diet Questionnaire 2 (CDQ-2) and Single-Center Cross-Sectional Insights into the Dietary Habits of Cardiovascular Patients

**Konstantinos Giakoumidakis [1,*], Evridiki Patelarou [1], Anastasia A. Chatziefstratiou [2], Dimitra Aloizou [3], Nikolaos Vaitsis [4], Hero Brokalaki [2], Nikolaos V. Fotos [2], Elisabeth Geniataki [1] and Athina E. Patelarou [1]**

1 Department of Nursing, School of Health Sciences, Hellenic Mediterranean University, 71410 Heraklion, Greece; epatelarou@hmu.gr (E.P.); ddk266@edu.hmu.gr (E.G.); apatelarou@hmu.gr (A.E.P.)
2 Department of Nursing, School of Health Sciences, National and Kapodistrian University of Athens, 11527 Athens, Greece; a.chatziefstratiou@yahoo.gr (A.A.C.); heropan@nurs.uoa.gr (H.B.); nikfotos@nurs.uoa.gr (N.V.F.)
3 ICU Department, IASO General and Maternity Hospital, 15123 Athens, Greece; dimitraloi@yahoo.gr
4 Primary Healthcare, 40300 Farsala, Greece; vaitsis@hotmail.com
* Correspondence: kongiakoumidakis@hmu.gr; Tel.: +30-2810379549

**Abstract: Background/Objectives**: Dietary recommendations are an essential part of guidelines for the best management of chronic cardiovascular diseases. The present study aimed to validate the Greek version of Cardiovascular Diet Questionnaire 2 (CDQ-2) and to assess the dietary habits among cardiovascular patients. **Methods**: A single-center cross-sectional observational study was conducted. The study population was cardiovascular patients that were users of a private primary healthcare clinic. The data were collected between December 2024 and January 2025. The questionnaire was translated from French, back-translated, and reviewed by a committee of experts. The MEDAS was used as a gold standard. The psychometric measurements that were performed included reliability coefficients and Explanatory Factor Analysis (EFA). **Results**: The total sample comprised 90 individuals. The Cronbach's $\alpha$ was 0.97. A bivariate Pearson's correlation established that there was a strong, statistically significant linear relationship between the CDQ-2 and MEDAS scores, with $r(90) = 0.962$ and $p < 0.001$. Cardiovascular patients seemed to have suboptimal dietary patterns, as indicated by the relatively low mean CDQ-2 score of 2.9 (SD = 17.2), along with a mean MEDAS score of 8 (SD = 5.2), where younger individuals ($p < 0.001$), males ($p = 0.042$), single/divorced/widowed individuals ($p < 0.001$), individuals with lower physical activity ($p = 0.001$), and active smokers ($p = 0.022$) demonstrated significantly poorer adherence to the optimal cardiovascular dietary status. **Conclusions**: The survey indicated that CDQ-2 was a valid and reliable scale to use in cardiovascular patients in Greece. Also, the patients were characterized by suboptimal dietary habits, indicating the need for personalized interventions to improve their dietary habits.

**Keywords:** cardiovascular disease; cross-sectional study; diet; questionnaire; validation study

## 1. Introduction

Cardiovascular disease (CVD) is the foremost cause of death all over the world, contributing to approximately 18 million deaths annually [1]. In Greece, CVD continues to be the leading cause of mortality and morbidity, despite the low rates recorded in the 1950s and 1960s, when the country was considered privileged in terms of cardiovascular health. According to the ATTICA epidemiological study, the incidence of cardiovascular



https://doi.org/10.3390/nu17101649

disease in Greece reached 360 cases per 10,000 individuals over a 20-year follow-up period (2002–2022), indicating a high lifetime risk of developing cardiovascular disease [2]. Beyond the estimation of cardiovascular disease-related deaths, there is growing concern about its substantial burden, as it ranks first compared with other diseases. In 2021, CVD was responsible for 14.9% of the total loss of healthy life years due to either premature mortality or disability [3,4].

Dietary modifications play a pivotal role in the secondary and tertiary prevention of cardiovascular disease. According to the literature, a diet rich in unsaturated fats and low in saturated fats is highly beneficial for patients with cardiovascular diseases, including those who have undergone Coronary Artery Bypass Grafting (CABG), as well as those with other forms of CVD, such as heart failure, hypertension, and ischemic heart disease. Many studies have documented the value of a well-balanced diet in beneficial patient outcomes, including healthier metabolic profiles, reduced inflammation, enhanced overall cardiovascular function, and diminished mortality rates [5,6].

For instance, a diet rich in fruits, vegetables, whole-grain cereals, and lean proteins has been consistently associated with better clinical outcomes and fewer complications in patients with cardiovascular diseases. These dietary patterns help regulate blood pressure, improve lipid profiles, and reduce the risk of recurrent cardiovascular events [7]. The Mediterranean diet is widely considered to be the most appropriate dietary model for cardiovascular patients due to its emphasis on plant-based foods, healthy fats (such as olive oil), and the moderate consumption of fish and poultry. This diet has been shown to significantly reduce mortality; morbidity; and complications, such as angina and acute myocardial infarction [8,9].

Beyond its physical health benefits, the Mediterranean diet also positively impacts psychological well-being. Unsanitary dietary habits, such as the high consumption of processed foods and saturated fats, have been linked to increased levels of anxiety, stress, and depression, which can deteriorate cardiovascular outcomes [10,11]. For instance, patients with heart failure who adhere to a poor diet pattern often experience higher levels of psychological distress, which can worsen their condition, lessening their quality of life [12]. Additionally, cognitive impairments, such as delirium and mild cognitive decline, are more frequent among cardiovascular patients with improper dietary habits, further underscoring the importance of a healthy diet in maintaining both physical and mental health [12].

Despite the well-documented benefits of a healthy diet, adherence to dietary recommendations remains suboptimal for individuals with various forms of cardiovascular disease. Studies have identified several barriers to dietary adherence, such as a lack of patient education, limited access to healthy foods, socioeconomic challenges, cultural factors, and insufficient follow-up care [13,14]. The first and crucial step to confront this issue is the reliable estimation of the nutritional status of these patients to plan and perform specific and systematic interventions to try to reverse the existing problematic situation and alleviate all the associated obstacles that impede the adoption of a healthy diet pattern among cardiovascular patients.

Cardiovascular Diet Questionnaire 2 (CDQ-2) is a validated dietary assessment tool originally developed for the French population by Paillard et al. [15] and designed to evaluate dietary habits in patients with cardiovascular diseases. According to its nature and content, it provides a comprehensive assessment of nutrient intake based on a seven-day dietary history and biomarkers. Additionally, this tool captures both qualitative and quantitative aspects of a diet, making it a robust tool for clinical and research settings [15].

The purpose of the present study was (a) to translate CDQ-2 into the Greek language and validate it for the Greek-speaking population of cardiovascular patients and (b) to assess their dietary status, identifying the factors influencing it. This study intended to add useful new data to the existing body of literature by providing a culturally adapted and validated dietary tool for the Greek-speaking population, which can serve many research and clinical purposes in the field of cardiovascular prevention and holistic care. Additionally, it could provide a comprehensive understanding of the current dietary status of cardiovascular patients and the influencing factors, offering insights into tailoring personalized interventions and policies.

## 2. Materials and Methods

### 2.1. Study Design

This was a single-center cross-sectional observational study. The study population was cardiovascular disease patients that were users of a private primary healthcare clinic. The convenience sampling method was used to collect data from December 2024 to January 2025. Participants who were eligible to take part in this study needed to be men or women aged 18 years and above who had been diagnosed with cardiovascular disease. Moreover, they needed to be able to read and write in Greek to ensure they could understand the study materials and take part in the related assessments effectively. Only individuals who willingly agreed to participate in this study were included in the enrollment process. As exclusion criteria, we used a history of psychiatric illness, a recent history of alcohol and/or drug abuse, dementia, and Alzheimer's disease (Figure 1).

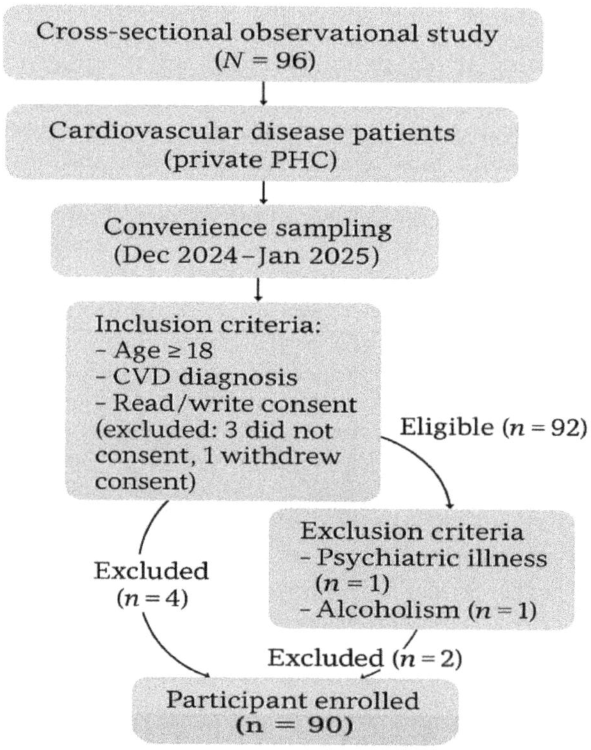


**Figure 1.** Participant flowchart. CVD: cardiovascular disease, PHC: primary healthcare.

### 2.2. Translation of CDQ-2

The process involved an independent translation of the original French as a forward translation by two separate individuals. After this phase, a third individual compared the two translations and was able to determine an agreed-upon translation (1st reconciliation version). A bilingual individual, whose mother tongue was French and was a professional translator, later translated the agreed-upon version into the original questionnaire's language (backward translation). However, the individual was unaware of the questionnaire's standard format.

Twenty patients with cardiovascular disease completed the translated version of the questionnaire to evaluate its apparent validity (face validity), which verified that the scale included questions that were relevant to the characteristic being measured and did not lead to inaccurate or incomplete responses. Additionally, three eHealth specialists reviewed the questionnaire as part of a cognitive debriefing to assess the tool and suggest ways to make it better (Content Validity). In the final version of the instrument (Supplementary Materials), items with a Coefficient Validity Ratio (CVR) greater than 0.70 were retained.

### 2.3. Reliability

To measure a scale's reliability, the internal consistency coefficient, Cronbach's alpha, was calculated. This coefficient evaluates the degree to which the questions that make up a scale measure the same concept. Values greater than or close to 0.70 (70%) are acceptable. An internal consistency coefficient between 0.50 and 0.60 (50–60%) is considered sufficient in the early stages of a study. If the value exceeds 0.80 (80%), then it is considered a particularly good reliability analysis.

### 2.4. Validity

Confirmatory factor analysis (CFA) was conducted to determine the model's fitness. An adequate or good fit was indicated by a Standardized Root-Mean-Squared Residual (SRMR) less than or equal to 0.08, a Coefficient of Determination (CD) greater than or equal to 0.90, and a Comparative Fit Index (CFI) greater than or equal to 0.90.

The construct validity was determined using Pearson's correlation between CDQ-2 and the selected gold standard questionnaire.

### 2.5. Translation and Weighting Questionnaire

Data were collected using an anonymous self-report questionnaire that consisted of three sub-sections:

- The first concerned the following demographic characteristics: (a) age, (b) biological sex, (c) educational level, (d) subjective economic situation, and (e) family situation.
- CDQ-2 includes 17 closed-ended questions designed to identify major sources of nutrients. For each of the 9 questions related to the saturated fatty acid (SFA) intake, the total score ranges from 0 to 27. The monounsaturated fatty acid (MUFA) intake is investigated with one question (total score range 0–6). Omega-3 fatty acid (ω3FA) intake is investigated with 3 questions (total score range 0–10). Finally, there are 4 questions on fruit and vegetable (FV) consumption (range 0–14). The total nutritional score is calculated as [(FV + MUFA + ω3FA) − SFA], fluctuating from −27 to +30. Higher scores indicate better nutrition, whereas the existing literature does not provide universal cut-off points.

MEDAS was created by Spanish researchers [16] and has been weighted and translated by Greek researchers [17]. This tool consists of 14 questions (total score range 0–14) about the main food groups consumed as part of the Mediterranean Diet, which is a valid means of rapidly assessing adherence to it. Higher scores indicate the healthiest dietary pattern, while a score $\geq 10$ is considered indicative of high adherence [18]. It is known that the dietary pattern associated with the Mediterranean Diet is characterized by the daily consumption of olive oil (mainly extra virgin), whole grains, fruits, and vegetables. The Mediterranean diet is a rich source of essential minerals, vitamins, and fiber and is considered one of the healthiest dietary patterns.

*2.6. Statistical Methodology*

We performed the statistical analysis using STATA software (version 12.0; Stata Corporation, College Station, TX, USA) for the confirmatory factor analysis and SPSS statistical software (version 27; SPSS, Chicago, IL, USA) for the remainder. For the descriptive statistical analysis, the continuous variables are given as the mean value and standard deviation, while the discrete ones are given as the absolute and relative frequencies. Multiple Logistic Regression was used to investigate the independent variables (age, biological sex, higher level of education, economic level, marital status, physical activity, smoking, and alcohol consumption) that can predict the dependent variable (CDQ-2). The minimum value of the statistical significance level was set at 5%. To weigh the CDQ-2 questionnaire, the following steps were followed: (a) bilingual translation (forward translation, reconciliation report, backward translation), (b) cognitive debriefing process of the questionnaire through the pilot data collection of a small sample of participants (10–15 people) to fully oversee the formation of the final form of the translated questionnaire, (c) calculation of the questionnaire reliability using the repeatability method, (d) calculation of the concurrent validity (the MEDAS questionnaire was used as the gold standard), and (e) calculation of validity through confirmatory factor analysis. For the confirmatory factor analysis, the calculation of the minimum required sample size showed that for 17 items, a single-factor model, a type I error ($\alpha$) of 5%, a statistical power of 80%, and an expected effect size of 0.1, at least 87 participants were required. This requirement was met, as the total sample size enrolled in the present study was 90 individuals.

## 3. Results

The total sample comprised 90 individuals, where 13 (14.4%) were female and 77 (85.6%) were male; the mean age was 63.8 $\pm$ 9.6 years. A total of 30 (33.3%) participants were single, divorced, or widowed, and 60 (66.7%) were married or cohabited. Regarding the education level, 21 (23.3%), 41 (45.6%), 21 (23.3%), and 7 (7.8%) participants had up to secondary education, post-secondary non-tertiary education, tertiary education, and held an MSc or PhD, respectively. A total of 24 (26.7%) participants reported a low economic level, while 50 (55.6%) and 16 (17.8%) reported middle and high economic levels, respectively. In terms of physical activity, 32 (35.6%) participants had a low level, 43 (47.8%) a middle level, and 15 (16.7%) a high level. Regarding alcohol consumption, 19 (21.1%) reported no consumption of alcohol, 55 (61.1%) moderate consumption, and 16 (17.8%) high consumption (Table 1). The CVR results for CDQ-2 showed that 100% of the items (n = 17) were acceptable, and the Cronbach's $\alpha$ was 0.97. A one-factor model conducted by CFA yielded acceptable global fit indices (SRMR = 0.08, CD = 0.99, CFI = 0.99), indicating that the 17 items in the one-factor solution proposed by the principal investigators should be accepted for the Greek version of CDQ-2 (Figure 2). The mean score of CDQ-2 was 2.9 (SD = 17.2), and the mean MEDAS score was 8 (SD = 5.2). A bivariate Pearson's correlation established that there was a strong, statistically significant linear relationship between the CDQ-2 and MEDAS scores, with r (90) = 0.962 and $p < 0.001$.

A multivariate analysis was performed to ascertain the effects of the independent variables, namely, age, biological sex, level of education, economic level, marital status, physical activity, smoking, and alcohol consumption, on the CDQ-2 score. The multiple linear regression model was statistically significant, with F (8, 81) = 75.4 and $p < 0.001$. The model explained 87% (Adjusted R-Square) of the variance in the score of CDQ-2. As shown in Table 2, of the eight predictor variables, only the following five were statistically significant: (1) age ($p < 0.001$), (2) biological sex ($p = 0.042$), (3) marital status ($p < 0.001$), (4) physical activity ($p = 0.001$), and (5) smoking ($p = 0.022$). Specifically, younger age, male sex, being single/divorced/widowed, lower physical activity levels, and active smoking status were strongly associated with lower CDQ-2 scores (Table 2). Table 3 displays the distribution of CDQ-2 scores according to the categories of the categorical variables.

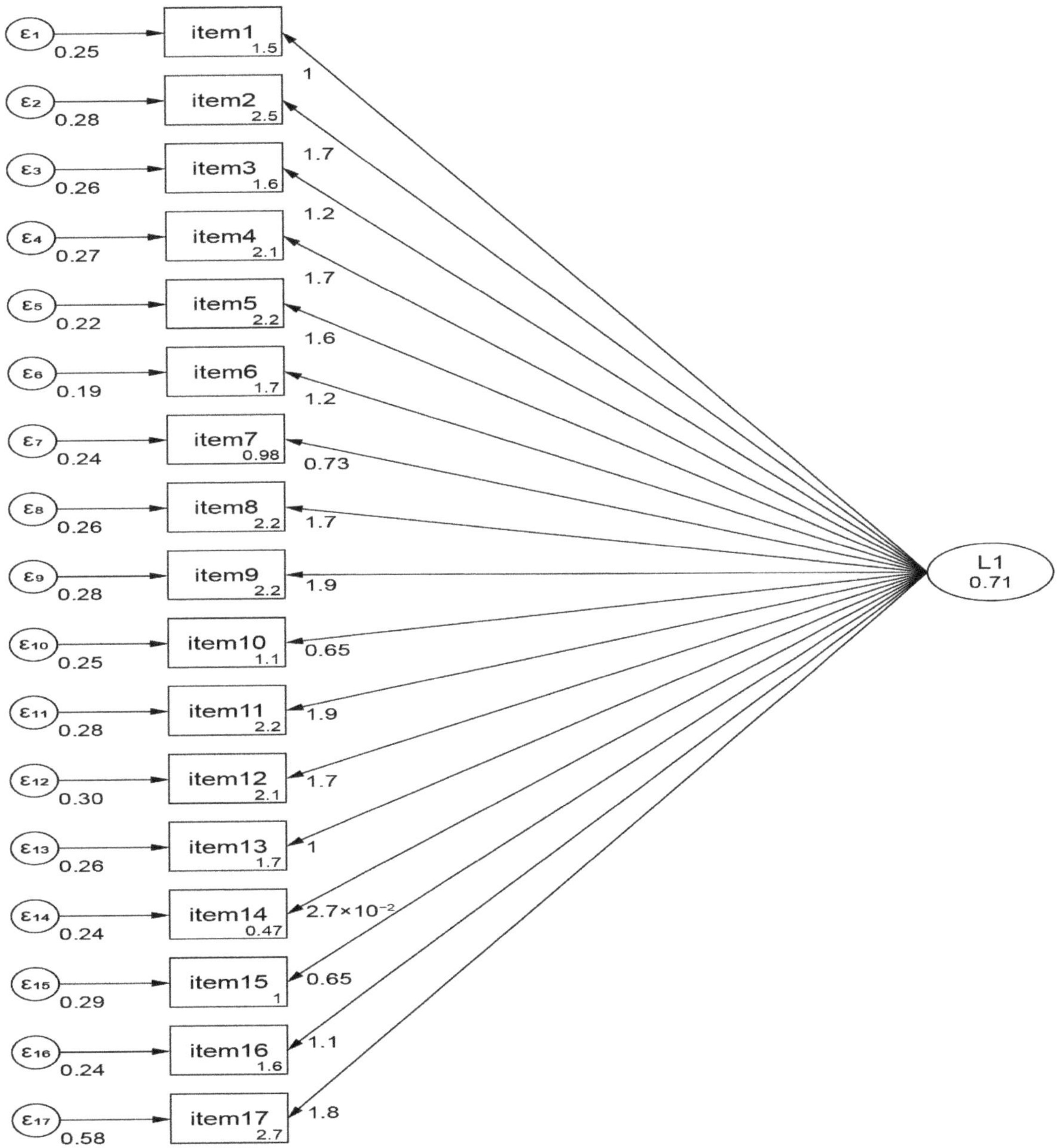


**Figure 2.** Confirmatory factor analysis of CDQ-2.

**Table 1.** Sample characteristics.

| | | N | N % |
|---|---|---|---|
| | Age (years) | 63.8 ± 9.6 * | |
| Biological sex | Female | 13 | 14.4% |
| | Male | 77 | 85.6% |
| Higher level of education | Up to secondary education | 21 | 23.3% |
| | Post-secondary non-tertiary education | 41 | 45.6% |
| | Tertiary education | 21 | 23.3% |
| | MSc/PhD | 7 | 7.8% |
| Economic level | Low | 24 | 26.7% |
| | Middle | 48 | 53.3% |
| | High | 18 | 20.0% |
| Marital status | Single, divorced, or widowed | 30 | 33.3% |
| | Married or cohabiting | 60 | 66.7% |
| Physical activity | Low | 32 | 35.6% |
| | Middle | 43 | 47.8% |
| | High | 15 | 16.7% |
| Smoking | Smoker | 17 | 18.9% |
| | Ex-smoker | 54 | 60.0% |
| | Non-smoker | 19 | 21.1% |
| Alcohol consumption | Medium consumption | 19 | 21.1% |
| | Social consumption | 55 | 61.1% |
| | No consumption | 16 | 17.8% |

(*) mean ± standard deviation.

**Table 2.** Contribution of each independent variable to the model and its statistical significance.

| | Unstandardized Coefficients | | Standardized Coefficients | t | Sig. | 95.0% Confidence Interval for B | |
|---|---|---|---|---|---|---|---|
| | B | Std. Error | Beta | | | Lower Bound | Upper Bound |
| (Constant) | 63.665 | 20.479 | | 3.109 | 0.003 | 22.918 | 104.412 |
| Age | −1.181 | 0.234 | −0.660 | −5.052 | 0.000 | −1.647 | −0.716 |
| Biological sex | 5.041 | 2.438 | 0.104 | 2.068 | 0.042 | 0.191 | 9.891 |
| Higher level of education | −0.564 | 1.647 | −0.029 | −0.342 | 0.733 | −3.842 | 2.714 |
| Economic level | 1.161 | 2.202 | 0.046 | 0.527 | 0.600 | −3.221 | 5.543 |
| Marital status | 10.905 | 2.118 | 0.301 | 5.149 | 0.000 | 6.691 | 15.120 |
| Physical activity | 4.500 | 1.355 | 0.184 | 3.321 | 0.001 | 1.804 | 7.196 |
| Smoking | −6.399 | 2.733 | −0.237 | −2.341 | 0.022 | −11.837 | −0.960 |
| Alcohol | 3.473 | 2.496 | 0.127 | 1.391 | 0.168 | −1.493 | 8.439 |

Dependent variable: CDQ-2.

**Table 3.** The mean score of CDQ-2 for a studied factor.

| | | CDQ-2 | |
|---|---|---|---|
| | | Mean | Standard Deviation |
| Biological sex | Female | 19.3 | 5.4 |
| | Male | 0.1 | 16.9 |
| Higher level of education | Up to secondary education | −19.1 | 1.8 |
| | Post-secondary non-tertiary education | 2.5 | 13.9 |
| | Tertiary education | 19.6 | 1.2 |
| | MSc/PhD | 21.1 | 1.7 |
| Economic level | Low | −15.6 | 10.3 |
| | Middle | 6.9 | 13.6 |
| | High | 16.8 | 12.5 |
| Marital status | Single, divorced, or widowed | −16.7 | 4.8 |
| | Married or cohabiting | 12.7 | 11.8 |
| Physical activity | Low | −14.2 | 7.3 |
| | Middle | 9.7 | 14.5 |
| | High | 19.9 | 1.4 |
| Smoking | Smoker | −14.0 | 12.5 |
| | Ex-smoker | 3.9 | 15.2 |
| | Non-smoker | 15.1 | 14.3 |
| Alcohol consumption | Medium consumption | −13.6 | 11.8 |
| | Social consumption | 3.3 | 15.7 |
| | No consumption | 21.1 | 0.9 |

## 4. Discussion

The present study contributed two main points: first, it documented the suboptimal adherence to healthy dietary patterns among patients with cardiovascular disease, as demonstrated in the low mean scores of both the MEDAS and CDQ-2 tools, and second, it validated the Greek version of CDQ-2 as a culturally adapted, valid, and reliable instrument for assessing the diet quality in this patient population. Moreover, the multivariate analysis revealed several socio-demographic variables, namely, age, sex, marital status, physical activity levels, and smoking status, that were substantial predictors of lower CDQ-2 scores and poor dietary adherence.

Specifically, the participants were not characterized by optimal adherence to proper diet habits. Despite the benefits of optimal diet habits for patients with cardiovascular diseases being distinct and well-documented in terms of lower morbidity [19,20] and mortality rates [20,21], many studies were in line with our findings, revealing inadequate adherence observed, even to the Mediterranean Diet among the inhabitants of Mediterranean countries [22–24]. This finding is indicative of poor self-management and self-care behavior, jeopardizing the secondary and tertiary prevention of cardiovascular disease. Adopting suboptimal adherence to a well-known advantageous diet archetype constitutes a global issue that may be attributed to systemic problems in patient education, nutritional counseling, low healthcare literacy, and limited access to structured and well-organized supportive services.

The low mean scores observed in the MEDAS (8, SD = 5.2) and CDQ-2 (2.9, SD = 17.2), even in a population thought to be highly motivated to change their lifestyle, have important clinical implications, underscoring the clinical importance of the early identification of patients with inadequate dietary habits and the need for tailored nutritional interventions to improve long-term cardiovascular outcomes [8,20]. Furthermore, these findings highlight the urgent need for more systematic, personalized, and non-generic nutritional interventions targeting high-risk patient groups [9,19].

Additionally, younger patients exhibited lower CDQ-2 scores, suggesting diminished adherence to the recommended eating patterns. This finding is in line with prior studies indicating that older individuals are generally more compliant with healthy dietary recommendations and guidelines, potentially due to increased awareness of secondary prevention measures and existing comorbidities [1,2]. Younger patients, even those already diagnosed with cardiovascular disease, may underestimate their risk, leading to a false sense of security, which impedes them from activating healthier diet habits. In contrast, older patients are more likely to adhere to healthier dietary patterns, possibly motivated by the presence of multiple health disorders and concerns about severe cardiovascular events.

Similarly, male sex was found to be significantly associated with lower CDQ-2 scores, suggesting a gender gap in dietary adherence among cardiovascular patients. This is consistent with findings from previous studies indicating that women are more likely to engage in health-promoting behaviors, including healthier eating habits and greater compliance with dietary recommendations [25,26]. Possible explanations for this disparity include higher health literacy levels among women, increased involvement in food preparation, and greater concern for long-term health outcomes. Additionally, traditional gender roles and sociocultural perceptions around masculinity may discourage men from prioritizing dietary changes, especially in older age groups [27].

Regarding marital status, being single, divorced, or widowed was associated with significantly lower adherence to cardiovascular dietary guidelines. Several studies have highlighted the protective effect of marriage or cohabitation on health behaviors and outcomes, including diet quality [28,29]. Living with a partner may provide emotional support, shared responsibility in meal planning, and accountability, which contribute to better adherence. Conversely, individuals who live alone may experience lower motivation to maintain structured eating habits or may resort to convenience and processed foods, especially in the context of older age and chronic illness [30].

The physical activity level was another significant determinant of CDQ-2 scores, with lower activity levels correlating with poorer dietary patterns. This finding aligns with literature suggesting that health-related behaviors tend to cluster together, with physically active individuals more likely to engage in healthy eating [31]. It has been proposed that physical activity improves self-regulation and health consciousness, which may influence dietary decisions. Additionally, individuals who exercise regularly are often exposed to health promotion environments or programs that reinforce positive dietary habits [32].

Active smoking was independently associated with lower CDQ-2 scores. Smokers are generally less likely to follow health guidelines, possibly due to a lower perceived vulnerability to disease or a higher tendency toward risk-taking behavior [33]. Moreover, smoking often co-occurs with other unhealthy lifestyle choices, including poor dietary habits, low physical activity, and high alcohol consumption [34]. This behavioral clustering underlines the importance of integrated lifestyle interventions that address multiple modifiable risk factors simultaneously in cardiovascular patients.

Additionally, this was a clinical study aimed at translating and validating a disease-specific dietary tool, namely, CDQ-2, for assessing dietary habits among patients with cardiovascular disease, based on a seven-day dietary history and biomarkers. The Greek version of CDQ-2 demonstrated good construct and face validity. The Cronbach's alpha was 0.97 for the entire scale, which confirmed the internal consistency of the tool in line with the validation analysis. According to the CFA, a one-factor solution that comprised all 17 items was proposed and accepted for the Greek version of CDQ-2. Therefore, CDQ-2 is a valid and reliable tool that is recommended for use as an overall scale. Moreover, CFA indicated acceptable global fit indices (SRMR = 0.08, CD = 0.99, CFI = 0.99).

We used the MEDAS questionnaire as the gold standard to calculate the concurrent validity of CDQ-2. The MEDAS assessed the main food groups consumed in the Mediterranean Diet. The analysis showed that the mean CDQ-2 total score was 2.9 (SD = 17.2), while the mean MEDAS total score was 8 (SD = 5.2). A bivariate Pearson's correlation revealed a strong, statistically significant linear relationship between the CDQ-2 and MEDAS total scores, with r (90) = 0.962 and $p < 0.001$. This finding underscores the robustness of CDQ-2 in estimating dietary adherence within the cardiovascular setting.

*Study's Strengths and Limitations*

Beyond the strengths outlined above and its contribution of new knowledge to the current body of literature by offering a culturally adapted and validated tool for the dietary assessment of Greek-speaking patients suffering from cardiovascular disorders, the present study had some limitations. First, the cross-sectional design and the single-center nature pose significant threats to the generalizability of the findings to a broader cardiovascular population, as well as to the establishment of causal relationships between dietary habits and patient characteristics or outcomes. Second, the convenience sampling method, combined with the existence of a gender-unbalanced sample, with a greater proportion of males, raises concerns regarding the generalization of the dietary assessment and adherence findings. Last but not least, the potential overestimation or underestimation of participants' dietary habits due to self-report bias may represent an additional issue of the present study.

## 5. Conclusions

This survey supported the validity and reliability of CDQ-2 among cardiovascular patients in Greece, while the strong correlation between the CDQ-2 and MEDAS scores underscored the robustness of CDQ-2 in assessing dietary adherence within this population group. The cardiovascular patients seemed to have suboptimal dietary patterns, as indicated by the relatively low mean CDQ-2 score of 2.9 (SD = 17.2), along with a mean MEDAS score of 8 (SD = 5.2), with younger individuals, males, single/divorced/widowed individuals, individuals with lower physical activity, and active smokers demonstrating poorer adherence to the optimal and beneficial cardiovascular dietary status. Healthcare providers could incorporate CDQ-2 in routine clinical practice to identify patients with a lower capacity to follow and adopt the recommended dietary modifications. Future research is needed to inform clinical practitioners and support the design of tailored and personalized interventions for improving dietary behaviors among cardiovascular patients. Also, future validation efforts should aim to include more gender-balanced and representative samples from multiple centers to confirm the applicability of CDQ-2, which would be more informative in terms of the generalization and exportation of the causal associations between variables.

**Supplementary Materials:** The following supporting information can be downloaded at: https://www.mdpi.com/article/10.3390/nu17101649/s1, CDQ-2 (in Greek).

**Author Contributions:** Conceptualization, K.G., E.P., A.A.C., D.A., N.V., H.B., N.V.F., E.G. and A.E.P.; methodology, K.G., E.P., A.A.C., D.A., N.V., H.B., N.V.F., E.G. and A.E.P.; software, K.G., E.P., A.A.C. and A.E.P.; validation, K.G., E.P., D.A., N.V., H.B. and A.E.P.; formal analysis, K.G., E.P., A.A.C., D.A., N.V.F. and A.E.P.; investigation, K.G., E.P., A.A.C., D.A. and A.E.P.; resources, K.G., E.P., N.V.F., E.G. and A.E.P.; writing—original draft preparation, K.G., E.P., A.A.C., D.A. and A.E.P.; writing—review and editing, K.G., E.P., A.A.C., D.A., N.V., H.B., N.V.F., E.G. and A.E.P.; supervision, K.G. and A.E.P. All authors have read and agreed to the published version of the manuscript.

**Funding:** This research received no external funding.

**Institutional Review Board Statement:** This study was conducted in accordance with the Declaration of Helsinki and approved by the relevant Research Ethics Committees of the Hellenic Mediterranean University (protocol code 29563, approved 8 November 2024). Permission was obtained from the creators to translate, validate, and use CDQ-2. Similarly, to use the MEDAS tool, permission was obtained from both its developers and the researchers who validated the Greek version.

**Informed Consent Statement:** Written informed consent has been obtained from the patients to publish this paper.

**Data Availability Statement:** The data that support the findings of this study are available from the corresponding author upon reasonable request due to privacy restrictions.

**Acknowledgments:** The authors would like to thank all participants for their voluntary participation.

**Conflicts of Interest:** The authors declare no conflicts of interest.

## References

1. Vanzella, L.M.; Rouse, V.; Ajwani, F.; Deilami, N.; Pokosh, M.; Oh, P.; Ghisi, G.L.M. Barriers and facilitators to participant adherence of dietary recommendations within comprehensive cardiac rehabilitation programmes: A systematic review. *Public Health Nutr.* **2021**, *24*, 4823–4839. [CrossRef] [PubMed]
2. Panagiotakos, D.; Sigala, E.G.; Damigou, E.; Loukina, A.; Dalmyras, D.; Mentzantonakis, G.; Barkas, F.; Adamidis, P.S.; Kravvariti, E.; Liberopoulos, E. The burden of cardiovascular disease and related risk factors in Greece: The ATTICA epidemiological study (2002–2022). *Hellenic J. Cardiol.* 2024. [CrossRef] [PubMed]
3. Vervoort, D.; Tchienga, D.; Ouzounian, M.; Mvondo, C.M. Thoracic aortic surgery in low- and middle-income countries: Time to bridge the gap? *JTCVS Open* **2024**, *19*, 210–214. [CrossRef]
4. Yang, G.-J.; Ouyang, H.-Q.; Zhao, Z.-Y.; Li, W.-H.; Fall, I.S.; Djirmay, A.G.; Zhou, X.-N. Discrepancies in neglected tropical diseases burden estimates in China: Comparative study of real-world data and Global Burden of Disease 2021 data (2004—2020). *BMJ* **2025**, *388*, e080969. [CrossRef]

5. Coyan, G.N.; Reeder, K.M.; Vacek, J.L. Diet and exercise interventions following coronary artery bypass graft surgery: A review and call to action. *Phys. Sportsmed.* **2014**, *42*, 119–129. [CrossRef]
6. Casquel De Tomasi, L.; Salomé Campos, D.H.; Grippa Sant'Ana, P.; Okoshi, K.; Padovani, C.R.; Masahiro Murata, G.; Nguyen, S.; Kolwicz, S.C., Jr.; Cicogna, A.C. Pathological hypertrophy and cardiac dysfunction are linked to aberrant endogenous unsaturated fatty acid metabolism. *PLoS ONE* **2018**, *13*, e0193553. [CrossRef]
7. Engelman, D.T.; Ben Ali, W.; Williams, J.B.; Perrault, L.P.; Reddy, V.S.; Arora, R.C.; Roselli, E.E.; Khoynezhad, A.; Gerdisch, M.; Levy, J.H.; et al. Guidelines for Perioperative Care in Cardiac Surgery: Enhanced Recovery After Surgery Society Recommendations. *JAMA Surg.* **2019**, *154*, 755–766. [CrossRef] [PubMed]
8. Estruch, R.; Ros, E.; Salas-Salvadó, J.; Covas, M.I.; Corella, D.; Arós, F.; Gómez-Gracia, E.; Ruiz-Gutiérrez, V.; Fiol, M.; Lapetra, J.; et al. Primary Prevention of Cardiovascular Disease with a Mediterranean Diet Supplemented with Extra-Virgin Olive Oil or Nuts. *N. Engl. J. Med.* **2018**, *378*, e34. [CrossRef]
9. Rees, K.; Takeda, A.; Martin, N.; Ellis, L.; Wijesekara, D.; Vepa, A.; Das, A.; Hartley, L.; Stranges, S. Mediterranean-style diet for the primary and secondary prevention of cardiovascular disease. *Cochrane Database Syst. Rev.* **2019**, *3*, Cd009825. [CrossRef]
10. Sansone, R.A.; Dittoe, N.; Hahn, H.S.; Wiederman, M.W. The prevalence of borderline personality disorder in a consecutive sample of cardiac stress test patients. *Prim. Care Companion CNS Disord.* **2011**, *13*, 27129. [CrossRef]
11. Elgazzar, E.; Ahmed, E.; Ahmed, S.A.; Karousa, M.M. Effects of betaine as feed additive on behavioral patterns and growth performance of Japanese quail. *Benha Vet. Med. J.* **2022**, *42*, 214–218. [CrossRef]
12. Saczynski, J.S.; Marcantonio, E.R.; Quach, L.; Fong, T.G.; Gross, A.; Inouye, S.K.; Jones, R.N. Cognitive trajectories after postoperative delirium. *N. Engl. J. Med.* **2012**, *367*, 30–39. [CrossRef] [PubMed]
13. Beirão, S.; Costa, J.G.; Ferreira-Pêgo, C. Assessing knowledge and awareness of Food and Drug Interactions among nutrition sciences students: Implications for education and clinical practice. *Nutr. Health* **2024**. [CrossRef]
14. Yancy, C.W.; Jessup, M.; Bozkurt, B.; Butler, J.; Casey, D.E., Jr.; Colvin, M.M.; Drazner, M.H.; Filippatos, G.S.; Fonarow, G.C.; Givertz, M.M. 2017 ACC/AHA/HFSA focused update of the 2013 ACCF/AHA guideline for the management of heart failure: A report of the American College of Cardiology/American Heart Association Task Force on Clinical Practice Guidelines and the Heart Failure Society of America. *J. Am. Coll. Cardiol.* **2017**, *70*, 776–803. [PubMed]
15. Paillard, F.; Flageul, O.; Mahé, G.; Laviolle, B.; Dourmap, C.; Auffret, V. Validation and reproducibility of a short food frequency questionnaire for cardiovascular prevention. *Arch. Cardiovasc. Dis.* **2021**, *114*, 570–576. [CrossRef]
16. Gregório, M.J.; Rodrigues, A.M.; Salvador, C.; Dias, S.S.; de Sousa, R.D.; Mendes, J.M.; Coelho, P.S.; Branco, J.C.; Lopes, C.; Martínez-González, M.A. Validation of the telephone-administered version of the mediterranean diet adherence screener (Medas) questionnaire. *Nutrients* **2020**, *12*, 1511. [CrossRef]
17. Michalis, A.; Costarelli, V. The Greek version of the Mediterranean diet adherence screener: Development and validation. *Nutr. Food Sci.* **2021**, *52*, 129–139. [CrossRef]
18. Vieira, L.M.; Gottschall, C.B.A.; Vinholes, D.B.; Martinez-Gonzalez, M.A.; Marcadenti, A. Translation and cross-cultural adaptation of 14-item Mediterranean Diet Adherence Screener and low-fat diet adherence questionnaire. *Clin. Nutr. ESPEN* **2020**, *39*, 180–189. [CrossRef]
19. Cangemi, R.; Miglionico, M.; D'Amico, T.; Fasano, S.; Proietti, M.; Romiti, G.F.; Corica, B.; Stefanini, L.; Tanzilli, G.; Basili, S.; et al. Adherence to the Mediterranean Diet in Preventing Major Cardiovascular Events in Patients with Ischemic Heart Disease: The EVA Study. *Nutrients* **2023**, *15*, 3150. [CrossRef]
20. Mertens, E.; Markey, O.; Geleijnse, J.M.; Lovegrove, J.A.; Givens, D.I. Adherence to a healthy diet in relation to cardiovascular incidence and risk markers: Evidence from the Caerphilly Prospective Study. *Eur. J. Nutr.* **2018**, *57*, 1245–1258. [CrossRef]
21. Furbatto, M.; Lelli, D.; Antonelli Incalzi, R.; Pedone, C. Mediterranean Diet in Older Adults: Cardiovascular Outcomes and Mortality from Observational and Interventional Studies—A Systematic Review and Meta-Analysis. *Nutrients* **2024**, *16*, 3947. [CrossRef] [PubMed]
22. Pant, A.; Chew, D.P.; Mamas, M.A.; Zaman, S. Cardiovascular Disease and the Mediterranean Diet: Insights into Sex-Specific Responses. *Nutrients* **2024**, *16*, 570. [CrossRef] [PubMed]
23. Martimianaki, G.; Peppa, E.; Valanou, E.; Papatesta, E.M.; Klinaki, E.; Trichopoulou, A. Today's Mediterranean Diet in Greece: Findings from the National Health and Nutrition Survey—HYDRIA (2013–2014). *Nutrients* **2022**, *14*, 1193. [CrossRef]
24. Obeid, C.A.; Gubbels, J.S.; Jaalouk, D.; Kremers, S.P.J.; Oenema, A. Adherence to the Mediterranean diet among adults in Mediterranean countries: A systematic literature review. *Eur. J. Nutr.* **2022**, *61*, 3327–3344. [CrossRef]
25. Wardle, J.; Haase, A.M.; Steptoe, A.; Nillapun, M.; Jonwutiwes, K.; Bellisle, F. Gender differences in food choice: The contribution of health beliefs and dieting. *Ann. Behav. Med.* **2004**, *27*, 107–116. [CrossRef] [PubMed]
26. Baker, A.H.; Wardle, J. Sex differences in health behaviours in young adults. *Psychol. Health* **2003**, *18*, 651–668.
27. Courtenay, W.H. Constructions of masculinity and their influence on men's well-being: A theory of gender and health. *Soc. Sci. Med.* **2000**, *50*, 1385–1401. [CrossRef]

28. Lee, H.J.; Ryu, H.; Kang, H.S. The effects of marital status on health behaviors in middle-aged and elderly Koreans. *Int. J. Environ. Res. Public Health* **2020**, *17*, 628.
29. Umberson, D. Gender, marital status and the social control of health behavior. *Soc. Sci. Med.* **1992**, *34*, 907–917. [CrossRef]
30. Hanna, K.L.; Collins, P.F. Relationship between living alone and food and nutrient intake. *Nutr. Rev.* **2015**, *73*, 594–611. [CrossRef]
31. Lenz, M.; Richter, T.; Mühlhauser, I. The morbidity and mortality associated with overweight and obesity in adulthood: A systematic review. *Dtsch. Arztebl. Int.* **2009**, *106*, 641–648. [PubMed]
32. Plotnikoff, R.C.; Costigan, S.A.; Karunamuni, N.; Lubans, D.R. Social cognitive theories used to explain physical activity behavior in adolescents: A systematic review and meta-analysis. *Prev. Med.* **2013**, *56*, 245–253. [CrossRef] [PubMed]
33. Spring, B.; Moller, A.C.; Coons, M.J. Multiple health behaviours: Overview and implications. *J. Public Health* **2012**, *34* (Suppl. S1), i3–i10. [CrossRef] [PubMed]
34. Poortinga, W. The prevalence and clustering of four major lifestyle risk factors in an English adult population. *Prev. Med.* **2007**, *44*, 124–128. [CrossRef]

nutrients

MDPI

*Article*

# Contribution of Food, Energy, Macronutrients and Fiber Consumption Patterns to Obesity and Other Non-Communicable Disease Risks in the Indonesian Population

**Fifi Retiaty [1,2], Nuri Andarwulan [1,3,*], Nurheni Sri Palupi [1,3], Fitrah Ernawati [2], Renata Kazimierczak [4] and Dominika Średnicka-Tober [4,*]**

1 Department of Food Science and Technology, Faculty of Agricultural Technology, IPB University, IPB Dramaga Campus, Bogor 16680, West Java, Indonesia; fifi007@brin.go.id (F.R.); hnpalupi@apps.ipb.ac.id (N.S.P.)
2 Center for Public Health and Nutrition Research, National Research and Innovation Agency, Cibinong Science Center, Bogor 16680, West Java, Indonesia; fitr043@brin.go.id
3 Southeast Asian Food and Agricultural Science and Technology (SEAFAST) Center, IPB University, IPB Dramaga Campus, Bogor 16680, West Java, Indonesia
4 Department of Functional and Organic Food, Institute of Human Nutrition Sciences, Warsaw University of Life Sciences, Nowoursynowska 159c, 02-776 Warsaw, Poland; renata_kazimierczak@sggw.edu.pl
* Correspondence: andarwulan@apps.ipb.ac.id (N.A.); dominika_srednicka-tober@sggw.edu.pl (D.Ś.-T.)

**Abstract:** Background: Obesity, characterized by excess body fat, has been recognized as one of the main global health problems of the current times. This article, based on the data from the Cohort study of risk factors for non-communicable diseases in Indonesia (FRPTM), aims to analyze the food consumption patterns and their association with the risk of obesity and related non-communicable diseases (NCDs) in the Indonesian population. Methods: The article presents data collected from 867 respondents aged 25 years and above observed for 5 years: 2011, 2013, 2015, 2017 and 2019. It includes sociodemographic characteristics, consumption (1 × 24-h recall), anthropometry, and biomedical data (lipid profile, blood glucose, blood pressure). Results: The study identified cereals as the food group consumed in the largest amount and the largest contributor to energy, protein, carbohydrates and fiber intake. The fats and oils group exceeded the recommended intake, while vegetable and fruit consumption, and consequently the fiber intake, were far below the recommendations. The energy and macronutrient intake, and the percentage of respondents with excessive intake levels, were consequently increasing during the studied years. The consumption patterns were associated with the incidence of obesity, which increased from 43.9% in 2011 to 69.9% (central obesity) and 67.9% (BMI-based obesity) in 2019. Conclusions: The dynamics of the consumption patterns clearly impacted the obesity prevalence. At the same time, the NCDs biomarkers measured remained relatively stable despite increasing obesity and macronutrient intake over the study period. The study provides important insights into diet-related risks for obesity in Indonesia, with a potential to inform public health policies and relevant intervention strategies.

**Keywords:** food pattern; diet; obesity; NCD; Indonesia

## 1. Introduction

Obesity, characterized by excess body fat, has been recognized as one of the main global health problems of the current times, with its prevalence reported to be dynamically increasing from year to year, including in lower- to middle-income countries [1]. In 2022, 43% of adults aged 18 years and over were overweight, and 16% were obese [2]. Obesity is a risk factor for a number of non-communicable diseases (NCDs), which impact 70% of deaths worldwide, with this figure being predicted to continue to increase in the next decades. Globally, the most common NCDs include cardiovascular disease (CVD) and type 2 diabetes [3]. One of the targets set in the Sustainable Development Goals (SDGs) is to reduce premature deaths from non-communicable diseases by one-third by 2030 [4].

The unbalanced consumption patterns, defined as the combination of foods that individuals and population groups consume, are among the main risk factors for obesity, and the associated NCDs biomarkers, such as increased blood pressure and dyslipidemia [5–7]. The macronutrient intake, but also the intake of energy and fiber, depending on the consumption patterns, has previously been suggested to be associated with the incidence of certain NCDs [8,9].

In Indonesia, which is the world's fourth most populous country, the prevalence of obesity in 2018 was estimated as 21.8% and increased to 23.4% in 2023 [10,11]. At the same time, the mortality rate due to obesity and other major NCDs risk factors has been on the rise in recent decades. For instance, CVDs were estimated to cause over 30% of deaths [12,13], giving Indonesia a fourth position worldwide with the highest rates of CVD-related mortality [13,14]. Although these alarming figures were clearly changing in tandem with a dietary transition [15], yet relatively few studies have looked into the associations between dietary intakes and patterns, and certain NCDs risk factors for the Indonesian population [16–19].

This article, based on the data from the Cohort study of risk factors for non-communicable diseases in Indonesia (FRPTM), aims to analyze the food consumption patterns of Indonesians and their association with the prevalence of obesity, as an early indication of other non-communicable diseases, including diabetes mellitus (DM), dyslipidemia, hypertension and coronary heart disease (CHD), with a potential to inform public health policies and to serve as a basis for relevant preventive and intervention strategies.

## 2. Materials and Methods

### 2.1. Study Design

This study used a quantitative method with a Secondary Data Analysis approach, using data from the Cohort Study of Non-Communicable Disease Risk Factors (FRPTM) in 2011, 2013, 2015, 2017 and 2019, conducted by the Health Research and Development Agency, Ministry of Health of the Republic of Indonesia. The FRPTM is a study with a prospective cohort design that examines various risk factors related to NCDs. FRPTM study (2011–2019) has been approved by the Health Research Ethics Commission of the Health Research and Development Agency, Ministry of Health of the Republic of Indonesia, with approvals no. KE.01.08/EC/485/2011 dated 10 August 2011, no. LB.02.01/5.2/KE.215/2013 dated 30 May 2013, no. LB.02.01/5.2/KE.135/2015 dated 9 March 2015, no. LB.02.01/2/KE.108/2017 dated 27 March 2017, no. LB.02.01/2/KE.102/2019 dated 8 April 2019.

### 2.2. Study Subjects

The population in this study were adults aged 25 years and above who participated in the Cohort study of risk factors for non-communicable diseases in Indonesia (FRPTM, 2011–2019). A purposive respondent sampling was applied, with the following eligibility criteria: respondents (both women and men) for whom all the data necessary for the purpose of this study's objectives were available, who consequently participated in the study since 2011 (baseline). This study included 867 respondents from FRTPM observed for 5 years: 2011, 2013, 2015, 2017, and 2019.

### 2.3. Data Collection and Measurements

The data analyzed in the study included sociodemographic data (age, gender, education, occupation), consumption data (1 × 24-h recall), anthropometry (body weight (BW), body height (BH), waist and abdominal circumference), biomedical data (blood lipid profile and blood glucose) and blood pressure data (systolic and diastolic). Sociodemographic data were collected using a questionnaire based on the WHO STEPS instrument (WHO 2024) [20]. Subjects were classified as hypertensive if their systolic blood pressure was ≥140 mmHg or diastolic blood pressure was ≥90 mmHg in two measurements with a 5-min interval. Anthropometric measurements included standard body mass index (BMI) and waist/abdominal circumference. The BMI was calculated as BW in kilograms divided by the square of BH in meters. Subjects were classified as overweight if their BMI was ≥23 $kg/m^2$ and as obese if their BMI was ≥25 $kg/m^2$, according to the WHO guidelines for Asian populations [21]. Central obesity was recorded if the waist circumference was >80 cm in women and >90 cm in men [21]. The diabetes mellitus (DM) status was determined by fasting blood glucose ≥ 126 mg/dL and blood glucose 2 h postprandial ≥ 200 mg/dL [22]. Dyslipidemia was determined based on the NCEP criteria (ATP III). Subjects with total cholesterol levels of ≥200 mg/dL, LDL cholesterol (LDL-C) levels of ≥130 mg/dL, triglyceride levels of ≥150 mg/dL, or HDL cholesterol (HDL-C) levels < 40 min mg/dL in men and <50 mg/dL in women were classified as dyslipidemic [23]. The LDL-C/HDL-C ratio value > 2.5 was considered a risk factor for hypertension, dyslipidemia and diabetes [24].

### 2.4. Data Analysis

The food consumption data were arranged based on the food group classification according to the ASEAN Food Composition Table [25] and analyzed using the Wilcoxon Paired Test, with $p$ values below 0.05 considered statistically significant. Nutrient intake data were analyzed using the Indonesian Food Composition Table (TKPI) [26], the ASEAN Food Composition Table, and the Nutri Survey [27]. The status (below RDA/appropriate/above RDA) was based on the recommendations of the Institute of Medicine (IOM) [28]. The obesity status based on the Body Mass Index (BMI) and the central obesity status were calculated using WHO guidelines [21]. The blood pressure, blood glucose, and lipid profile status referred to the limits set in the WHO guidelines [29].

## 3. Results

### 3.1. Sociodemographic Characteristics of Participants

The socio-demographic characteristics analyzed within the study included age, gender, education, and occupation. This study consisted of 867 respondents who were observed for 5 years. The age groups in this study consisted of adults aged 25 years and above, both females (67.7%) and males (33.3%). The most common occupation of respondents was a housewife/assistant (53.3%), and the least common occupation was a farmer (0.1%). The most common education level of respondents was high school (34.3%), and the least common was no school (1.4%).

### 3.2. Consumption Patterns

Consumption patterns during the 5 years of observation presented in Table 1 show that cereals and their processed products were the food group consumed in the greatest amount. In nearly every year of the observation, 100% of respondents consumed this food group, with the largest average of 259.61 ± 111.36 g in 2011. However, it was still slightly below the expected food pattern (PPH), with the recommended daily intake of 269 g. Fats and oils also belonged to the food groups consumed by almost 100% of respondents in each year of observation, with the largest consumption of 78.62 ± 71.68 g in 2019, far exceeding the expected food pattern (21 g). The main source of animal protein in the participants' diet was meat and processed meat, consumed by 58.24–74.27% of respondents, with the highest average consumption level of 71.68 ± 76.41 g in 2019. Nuts and their processed products were consumed by 79.58–87.19% of respondents, with the highest average of 94.19 ± 84.36 g in 2017, far exceeding PPH (37 g) [30]. The "sugar, syrup, and confectionery" group was consumed by 58.36–83.27% of respondents, with the highest average consumption of 34.19 ± 26.48 g in 2019. This average did not exceed the recommended limit of the Ministry of Health, which is 50 g/day. The vegetables were consumed by 83.73–90.19% of respondents, with the highest average consumption of 68.08 ± 58.82 g in 2017, while fruits and their processed products were consumed by 42.67–55.59%, with the highest average consumption of 85.88 ± 121.56 g in 2017. Vegetable and fruit consumption was still far below PPH (262 g). The non-alcoholic beverage group was consumed by 84.77–92.50% of respondents, with the highest average of 471.05 ± 411.44 g in 2019. Looking into the consumption dynamics in the studied period (between 2011 and 2019), there was a drop in the consumption of cereals, and a significant increase in the consumption of fats and oils, sugars, syrup and confectionery, non-alcoholic beverages, starchy roots and tubers, and animal-sourced products such as meat, eggs, and milk and dairy. At the same time, there was a significant increase in drinking water consumption, and a slight increase in vegetables and fruits consumption (Table 1).

### *3.3. Energy, Macronutrients and Fiber Intake*

The results on the energy, macronutrients and fiber intake are presented in Figures 1 and 2. The average energy intake showed an increasing trend within the period under investigation (2011–2019), but it was still below the adequate intake of 2250 kcal, except for 2019. At the same time, the percentage of participants with an excessive energy intake status has largely increased in the observed period, from 4.6% in 2011 to 41.2% in 2019.

The average protein intake also increased during the studied period, although it was still below the RDA (60 g), except for 2019. At the same time, the percentage of respondents with adequate or too high protein intake was consequently increasing during the studied period, reaching 13% (appropriate intake) and 22.4% (above RDA) in 2019.

Except for 2017 and 2019, the average fat intake was also below the RDA (65 g). However, as reported for total energy and protein, the percentage of participants with excessive fat intake has largely increased during the 5 years of observation, exceeding 55% of the studied population in 2017 and 2019.

The carbohydrate intake was also increasing during the course of the five years, but the average value was still below the RDA (360 g). At the same time, the percentage of participants showing an excessive carbohydrate intake appears to have been increasing from 2013 to 2019, with the largest increase between 2017 and 2019 (from 12% to 37%).

The average fiber intake was far below the RDA (32 g), with almost 100% of the studied population not reaching adequate intake levels.

**Table 1.** Food consumption patterns of the population of 867 respondents from FRTPM study in Indonesia during five years of observation (2011–2019).

| Food Groups | n | 2011 Mean ± SD (g) | n | 2013 Mean ± SD (g) | n | 2015 Mean ± SD (g) | n | 2017 Mean ± SD (g) | n | 2019 Mean ± SD (g) |
|---|---|---|---|---|---|---|---|---|---|---|
| Cereals and cereal products | 867 | 259.61 a ± 111.36 | 865 | 241.47 b ± 91.97 | 866 | 259.11 c ± 104.41 | 867 | 255.41 c ± 113.86 | 866 | 234.84 d ± 132.06 |
| Starchy roots and tubers and products | 389 | 16.33 a ± 31.95 | 298 | 16.51 b ± 37.33 | 526 | 24.66 a ± 45.26 | 543 | 34.03 c ± 52.13 | 598 | 43.37 c ± 65.82 |
| Legumes, nuts and seeds, and products | 690 | 76.02 a ± 76.60 | 743 | 67.39 b ± 58.18 | 756 | 83.79 c ± 78.71 | 751 | 94.14 d ± 84.36 | 737 | 83.29 e ± 78.10 |
| Vegetables and products | 742 | 48.13 a ± 42.46 | 726 | 48.72 b ± 47.29 | 747 | 49.71 c ± 46.19 | 773 | 68.08 d ± 58.81 | 782 | 61.15 e ± 52.77 |
| Fruits and products | 420 | 73.19 a ± 107.21 | 436 | 50.56 b ± 77.21 | 370 | 55.29 c ± 96.13 | 482 | 85.88 a ± 121.56 | 477 | 82.39 b ± 122.16 |
| Meat and products | 505 | 42.56 a ± 51.89 | 541 | 36.44 b ± 43.76 | 525 | 50.36 c ± 74.85 | 579 | 63.75 d ± 69.21 | 644 | 71.68 e ± 76.41 |
| Finfish, shellfish, other aquatic animals and products | 464 | 25.34 a ± 36.44 | 465 | 27.30 b ± 37.33 | 491 | 32.15 c ± 55.48 | 430 | 26.23 d ± 42.85 | 388 | 22.43 e ± 41.31 |
| Eggs and products | 470 | 29.93 a ± 40.70 | 594 | 36.10 b ± 40.18 | 464 | 30.82 c ± 41.65 | 516 | 35.73 d ± 44.30 | 577 | 37.22 e ± 45.99 |
| Milk and products | 145 | 6.27 a ± 26.69 | 74 | 3.57 b ± 20.08 | 101 | 6.78 c ± 37.11 | 325 | 10.83 d ± 46.95 | 384 | 13.13 e ± 43.59 |
| Fats and oils | 862 | 41.71 a ± 38.74 | 858 | 37.05 b ± 40.28 | 862 | 55.04 c ± 48.67 | 861 | 71.05 d ± 55.84 | 862 | 78.62 e ± 71.68 |
| Sugars, syrup and confectionery | 641 | 19.55 a ± 18.10 | 506 | 17.19 b ± 33.06 | 658 | 21.95 b ± 22.95 | 691 | 25.61 bc ± 27.09 | 722 | 34.19 c ± 26.48 |
| Spices and condiments | 859 | 11.43 a ± 10.33 | 850 | 12.58 b ± 13.81 | 864 | 15.12 c ± 17.78 | 866 | 19.66 a ± 21.50 | 860 | 13.47 d ± 15.05 |
| Alcoholic beverages | - | - | - | - | 1 | 0.21 a ± 6.28 | 2 | 0.27 b ± 7.65 | 4 | 1.51 c ± 43.47 |
| Nonalcoholic beverages | 735 | 205.70 a ± 231.26 | 788 | 421.15 b ± 357.41 | 791 | 426.35 c ± 369.04 | 802 | 442.09 d ± 347.95 | 794 | 471.06 e ± 411.44 |
| Fast foods | 1 | 0.12 a ± 3.40 | 2 | 0.10 b ± 2.17 | 2 | 0.23 c ± 4.80 | 3 | 0.33 d ± 7.79 | 5 | 0.76 e ± 10.46 |
| Mixed food dishes | 301 | 17.01 a ± 33.70 | 477 | 31.47 b ± 45.63 | 274 | 12.21 c ± 28.57 | 358 | 17.94 d ± 31.81 | 372 | 19.72 e ± 43.89 |
| Miscellaneous | - | - | - | - | - | - | - | - | 3 | 0.00 a ± 0.08 |
| Traditional herbs and supplements | 6 | 0.01 a ± 0.11 | 14 | 0.30 b ± 4.05 | 10 | 0.04 c ± 0.70 | 25 | 0.33 d ± 3.52 | 27 | 0.27 e ± 4.87 |
| Total | | 872.92 | | 1047.90 | | 1123.82 | | 1251.34 | | 1 69.11 e |
| Drinking water | 853 | 984.97 a ± 537.14 | 831 | 1005.10 a ± 598.61 | 853 | 1229.13 c ± 630.26 | 855 | 1297.88 d ± 657.42 | 855 | 1413.01 e ± 749.08 |
| Total with drinking water | | 1857.89 | | 2052.99 | | 2352.94 | | 2549.22 | | 2682.12 |

Different letters within the same row (a-e) show statistically significant differences between years (Wilcoxon Paired Test, $p < 0.05$).

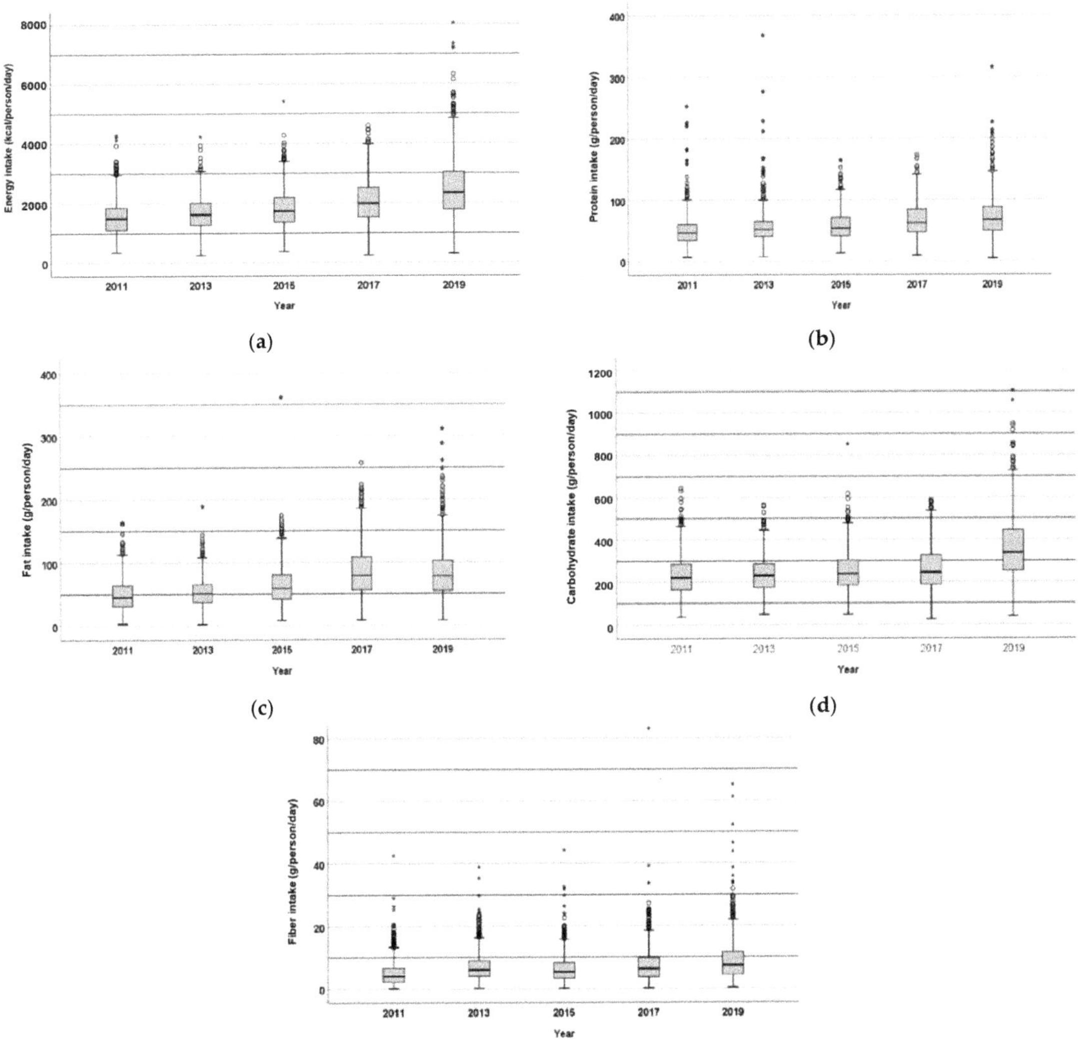


**Figure 1.** Daily intake of energy (kcal/person/day) (**a**), protein (**b**), fat (**c**), carbohydrates (**d**), and fiber (**e**) (g/person/day) by the population of 867 respondents from FRTPM study in Indonesia during five years of observation (2011–2019).

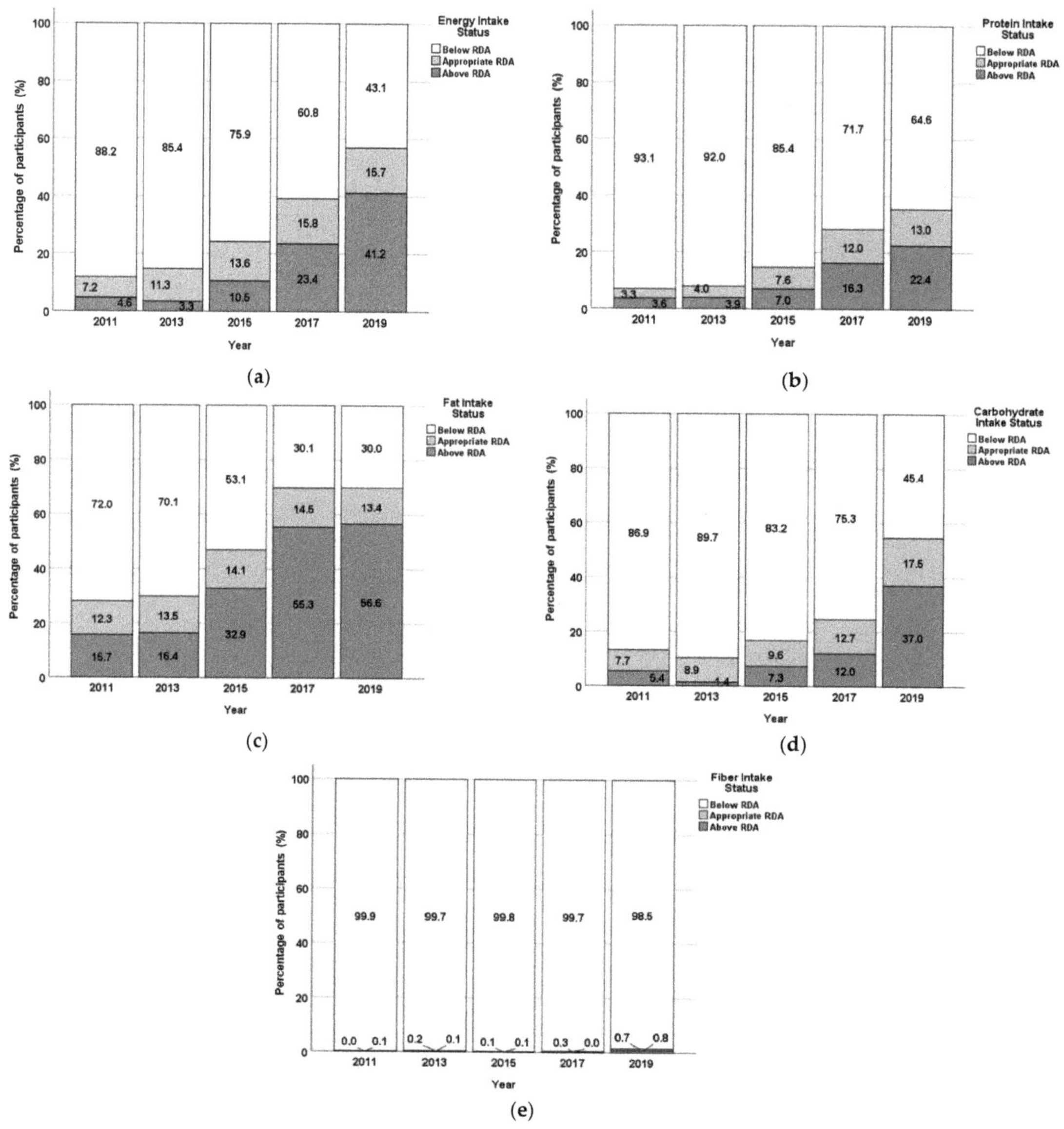


**Figure 2.** Energy (**a**), protein (**b**), fat (**c**), carbohydrates (**d**), and fiber (**e**) intake status of the population of 867 respondents from FRTPM study in Indonesia during five years of observation (2011–2019): percentage of participants with intake levels below RDA/appropriate/above RDA.

### *3.4. Contribution of Food Groups to Nutrient Intake*

The results on the contribution of food groups to nutrient intake are shown in Table 2. The cereals and processed cereal-based foods had the largest contribution to energy (47.71%), protein (37.20%), carbohydrates (71.57%), and fiber (28.03%) intake. The fats and oils group is the second largest contributor to energy intake (16.78%) and contributes the most to fat intake (50.69%). Other food groups that bring fat intake contribution of more than 10% are meat and processed meat-based products (14.88%) and nuts, seeds, and their processed products (10.56%).

Food groups that contribute quite significantly to protein intake are also nuts, seeds, and their products (18.02%) and meat and processed meat-based products (16.4%). Other animal protein source food groups, such as fish, shellfish, and other aquatic animals, contribute 9.56%, and eggs and their processed products contribute 7.11%. The average carbohydrate intake has increased during the 5 years of observation, allegedly due to the consumption of sugars from the high-sugar non-alcoholic beverage group, such as sweet drinks made at home, manufactured sweet drinks, and carbonated drinks. The sugar, syrup, and confectionery food group contributes to carbohydrate intake by 8.04%. Food groups that contribute to fiber intake are vegetables and their processed products (18.54%), nuts, grains, and their products (17.82%), and fruit and processed products (17.67%).

### *3.5. Obesity as an Early Indication of Non-Communicable Diseases*

Central obesity is determined based on waist circumference (WC) (Figure 3). The average value of WC and the central obesity status (% of participants with identified central obesity) increased in the period under investigation, from 43.9% in 2011 to 69.9% in 2019. The obesity status based on BMI (Figure 4) also shows an increase in the percentage of obese subjects, from 43.9% in 2011 to 67.9% in 2019 (although there was a slight decrease between 2015 and 2017).

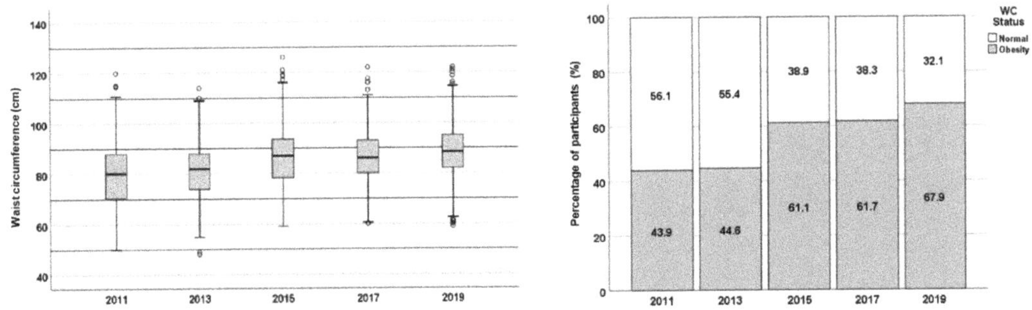


(a) (b)

**Figure 3.** Central obesity status of the population of 867 respondents from FRTPM study in Indonesia during five years of observation (2011–2019), (**a**)—boxplot (waist circumference—WC, cm); (**b**)—percentage of participants with/without central obesity.

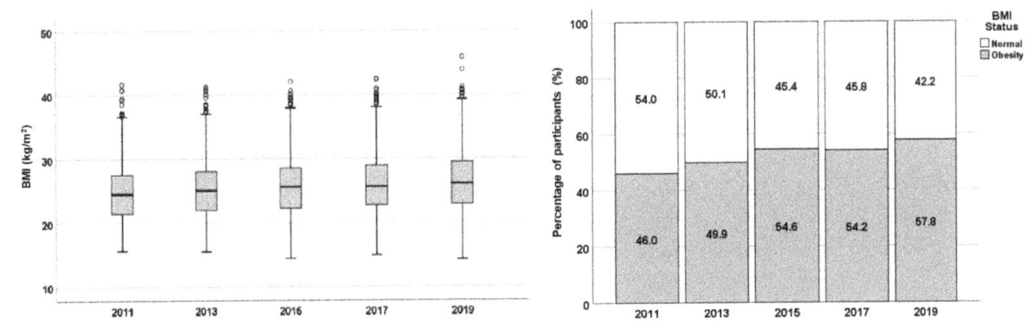


(a) (b)

**Figure 4.** The BMI-based obesity status of the population of 867 respondents from FRTPM study in Indonesia during five years of observation (2011–2019), (**a**)—boxplot (BMI, kg/m$^2$); (**b**)—percentage of participants with/without BMI-based obesity.

**Table 2.** Food group contributions to energy, macronutrients and fiber intake per capita/day of the population of 867 respondents from FRTPM study in Indonesia during five years of observation (2011–2019) (mean ± SD).

| Food Groups | Energy Contribution | | Protein Contribution | | Fat Contribution | | Carbohydrate Contribution | | Fiber Contribution | |
|---|---|---|---|---|---|---|---|---|---|---|
| | kcal/Day | % | g/Day | % | g/Day | % | g/Day | % | g/Day | % |
| Cereals and products | 868.43 ± 389.20 | 47.71 ± 13.75 | 20.96 ± 9.50 | 37.20 ± 13.98 | 5.04 ± 3.40 | 9.21 ± 8.11 | 176.63 ± 79.96 | 71.57 ± 14.42 | 1.70 ± 2.08 | 28.03 ± 22.83 |
| Starchy roots, tubers and products | 33.75 ± 81.15 | 1.78 ± 3.97 | 0.34 ± 0.69 | 0.63 ± 1.79 | 0.40 ± 2.24 | 0.57 ± 2.62 | 7.24 ± 16.57 | 2.92 ± 6.16 | 0.23 ± 0.71 | 3.82 ± 9.50 |
| Legumes, nuts and seeds, and products | 125.60 ± 127.12 | 6.81 ± 6.11 | 10.75 ± 10.14 | 18.02 ± 14.86 | 7.06 ± 8.20 | 10.56 ± 10.23 | 7.22 ± 8.50 | 3.06 ± 3.49 | 1.04 ± 1.23 | 17.82 ± 17.70 |
| Vegetables and products | 16.28 ± 16.35 | 0.92 ± 0.94 | 0.99 ± 1.11 | 1.76 ± 2.10 | 0.26 ± 0.37 | 0.44 ± 0.65 | 3.05 ± 3.12 | 1.31 ± 1.37 | 1.17 ± 1.59 | 18.54 ± 17.17 |
| Fruits and products | 48.84 ± 74.86 | 2.66 ± 3.99 | 0.58 ± 0.91 | 1.05 ± 1.75 | 1.08 ± 4.27 | 1.53 ± 5.47 | 11.86 ± 18.06 | 4.79 ± 7.02 | 1.43 ± 2.64 | 17.67 ± 22.97 |
| Meat and products | 150.13 ± 191.12 | 7.79 ± 9.04 | 11.51 ± 15.12 | 16.94 ± 18.14 | 11.03 ± 14.73 | 14.88 ± 16.75 | 0.92 ± 3.14 | 0.38 ± 1.33 | 0.01 ± 0.14 | 0.21 ± 2.27 |
| Finfish, shellfish, other aquatic animals and products | 34.66 ± 58.00 | 1.97 ± 3.09 | 5.89 ± 10.23 | 9.56 ± 13.07 | 0.81 ± 2.03 | 1.43 ± 3.26 | 0.78 ± 2.06 | 0.33 ± 0.88 | 0.00 ± 0.00 | 0.00 ± 0.07 |
| Eggs and products | 56.38 ± 71.16 | 3.12 ± 4.04 | 4.06 ± 5.24 | 7.11 ± 9.33 | 3.63 ± 4.69 | 5.75 ± 7.83 | 1.47 ± 5.86 | 0.63 ± 2.25 | 0.01 ± 0.06 | 0.26 ± 1.40 |
| Milk and products | 17.49 ± 51.44 | 0.93 ± 2.70 | 1.11 ± 3.06 | 1.8 ± 4.70 | 0.69 ± 2.64 | 1.01 ± 3.89 | 1.71 ± 4.83 | 0.73 ± 2.12 | 0.00 ± 0.00 | 0.00 ± 0.00 |
| Fats and oils | 321.26 ± 237.12 | 16.78 ± 8.16 | 0.50 ± 0.96 | 0.82 ± 1.59 | 35.43 ± 26.32 | 50.69 ± 17.46 | 1.82 ± 3.57 | 0.73 ± 1.44 | 0.34 ± 0.67 | 5.29 ± 10.01 |
| Sugars, syrup and confectionery | 85.28 ± 97.58 | 4.76 ± 5.15 | 0.29 ± 1.30 | 0.49 ± 2.10 | 0.40 ± 1.68 | 0.65 ± 2.76 | 19.43 ± 21.11 | 8.04 ± 8.15 | 0.07 ± 0.55 | 0.78 ± 5.05 |
| Spices and condiments | 8.05 ± 13.29 | 0.44 ± 0.66 | 0.60 ± 2.01 | 0.96 ± 1.82 | 0.10 ± 0.25 | 0.16 ± 0.41 | 1.18 ± 1.72 | 0.52 ± 0.83 | 0.11 ± 0.34 | 2.06 ± 5.14 |
| Alcoholic beverages | 0.80 ± 34.03 | 0.01 ± 0.52 | 0.00 ± 0.13 | 0.00 ± 0.09 | 0.00 ± 0.00 | 0.00 ± 0.00 | 0.03 ± 1.28 | 0.01 ± 0.23 | 0.00 ± 0.00 | 0.00 ± 0.00 |
| Nonalcoholic beverages | 27.55 ± 68.20 | 1.52 ± 3.63 | 0.73 ± 3.42 | 1.22 ± 3.46 | 0.12 ± 0.56 | 0.24 ± 1.31 | 4.62 ± 12.88 | 1.92 ± 5.12 | 0.19 ± 1.25 | 2.42 ± 8.56 |
| Fast foods | 0.87 ± 18.17 | 0.05 ± 1.09 | 0.07 ± 1.58 | 0.09 ± 1.89 | 0.05 ± 1.21 | 0.08 ± 1.71 | 0.02 ± 0.57 | 0.01 ± 0.34 | 0.00 ± 0.04 | 0.02 ± 0.77 |
| Mixed food dishes | 48.98 ± 88.27 | 2.78 ± 5.03 | 1.30 ± 2.48 | 2.33 ± 4.51 | 1.67 ± 3.34 | 2.78 ± 5.68 | 7.23 ± 13.51 | 3.10 ± 5.77 | 0.17 ± 0.48 | 3.07 ± 8.09 |
| Miscellaneous | - | - | - | - | - | - | - | - | - | - |
| Traditional herbs and supplements | 0.01 ± 0.87 | 0.001 ± 0.09 | 0.001 ± 0.06 | 0.002 ± 0.14 | - | - | 0.003 ± 0.18 | 0.01 ± 0.36 | - | - |
| Drinking water | - | - | - | - | - | - | - | - | - | - |
| Total | 1844.36 | 100.30 | 59.68 | 99.99 | 67.77 | 99.98 | 245.20 | 100.05 | 6.49 | 100.00 |

### 3.6. Observation of Biomedical Parameters of Non-Communicable Diseases

Biomedical parameters associated with non-communicable diseases, such as diabetes and cardiovascular disease, include glycemic control (fasting blood glucose/FBG and 2-h postprandial blood glucose), blood pressure (systolic and diastolic), and lipid profile (cholesterol, LDL-C, triglycerides, and HDL-C) [31]. The average values of biomedical parameters during the five years of observation in this study can be seen in Table 3 below.

**Table 3.** Biomedical parameter (selected NCDs biomarker) values of the population of 867 respondents from FRTPM study in Indonesia during five years of observation (2011–2019) (mean ± SD).

| Parameters | Year | | | | |
|---|---|---|---|---|---|
| | 2011 | 2013 | 2015 | 2017 | 2019 |
| Fasting blood glucose (mg/dL) | 92.04 ± 25.91 | 85.80 ± 24.25 | 95.73 ± 30.29 | 105.02 ± 44.80 | 105.88 ± 38.90 |
| Blood glucose 2-h postprandial (mg/dL) | 126.05 ± 53.66 | 123.23 ± 45.87 | 136.34 ± 55.04 | 144.39 ± 68.04 | 138.48 ± 63.25 |
| Total cholesterol (mg/dL) | 195.70 ± 34.81 | 200.23 ± 35.15 | 196.47 ± 35.78 | 199.13 ± 36.73 | 204.82 ± 38.54 |
| Triglycerides (mg/dL) | 106.96 ± 62.79 | 117.25 ± 71.05 | 116.73 ± 68.08 | 122.59 ± 78.52 | 128.60 ± 87.40 |
| LDL cholesterol (mg/dL) | 126.49 ± 30.49 | 128.09 ± 31.75 | 128.03 ± 32.65 | 123.64 ± 31.59 | 128.27 ± 33.54 |
| HDL cholesterol (mg/dL) | 51.37 ± 11.46 | 52.14 ± 12.35 | 52.89 ± 11.25 | 51.80 ± 12.35 | 48.86 ± 11.89 |
| LDL-C/HDL-C ratio | 2.58 ± 0.82 | 2.56 ± 0.82 | 2.52 ± 0.81 | 2.50 ± 0.82 | 2.75 ± 0.93 |
| Blood pressure, systolic (mmHg) | 129.79 ± 23.78 | 127.29 ± 22.29 | 127.80 ± 21.42 | 104.83 ± 29.54 | 128.01 ± 20.09 |
| Blood pressure, diastolic (mmHg) | 81.34 ± 13.24 | 80.76 ± 12.72 | 80.34 ± 12.05 | 83.97 ± 12.15 | 81.00 ± 11.08 |

The mean fasting blood glucose value ≥100 mg/dL was only recorded in 2017 (105.02 mg/dL) and 2019 (105.88 mg/dL), while blood glucose 2-h postprandial ≥140 mg/dL was only recorded in 2017 (144.39 mg/dL). The mean cholesterol levels exceeding the limit of 200 mg/mL were recorded in 2013 and 2019. The mean triglycerides (TG) values during the 5 years of observation have increased, but were still within normal limits (<150 mg/dL). The mean LDL cholesterol level during the 5 years of observation was nearly within the limits (100–128 mg/dL). The average HDL cholesterol concentrations during the 5 years of observation were all in the normal range (>40 mg/dL and <60 mg/dL). The LDL-C/HDL-C ratio during the 5 years of observation, except for 2017, exceeded 2.5, with the limit of 2.5 being recognized as an indicator of the risk of DM and cardiovascular disease [24]. In this study, both systolic and diastolic blood pressure were, on average, in the normal range during the 5 years of observation.

To summarize, the results obtained related to biomedical parameters in this study did not have the same pattern as changes in macronutrient intake, which tended to increase each year of observation.

## 4. Discussion

As previously mentioned, consumption patterns in the presented study showed that cereals and their processed products were the food group consumed in the greatest amount, by nearly 100% of respondents. A similar trend has previously been reported in other studies, focused on the European population [32]. Similarly, fats and oils belonged to the food groups consumed by almost all respondents in all study years, far exceeding the expected food pattern, which is also in agreement with other previous studies [33]. The observed vegetable and fruit consumption far below PPH also confirms global trends and proves the high importance of the intervention in this matter. The results on the energy and macronutrient intake were also mostly in agreement with other similar studies that reported protein and carbohydrate intake below the recommendations [34,35], the increased share of the population with fat intake exceeding nutritional adequacy [35], and the low fiber intakes, with almost 100% of the studied population not reaching adequate intake levels [36,37].

Similarly to the presented study, another study in Indonesia also reported that the main food groups that contribute to energy and protein intake in Indonesian households are cereals, especially rice, next to animal protein sources such as fish and chicken [38]. Another study in Indonesia stated that the main food groups that contribute to energy and protein intake in Indonesian households include carbohydrate staples and protein sources from food consumed outside homes, such as soups, satays, meatball noodles, cooked fish, and processed meat [39]. In another study, fish, poultry, red meat, eggs, milk, and plant sources such as cereals, nuts, and tubers were listed among the food groups that contributed the most to energy and protein intake in Indonesian households [40].

Research in Ireland has shown similar results to this study, reporting that cereal products make a significant contribution to the average daily intake of energy (26%), protein (21%), fat (13%), carbohydrates (41%), and fiber (45%) [41]. Food consumption survey data from five developed countries show that this food group contributes to the daily intake of energy, saturated fat, fiber, and certain nutrients with very similar percentages [42]. Research in the UK population also reported a large (47%) contribution of cereals and their processed foods to carbohydrate intake [43]. The results of this study and studies in several other countries show that the main food groups consumed in the country make the largest contribution to energy and nutrient intake. Other research in Indonesia reported that grain products provided the highest contribution to energy (67.2%) and protein (44.7%) consumption, while animal protein only contributed 38.7% [44].

Both the central obesity and the BMI-based obesity status (% of participants with identified obesity) increased in the period under investigation in the presented study, which was associated with excessive energy, carbohydrate, fat and protein intake and the fiber intake far below the RDA. A high-calorie and low-nutrient diet is known to contribute greatly to the incidence of obesity and NCDs [45], with the prevalence of these conditions significantly growing globally. Other studies also report that carbohydrate intake, especially from sweet foods, contributes significantly to obesity [7,46]. However, the increase in the obesity status in the present study is also suspected due to the increasing status of excess protein and fat intake each year of observation. The status of excessive protein intake in the subsequent years was as follows: 3.6%, 3.9%, 7.0%, 16.3%, 22.4%, while the status of excessive fat intake was 15.7%, 16.4%, 32.9%, 55.2%, 56.6%. Research in Australia has also shown an association between higher total protein intake and increased BMI and LP. Other studies have reported the associations between fiber intake and weight loss, improvement of lipid profiles, glucose metabolism, and blood pressure levels [47,48].

Even though excessive fat accumulation in the body is often attributed mainly to the energy intake exceeding energy expenditures, with excessive food consumption being identified as the primary cause of the imbalance, researchers also attribute the initial cause of obesity to an intrinsic metabolic defect that diverts fuel partitioning from pathways for mobilization and oxidation to pathways for synthesis and storage. The resulting reduction in fuel oxidation and energy capture in adipose tissue leads to a compensatory increase in energy intake [49]. It is generally believed that the primary cause of type 2 diabetes is obesity-induced insulin resistance in non-adipose tissues, combined with insufficient insulin secretion by pancreatic β-cells to overcome this resistance. High levels of circulating free fatty acids are deposited in insulin-sensitive non-adipose tissue cells, resulting in lip toxicity, which is an important cause of insulin resistance [50]. The increase in obesity status in this study can be an early indication of NCDs such as diabetes mellitus and CHD. This study found that excessive consumption patterns and nutrient intake, especially in fat, protein and carbohydrate intake, and lack of fiber intake, tended to increase obesity status, but did not show the same tendency in the diabetes mellitus and cardiovascular disease biomarkers such as blood glucose levels and lipid profile status (dyslipidemia).

Even though not only consumption patterns and nutrient intake are risk factors for NCDs, obesity can trigger diabetes mellitus, which is associated with an increased risk of CHD [51].

Other studies also reported that obesity is not limited to fat accumulation, but there are other risk factors related to hormones as controllers of energy homeostasis. The concept of "disturbed energy balance" is believed to be the beginning of obesity, but various other factors, such as lack of sleep, lack of physical activity, and psychological factors, are also reported to have an influence on the development of obesity [50].

Macronutrient imbalance, particularly due to overnutrition, is a significant risk factor for the development of insulin resistance and type 2 diabetes mellitus. The intake of various nutrients, such as fructose, dietary fiber, fatty acids, and amino acids, clearly affects insulin sensitivity and glucose homeostasis. Adjusting the intake of these macronutrients is essential to prevent insulin resistance, highlighting the importance of understanding their role in energy balance and metabolic health in individuals with diabetes [52]. The relationship between macronutrient proportions and insulin resistance is complex and not fully understood. A high-fat, low-carbohydrate diet significantly reduces insulin resistance compared to a low-fat, high-carbohydrate diet [53]. Fat accumulation, particularly in the abdominal area, can increase insulinemia, which inhibits fat mobilization and oxidation. In individuals prone to obesity, reduced fat oxidation exacerbates this imbalance, contributing to insulin resistance. Thus, macronutrient imbalance, particularly regarding fat, plays a significant role in the development of insulin resistance [54].

Biomedical parameters associated with non-communicable diseases, such as diabetes and cardiovascular disease, reported in this study, included glycemic control, blood pressure, and lipid profile [31]. These biomedical markers did not show the same pattern as changes in macronutrient intake, which tended to increase each year of observation. This is in line with the results of other studies that did not show significant relationships between macronutrient intake and NCDs [55–57]. Interestingly, a study in China concluded that a decreasing trend in high carbohydrate intake, combined with an increasing trend in low fat intake, was significantly associated with an increased risk of diabetes among adults [58]. High daily calorie intake from carbohydrates, protein, and fat significantly contributes to the risk of complications in patients with type 2 diabetes mellitus. Carbohydrate intake exceeding 65% is associated with an increased risk of cardiovascular disease [59].

The cross-sectional epidemiological International Study of Macro/Micronutrients and Blood Pressure (INTERMAP), involving respondents from Japan, China, England and America, found that higher intake of vegetable protein and polyunsaturated fatty acids were inversely associated with blood pressure, while high intake of sugar and animal protein were directly associated with increased blood pressure levels [60]. A study in Korea reported that macronutrient composition significantly affects the risk of hypertension. An unbalanced diet that is high in carbohydrates and sodium is associated with an increased risk of hypertension, especially in women [61].

A Dietary Approaches to Stop Hypertension (DASH) study reported that a carbohydrate-rich diet, combined with an emphasis on fruits, vegetables, and low-fat dairy products and reduced saturated fat, total fat, and cholesterol, substantially lowered blood pressure and low-density lipoprotein cholesterol. The Optimal Macro-Nutrient Intake to Prevent Heart Disease (Omni Heart) study, showed that replacing some carbohydrates with protein (about half from plant sources) or with unsaturated fat (mostly monounsaturated fat) further reduced blood pressure, low-density lipoprotein cholesterol, and the risk of coronary heart disease. The results of these trials highlight the importance of macronutrients as determinants of cardiovascular disease risk [62].

A 6-year cohort study in Tehran showed an association between macronutrient quality, regardless of quantity, and the risk of chronic diseases, especially MetS [63]. Data from the

Korean Genome and Epidemiology Study over 10 years found that a high glycemic load diet increased the risk of developing DM in middle-aged and older Korean men, but not in women [64]. Another 14-year cohort study concluded that higher energy, protein, and fat intake at dinner compared to breakfast increased the risk of DM [65].

The National Health and Nutrition Examination Survey (NHANES) in the United States, including a 15-year cohort study, reported that, in women, low fat (10%) and high carbohydrate (75%) consumption was associated with the least optimal TG and HDL-C. In men, HDL cholesterol was positively associated with fat and no association was detected with TG. The positive association of total cholesterol was especially in men in a diet consisting of 25% protein, 30% carbohydrate, and 45% fat. The highest positive association with systolic in both sexes was in a diet containing low fat (10%) combined with moderate protein (25%). The association with diastolic blood pressure was specific to women with higher values in those consuming fat in the upper range (55%). There was no association between macronutrient composition and glycemic control or adiposity. This study revealed a sex-specific association between macronutrient composition and cardiometabolic health. Further research is needed to explore this association across age groups [66].

A 17-year longitudinal study found that higher diet quality scores were associated with lower risk of MetS or its components among Tehran adults. Higher intake of healthy food group components and lower consumption of unhealthy food group components of the diet quality score predicted lower incident MetS and its risk factors [67]. In a prospective study over 18 years, a higher intake of plant protein was associated with lower total mortality and cardiovascular mortality. Although animal protein intake was not associated with mortality outcomes, replacing red meat or processed meat protein with plant protein was associated with lower total mortality, cancer-related mortality, and cardiovascular mortality [68]. However, another study that also took 18 years, concluded that there was no association between low carbohydrate and high protein consumption with cardiovascular disease [69]. Results of an 18-year study in China showed that both high and low carbohydrate percentages were associated with an increased risk of new-onset hypertension, with minimal risk at 50% to 55% carbohydrate intake. The increased risk was mainly found in those with a low intake of high-quality carbohydrates or a high intake of low-quality carbohydrates. These findings support high-quality carbohydrate intake, and replacement of low-quality carbohydrates with plant products, for hypertension prevention [70]. The 32-year Nurses' Health Study I, and 26-year Nurses' Health Study II, reported that carbohydrate quality plays an important role in the risk of type 2 diabetes. High-quality carbohydrates, especially those from whole grains, were associated with a lower risk of type 2 diabetes. Conversely, low-quality carbohydrates, such as those from refined grains and added sugars, were associated with a higher risk of type 2 diabetes [71].

The results of several studies described above suggest that explanation of the relationships between consumption patterns and NCDs and/or their respective biomarkers requires a long observation period, and taking into consideration the complexity of lifestyle and sociodemographic characteristics, as well as the complexity of dietary factors including, among others, the balance of energy and individual macronutrients but also their quality and dietary sources.

The presented study provides important insights into diet-related risks for obesity and non-communicable diseases in Indonesia, but it has its limitations. The self-reported 24-h dietary recall applied in the study, while valuable for assessing dietary intake, can be affected by recall bias and misreporting, and does not fully allow for capturing all habitual intake characteristics and for the identification of irregularly consumed foods in a typical diet. The accuracy of the undertaken estimations could therefore be enhanced by multiple 24-h recalls or validated food frequency questionnaires. Moreover, the adjustment of the outcomes for a number of potential lifestyle and sociodemographic factors, unexecuted in the study, could allow for further exploration and explanation of the observed trends.

Further research should consider the larger sample size, consumption data in the form of multiple 24-h recall or/and validated food frequency questionnaire, monitoring of a complexity of lifestyle and sociodemographic factors, the addition of other NCD risk factor variables, and, last but not least, a longer observation period.

## 5. Conclusions

To summarize, the study identified cereals as the food group consumed in the largest amount and the largest contributor to energy, protein, carbohydrates and fiber intake. The fats and oils group exceeded the recommended intake, while vegetable and fruit consumption, and consequently the fiber intake, were far below the recommendations, with almost 100% of the studied population not reaching adequate fiber intake levels.

The energy and macronutrient intake, and the percentage of respondents with excessive intake levels, were consequently increasing during the studied years. The consumption pattern of food groups, both in terms of type and quantity, and consequently specific macronutrients, was associated with the incidence of obesity, with the main indications being identified as high consumption of food groups that strongly contributed to overall energy, fat and carbohydrate intake, and fiber consumption below the RDA. At the same time, the biomedical parameters (NCDs biomarkers) measured remained relatively stable despite increasing obesity and macronutrient intake over the study period.

The presented study provides important insights into diet-related risks for obesity in Indonesia. Its results could inform public health policies and help design intervention strategies in Indonesia, such as developing targeted dietary education campaigns, to address excessive fat and insufficient fiber intake.

**Author Contributions:** Conceptualization, F.R., N.A., N.S.P., F.E., R.K. and D.Ś.-T.; methodology, F.R., N.A., N.S.P. and F.E.; validation, F.R., N.A., N.S.P. and F.E.; formal analysis, F.R., N.A., N.S.P. and F.E.; investigation, F.R., N.A., N.S.P. and F.E.; resources, F.R., N.A., N.S.P. and F.E.; data curation, F.R., N.A., N.S.P., F.E., R.K. and D.Ś.-T.; writing—original draft preparation, F.R., N.A., N.S.P., F.E. and D.Ś.-T.; writing—review and editing, F.R., N.A., N.S.P., F.E., R.K. and D.Ś.-T.; visualization, F.R., N.A., N.S.P. and F.E.; supervision, F.R., N.A., N.S.P. and F.E.; project administration, F.R., N.A., N.S.P. and F.E.; funding acquisition, F.R., N.A., N.S.P., F.E., R.K. and D.Ś.-T. All authors have read and agreed to the published version of the manuscript.

**Funding:** This research was funded by the National Research and Innovation Agency, Indonesia, grant number B-4637/II.5.4/SI.06.01/7/2024. The APC was funded with a grant from the Financial Support System for Scientists and Research Teams in the Warsaw University of Life Sciences, Poland (awarded in 2023 to Renata Kazimierczak, grant number 853-2-80-45-780400-S23017).

**Institutional Review Board Statement:** The Cohort study of risk factors for non-communicable diseases in Indonesia has been approved by the Health Research Ethics Commission of the Health Research and Development Agency, Ministry of Health of the Republic of Indonesia (approvals no. KE.01.08/EC/485/2011 dated 10 August 2011; No. LB.02.01/5.2/KE.215/2013 dated 30 May 2013; No. LB.02.01/5.2/KE.135/2015 dated 9 March 2015; No. LB.02.01/2/KE.108/2017 dated 27 March 2017; No. LB.02.01/2/KE.102/2019 dated 8 April 2019.

**Informed Consent Statement:** Informed consent was obtained from all subjects involved in the study.

**Data Availability Statement:** Data will be made available upon request by the author Nuri Andarwulan.

**Acknowledgments:** The authors would like to thank the Health Development Policy Agency for providing secondary data from the FRPTM Cohort Study.

**Conflicts of Interest:** The authors declare no conflicts of interest. The funders had no role in the design of the study; in the collection, analyses, or interpretation of data; in the writing of the manuscript; or in the decision to publish the results.

## References


1. Mohajan, D.; Mohajan, H.K. Obesity and Its Related Diseases: A New Escalating Alarming in Global Health. *J. Innov. Med Res.* **2023**, *2*, 12–23. [CrossRef]
2. World Health Organization. Obesity and Overweight. Available online: https://www.who.int/news-room/fact-sheets/detail/obesity-and-overweight (accessed on 14 March 2025).
3. Gołacki, J.; Matyjaszek-Matuszek, B. Obesity—Standards, Trends and Advances. *Adv. Med. Sci.* **2024**, *69*, 208–215. [CrossRef]
4. Kaptoge, S.; Pennells, L.; De Bacquer, D.; Cooney, M.T.; Kavousi, M.; Stevens, G.; Riley, L.M.; Savin, S.; Khan, T.; Altay, S.; et al. World Health Organization Cardiovascular Disease Risk Charts: Revised Models to Estimate Risk in 21 Global Regions. *Lancet Glob. Health* **2019**, *7*, e1332–e1345. [CrossRef] [PubMed]
5. Damasceno, A. Noncommunicable Disease. In *Heart of Africa: Clinical Profile of an Evolving Burden of Heart Disease in Africa*; Stewart, S.S., Sliwa, K., Mocumbi, A., Damasceno, A., Ntsekhe., M., Eds.; John Wiley & Sons, Ltd.: Hoboken, NJ, USA, 2016; pp. 155–157, ISBN 9781118336960.
6. Kelly, B.; Silveira, S.; Moreira, T.; Oliveira, S.; Andrade, A.; Hermana, H.; Hermsdorff, M.; Oliveira, C.D.; Rosa, B.; Castro, C. Dietary Pattern and Macronutrients Profile on the Variation of Inflammatory Biomarkers: Scientific Update. *Cardiol. Res. Pract.* **2018**, *2018*, 4762575. [CrossRef]
7. Bestari, F.F.; Andarwulan, N.; Palupi, E. Synthesis of Effect Sizes on Dose Response from Ultra-Processed Food Consumption against Various Noncommunicable Diseases. *Foods* **2023**, *12*, 4457. [CrossRef]
8. Crovetto, M.; Sepúlveda, M.J. Relationship between Dietary Energy Intake, Nutritional Status and Cardiovascular Risk in Adults from the Communes of Quellón and Chonchi, Chiloé, Chile. *J. Prev. Med. Hyg.* **2022**, *63*, 435–441. [CrossRef]
9. Pereira, M.; Valado, A. Dietary Fiber in Preventing Non-Communicable Diseases: Predicting Prevented Deaths and Economic Impact through the Use of Algae as a Fiber Source. *Recent Prog. Nutr.* **2024**, *4*, 1–11. [CrossRef]
10. Health Development Policy Agency. *Indonesia Health Survey 2023 in Numbers*; Health Development Policy Agency: Jakarta, Indonesia, 2024.
11. Harbuwono, D.S.; Pramono, L.A.; Yunir, E.; Subekti, I. Obesity and Central Obesity in Indonesia: Evidence from a National Health Survey. *Med. J. Indones.* **2018**, *27*, 114–120. [CrossRef]
12. Ministry of Health Republic Indonesia. Hasil Utama Riset Kesehatan Dasar (Key Results of Basic Health Research). 2018. Available online: https://layanandata.kemkes.go.id/katalog-data/riskesdas/ketersediaan-data/riskesdas-2018 (accessed on 14 March 2025).
13. Ardiana, M.; Harsoyo, P.M.; Hermawan, H.O.; Sufiyah, I.M.; Firmanda, D.R.; Desita, S.R.; Paramitha, A.D.; Hariftyani, A.S.; Shabrina, F.A.; Triastuti, F. Higher Cardiovascular Risks and Atherogenic Index of Plasma Found in Police Officers of Developing Country in Surabaya, East Java, Indonesia. *Clin. Epidemiol. Glob. Health* **2022**, *17*, 101132. [CrossRef]
14. Roth, G.A.; Mensah, G.A.; Johnson, C.O.; Addolorato, G.; Ammirati, E.; Baddour, L.M.; Barengo, N.C.; Beaton, A.; Benjamin, E.J.; Benziger, C.P.; et al. Global Burden of Cardiovascular Diseases and Risk Factors, 1990-2019: Update From the GBD 2019 Study. *J. Am. Coll. Cardiol.* **2020**, *76*, 2982–3021. [CrossRef]
15. Lipoeto, N.I.; Wattanapenpaiboon, N.; Malik, A.; Wahlqvist, M.L. The Nutrition Transition in West Sumatra, Indonesia. *Asia Pac. J. Clin. Nutr.* **2004**, *13*, 312–316. [PubMed]
16. Pengpid, S.; Peltzer, K. The Prevalence of Underweight, Overweight/Obesity and Their Related Lifestyle Factors in Indonesia, 2014–2015. *AIMS Public Health* **2017**, *4*, 633–649. [CrossRef] [PubMed]
17. Mahiroh, H.; Astutik, E.; Pratama, R.A. The Association of Body Mass Index, Physical Activity and Hypertension in Indonesia. *Jurnal Ners* **2019**, *14*, 16–22. [CrossRef]
18. Peltzer, K.; Pengpid, S. The Prevalence and Social Determinants of Hypertension among Adults in Indonesia: A Cross-Sectional Population-Based National Survey. *Int. J. Hypertens.* **2018**, *2018*, 5610725. [CrossRef]
19. Anyanwu, O.A.; Folta, S.C.; Zhang, F.F.; Chui, K.; Chomitz, V.R.; Kartasurya, M.I.; Naumova, E.N. A Cross-Sectional Assessment of Dietary Patterns and Their Relationship to Hypertension and Obesity in Indonesia. *Curr. Dev. Nutr.* **2022**, *6*, nzac091. [CrossRef] [PubMed]
20. World Health Organization. Standard STEPS Instrument. Available online: https://www.who.int/teams/noncommunicable-diseases/surveillance/systems-tools/steps/instrument (accessed on 28 March 2025).
21. World Health Organization. Regional Office for the Western Pacific. *The Asia-Pacific Perspective: Redefining Obesity and Its Treatment*; Health Communications Australia: Sydney, Australia, 2000. Available online: https://iris.who.int/handle/10665/206936 (accessed on 14 March 2025).

22. American Diabetes Association Professional Practice Committee. 2. Classification and Diagnosis of Diabetes: Standards of Medical Care in Diabetes—2022. *Diabetes Care* **2022**, *45*, 17–38. [CrossRef]
23. National Cholesterol Education Program (NCEP) Expert Panel on Detection, Evaluation, and Treatment of High Blood Cholesterol in Adults (Adult Treatment Panel III). Third Report of the National Cholesterol Education Program (NCEP) Expert Panel on Detection, Evaluation, and Treatment of High Blood Cholesterol in Adults (Adult Treatment Panel III). *Circulation* **2002**, *106*, 3143–3421. [CrossRef]
24. Chen, Q.J.; Lai, H.M.; Chen, B.D.; Li, X.M.; Zhai, H.; He, C.H.; Pan, S.; Luo, J.Y.; Gao, J.; Liu, F.; et al. Appropriate LDL-C-to-HDL-C Ratio Cutoffs for Categorization of Cardiovascular Disease Risk Factors among Uygur Adults in Xinjiang, China. *Int. J. Environ. Res. Public Health* **2016**, *13*, 235. [CrossRef]
25. Institute of Nutrition, Mahidol University. *ASEAN Food Composition Database ASEANFOODS Regional Centre and INFOODS Regional Database Centre*; Institute of Nutrition, Mahidol University: Nakhon Pathom, Thailand, 2014; ISBN 9746644807.
26. Direktorat Jenderal Kesehatan Masyarakat. *Tabel Komposisi Pangan Indonesia 2017*; Kementerian Kesehatan RI: Jakarta, Indonesia, 2018. Available online: https://repository.stikespersadanabire.ac.id/assets/upload/files/docs_1634523137.pdf (accessed on 14 March 2025).
27. NutriSurvey. Available online: https://nutrisurvey.de/nbs.htm (accessed on 14 March 2025).
28. Trumbo, P.; Schlicker, S.; Yates, A.A.; Poos, M. Food and Nutrition Board of the Institute of Medicine, The National Academies. Dietary reference intakes for energy, carbohydrate, fiber, fat, fatty acids, cholesterol, protein and amino acids. *J. Am. Diet. Assoc.* **2002**, *102*, 1621–1630. [CrossRef]
29. Khatib, O.M.N. (Ed.) *Guidelines for the Prevention, Management and Care of Diabetes Mellitus*; (EMRO Technical Publications Series No. 32); World Health Organization Regional Office for the Eastern Mediterranean: Cairo, Egypt, 2006.
30. Peraturan Badan Pangan Nasional Nomor 11 Tahun 2023 Tentang Pola Pangan Harapan. Available online: https://peraturan.bpk.go.id/Details/307661/peraturan-bapanas-no-11-tahun-2023 (accessed on 14 March 2025).
31. Fridman, D.; Makaryus, A.N.; Makaryus, J.N.; Bhanvadia, A.; Erion Qaja, A.M.; McFarlaneQaj, S.I. Diabetes and Coronary Artery Disease—Pathophysiologic Insights and Therapeutic Implications. *Intech* **2016**, *11*, 247–260. [CrossRef]
32. Koch, W.; Karim, M.R.; Marzec, Z.; Miyataka, H.; Himeno, S.; Asakawa, Y. Dietary Intake of Metals by the Young Adult Population of Eastern Poland: Results from a Market Basket Study. *J. Trace Elem. Med. Biol.* **2016**, *35*, 36–42. [CrossRef] [PubMed]
33. Schwingshackl, L.; Zähringer, J.; Beyerbach, J.; Werner, S.W.; Heseker, H.; Koletzko, B.; Meerpohl, J.J. Total Dietary Fat Intake, Fat Quality, and Health Outcomes: A Scoping Review of Systematic Reviews of Prospective Studies. *Ann. Nutr. Metab.* **2021**, *77*, 4–15. [CrossRef]
34. Khanam, Z.; Shankar, H.; Mishra, C. Macro-Nutrient Intake of Reproductive Age Group Women: Findings of a Community Based Study from Rural Varanasi. *Int. J. Community Med. Public Health* **2016**, *3*, 566–575. [CrossRef]
35. Zhao, Y.; Araki, T. Evaluation of Disparities in Adults' Macronutrient Intake Status: Results from the China Health and Nutrition 2011 Survey. *Nutrients* **2021**, *13*, 3044. [CrossRef]
36. González-Torres, S.; González-Silva, N.; Pérez-Reyes, Á.; Anaya-Esparza, L.M.; Sánchez-Enríquez, S.; Vargas-Becerra, P.N.; Villagrán, Z.; García-García, M.R. Food Consumption and Metabolic Risks in Young University Students. *Int. J. Environ. Res. Public Health* **2022**, *19*, 449. [CrossRef]
37. Carlsen, H.; Pajari, A.M. Dietary Fiber—A Scoping Review for Nordic Nutrition Recommendations 2023. *Food Nutr. Res.* **2023**, *67*, 1–14. [CrossRef] [PubMed]
38. Baladina, N.; Toiba, H.; Hanani, N.; Suhartini, S.; Widarjono, A. Do Income Levels Affect the Food Consumption Pattern of Households? Evidence from Indonesia. *AEFR* **2024**, *14*, 695–711. [CrossRef]
39. Anindita, R.; Khoiriyah, N.; Sa'Diyah, A.A. Food Consumption Pattern Far Away from Home as a Source of Household Food Protein in Indonesia. *IOP Conf. Ser. Earth Environ. Sci.* **2022**, *1107*, 012118. [CrossRef]
40. Khusun, H.; Februhartanty, J.; Anggraini, R.; Mognard, E.; Alem, Y.; Noor, M.I.; Karim, N.; Laporte, C.; Poulain, J.P.; Monsivais, P.; et al. Animal and Plant Protein Food Sources in Indonesia Differ Across Socio-Demographic Groups: Socio-Cultural Research in Protein Transition in Indonesia and Malaysia. *Front. Nutr.* **2022**, *9*, 762459. [CrossRef]
41. Burke, S.J.; Gibney, M.J.; Dwyer, N.A.O.; Mccarthy, S.N. The Influence of Cereal and Dairy Consumption on the Irish Diet: Implications for Developing Food-Based Dietary Guidelines. *Public Health Nutr.* **2005**, *8*, 227–237. [CrossRef]
42. Auestad, N.; Hurley, J.S.; Fulgoni, V.L.; Schweitzer, C.M. Contribution of Food Groups to Energy and Nutrient Intakes in Five Developed Countries. *Nutrients* **2015**, *7*, 4593–4618. [CrossRef] [PubMed]
43. Laskowski, W.; Górska-Warsewicz, H.; Rejman, K.; Czeczotko, M.; Zwolińska, J. How Important Are Cereals and Cereal Products in the Average Polish Diet? *Nutrients* **2019**, *11*, 679. [CrossRef] [PubMed]
44. Prihatini, S.; Jahari, A.B. Kontribusi Golongan Bahan Makanan Terhadap Konsumsi Energi Dan Protein Rumah Tangga Di Indonesia. *Puslitbang Gizi Dan Makanan* **2010**, *33*, 30–41.
45. Isaura, E.R.; Chen, Y.C.; Yang, S.H. Pathways from Food Consumption Score to Cardiovascular Disease: A Seven-Year Follow-up Study of Indonesian Adults. *Int. J. Environ. Res. Public Health* **2018**, *15*, 1567. [CrossRef]

46. Willems, A.E.M.; Sura-De Jong, M.; Van Beek, A.P.; Nederhof, E.; Van Dijk, G. Effects of Macronutrient Intake in Obesity: A Meta-Analysis of Low-Carbohydrate and Low-Fat Diets on Markers of the Metabolic Syndrome. *Nutr. Rev.* **2021**, *79*, 429–444. [CrossRef]
47. Almaraz, R.S.; Fuentes, M.M.; Milla, S.P.; Plaza, B.L.; Bermejo López, L.M.; Candela, C.G. Indicaciones de Diferentes Tipos de Fibra En Distintas Patologías. *Nutr. Hosp.* **2015**, *31*, 2372–2383. [CrossRef]
48. Karimi, E.; Yarizadeh, H.; Setayesh, L.; Sajjadi, S.F.; Ghodoosi, N.; Khorraminezhad, L.; Mirzaei, K. High Carbohydrate Intakes May Predict More Inflammatory Status than High Fat Intakes in Pre-Menopause Women with Overweight or Obesity: A Cross-Sectional Study. *BMC Res. Notes* **2021**, *14*, 279. [CrossRef]
49. Friedman, M.I.; Sørensen, T.I.A.; Taubes, G.; Lund, J.; Ludwig, D.S. Trapped Fat: Obesity Pathogenesis as an Intrinsic Disorder in Metabolic Fuel Partitioning. *Obes. Rev.* **2024**, *25*, e13795. [CrossRef]
50. Ghanemi, A.; Yoshioka, M.; St-Amand, J. Broken Energy Homeostasis and Obesity Pathogenesis: The Surrounding Concepts. *J. Clin. Med.* **2018**, *7*, 453. [CrossRef]
51. Fatade, Y.A.; Dave, E.K.; Vatsa, N.; Crumbs, T.; Calhoun, A.; Sharma, A.; Shufelt, C.L.; Mehta, P.K. Obesity and Diabetes in Heart Disease in Women. *Metab Target Organ Damage M&TOD* **2024**, *4*, 22. [CrossRef]
52. Yang, K.; Yang, Y.; Xie, Y.; Mao, Y.; Li, X.; Guo, Q. Impact of Macronutrient Composition in Nutrition Shakes on Postprandial Glycemic Response, Appetite, and Food Intake. *Food Hydrocoll.* **2023**, *141*, 108685. [CrossRef]
53. Hasan Entezari, M.; Salehi, M.; Rafieian-Kopaei, M.; Kafeshani, M. Fat and Carbohydrate Proportions Influence on the Insulin Resistance; a Systematic Review and Meta-Analysis on Controlled Clinical Trials. *J. Prev. Epidemiol.* **2017**, *2*, e02.
54. Ailshul, M.D. Energy Balance and Obesity in Man. *Nutr. Today* **1975**, *10*, 29–30. [CrossRef]
55. Temesgen, M.; Ratta, N. Adverse Effect of Fat Intake on Insulin Sensitivity and Associated Risk of Non-Communicable Diseases (NCD): A Review. *Adv. Life Sci. Technol.* **2015**, *29*, 23–40.
56. McKenzie, M.R.; Illingworth, S. Should a Low Carbohydrate Diet Be Recommended for Diabetes Management? *Proc. Nutr. Soc.* **2017**, *76*, 91027. [CrossRef]
57. Wikarek, T.; Kocełak, P.; Owczarek, A.J.; Chudek, J.; Olszanecka-Glinianowicz, M. Effect of Dietary Macronutrients on Postprandial Glucagon and Insulin Release in Obese and Normal-Weight Women. *Int. J. Endocrinol.* **2020**, *2020*, 4603682. [CrossRef] [PubMed]
58. Wang, S.; Ruirui, G.; Li, X.; Wang, F.; Wu, Z.; Liu, Y.; Dong, Y.; Li, B. The Association between Multiple Trajectories of Macronutrient Intake and the Risk of New-Onset Diabetes in Chinese Adults. *J. Diabetes* **2024**, *16*, e13555. [CrossRef]
59. El-Alameey, I.R.; Aljohani, R.N.; Allhebi, S.A.; Alahmadi, H.A.; Alsakrani, R.K. Macronutrient Intake and Association with the Risk Factors of Diabetic Complications among People with Type 2 Diabetes. *Maced. J. Med. Sci.* **2024**, *12*, 73–82. [CrossRef]
60. Chan, Q.; Stamler, J.; Oude Griep, L.M.; Daviglus, M.L.; Van Horn, L.; Elliott, P. An Update on Nutrients and Blood Pressure Summary of INTERMAP Study Findings. *J. Atheroscler. Thromb.* **2016**, *23*, 276–289. [CrossRef]
61. Oh, H.Y.; Kim, M.K.; Lee, M.; Kim, Y.O. Macronutrient Composition and Sodium Intake of Diet Are Associated with Risk of Metabolic Syndrome and Hypertension in Korean Women. *PLoS ONE* **2013**, *8*, e78088. [CrossRef]
62. Miller, V.; Mente, A.; Dehghan, M.; Rangarajan, S.; Zhang, X.; Swaminathan, S.; Dagenais, G.; Gupta, R.; Mohan, V.; Lear, S.; et al. Fruit, Vegetable, and Legume Intake, and Cardiovascular Disease and Deaths in 18 Countries (PURE): A Prospective Cohort Study. *Lancet* **2017**, *390*, 2037–2049. [CrossRef] [PubMed]
63. Farhadnejad, H.; Mokhtari, E.; Teymoori, F.; Jahromi, M.K.; Saber, N.; Ahmadirad, H.; Norouzzadeh, M.; Mirmiran, P.; Azizi, F. Macronutrients Quality Indices and Risk of Metabolic Syndrome and Its Components in Iranian Adults. *BMC Cardiovasc. Disord.* **2024**, *24*, 126. [CrossRef]
64. Lee, S.W.; Kim, H.C.; Nam, C.; Lee, H.Y.; Ahn, S.V.; Oh, Y.A.; Suh, I. Age-Differential Association between Serum Uric Acid and Incident Hypertension. *Hypertens. Res.* **2019**, *42*, 428–437. [CrossRef]
65. Ren, X.; Yang, X.; Jiang, H.; Han, T.; Sun, C. The Association of Energy and Macronutrient Intake at Dinner vs Breakfast with the Incidence of Type 2 Diabetes Mellitus in a Cohort Study: The China Health and Nutrition Survey, 1997–2011. *J. Diabetes* **2021**, *13*, 882–892. [CrossRef] [PubMed]
66. Koemel, N.A.; Senior, A.M.; Laouali, N.; Celermajer, D.S.; Grech, A.; Parker, H.M.; Simpson, S.J.; Raubenheimer, D.; Gill, T.P.; Skilton, M.R. Associations between Dietary Macronutrient Composition and Cardiometabolic Health: Data from NHANES 1999–2014. *Eur. J. Nutr.* **2025**, *64*, 68. [CrossRef] [PubMed]
67. Mirmiran, P.; Hosseini-Esfahani, F.; Esfandiar, Z.; Hosseinpour-Niazi, S.; Azizi, F. Associations between Dietary Antioxidant Intakes and Cardiovascular Disease. *Sci. Rep.* **2022**, *12*, 1504. [CrossRef]
68. Budhathoki, S.; Sawada, N.; Iwasaki, M.; Yamaji, T.; Goto, A.; Kotemori, A.; Ishihara, J.; Takachi, R.; Charvat, H.; Mizoue, T.; et al. Association of Animal and Plant Protein Intake with All-Cause and Cause-Specific Mortality in a Japanese Cohort. *JAMA Intern. Med.* **2019**, *179*, 1509–1518. [CrossRef]

69. Nilsson, L.M.; Winkvist, A.; Eliasson, M.; Jansson, J.H.; Hallmans, G.; Johansson, I.; Lindahl, B.; Lenner, P.; Van Guelpen, B. Low-Carbohydrate, High-Protein Score and Mortality in a Northern Swedish Population-Based Cohort. *Eur. J. Clin. Nutr.* **2012**, *66*, 694–700. [CrossRef]
70. Li, X.; Yu, J.; Wen, L.; Li, Q.; Yan, J.; Tian, J.; Tong, C.; Tong, Q.; Qi, H.; Saffery, R.; et al. Vitamin D Status in Women with Dichorionic Twin Pregnancies and Their Neonates: A Pilot Study in China. *BMC Pregnancy Childbirth* **2021**, *21*, 279. [CrossRef]
71. Braun, K.; Guasch-Ferré, M.L.; Malik, V.; Alessa, H.; Willett, W.; Hu, F.B.; Voortman, T.; Bhupathiraju, S. Carbohydrate Quantity and Quality and Risk of Type 2 Diabetes: Results from Three Large Prospective US Cohorts. *Curr. Dev. Nutr.* **2020**, *4*, 1380. [CrossRef]

nutrients

MDPI

*Article*

# Assessment of the Risk of Insulin Resistance in Workers Classified as Metabolically Healthy Obese

**Miguel García Samuelsson [1,2], Pedro Juan Tárraga López [3], Ángel Arturo López-González [1,2,4,5,*], Hernán Paublini [1,2], Emilio Martínez-Almoyna Rifá [1,2] and José Ignacio Ramírez-Manent [1,4,5,6]**

1 ADEMA-Health Group, University Institute of Health Sciences (IUNICS), 07120 Palma de Mallorca, Balearic Islands, Spain; miguelsamuelsson@gmail.com (M.G.S.); h.paublini@eua.edu.es (H.P.); emilio@mompra.com (E.M.-A.R.); jignacioramirez@telefonica.net (J.I.R.-M.)
2 Faculty of Dentistry, ADEMA-UIB University School, 07009 Palma de Mallorca, Balearic Islands, Spain
3 Faculty of Medicine, University of Castilla-La Mancha, 02071 Albacete, Spain; pjtarraga@sescam.jccm.es
4 Balearic Islands Health Research Institute Foundation (IDISBA), 07004 Palma de Mallorca, Balearic Islands, Spain
5 Balearic Islands Health Service, 07003 Palma de Mallorca, Balearic Islands, Spain
6 Faculty of Medicine, University of the Balearic Islands, 07122 Palma de Mallorca, Balearic Islands, Spain
* Correspondence: angarturo@gmail.com

**Abstract: Introduction and Objectives**: Obesity constitutes a significant public health concern and is frequently linked to metabolic dysfunctions, particularly insulin resistance (IR). Nevertheless, a subset of obese individuals, referred to as metabolically healthy obese (MHO), do not exhibit overt metabolic abnormalities. The present study aims to assess the risk of developing IR among MHO workers and to explore the determinants contributing to this risk. **Methods**: This cross-sectional investigation utilized data from a cohort of 68,884 obese workers across multiple occupational sectors in Spain. The classification of participants as MHO was based on the number of metabolic syndrome components, in accordance with the criteria established by the National Cholesterol Education Program Adult Treatment Panel III (NCEP-ATPIII). Anthropometric, clinical, and biochemical parameters—including body mass index (BMI), waist circumference, lipid profile, glycemic levels, and blood pressure—were systematically assessed. The likelihood of developing IR was estimated through various validated risk assessment models. **Results**: The analysis indicates that, despite having a relatively favorable metabolic profile, individuals classified as MHO also show signs of metabolic deterioration, such as an increased risk of insulin resistance. Key risk factors such as physical inactivity, low adherence to the Mediterranean diet, and socioeconomic disparities were identified as significant contributors to the transition from the MHO phenotype to a metabolically unhealthy state. Logistic regression analyses corroborated that insufficient physical activity and suboptimal dietary habits were strongly associated with an elevated risk of IR. **Conclusions**: The findings underscore the dynamic and potentially transient nature of the MHO phenotype, emphasizing the necessity of proactive monitoring and early preventive strategies. Encouraging physical activity, promoting adherence to a nutritionally balanced diet, and implementing workplace health initiatives emerge as critical measures to attenuate the risk of IR and metabolic deterioration in MHO individuals. Future longitudinal studies are warranted to enhance risk stratification and to formulate tailored preventive interventions.

**Keywords:** metabolically healthy obese; insulin resistance; Mediterranean diet; physical activity; sociodemographic variables; tobacco consumption

## 1. Introduction

Obesity represents one of the major public health challenges of the 21st century [1], frequently associated with various metabolic comorbidities, among which insulin resistance (IR) stands out [2]. However, a subgroup of obese individuals, referred to as "metabolically healthy obese" (MHO), appears not to exhibit the typical metabolic dis-turbances associated with excess adiposity [3]. This apparent paradox has garnered in-creasing interest within the scientific community, particularly concerning the risk of de-veloping IR in this population [4,5].

MHO individuals are defined as those with a body mass index (BMI) greater than 30 kg/m$^2$ who, despite being obese, do not exhibit insulin resistance or other associated metabolic risk factors such as hypertension or hyperglycemia [6]. The most distinctive characteristic of these individuals is their higher insulin sensitivity compared to metabolically unhealthy obese (NMHO) individuals [7]. Additionally, they tend to have a more favorable lipid profile [8], lower levels of inflammatory markers [9], and a fat distribution that favors subcutaneous rather than visceral storage. This adipose tissue distribution may play a protective role against the development of metabolic disorders [10]. Epidemiological studies estimate that this phenotype accounts for approximately 10% to 30% of the obese population, depending on the diagnostic criteria employed and the demographic characteristics of the analyzed cohorts [11].

Insulin resistance is a condition in which muscle, fat, and liver cells do not respond adequately to insulin, hindering glucose uptake and leading to elevated blood sugar levels [12]. This dysfunction is a key factor in the pathogenesis of type 2 diabetes mellitus [13] and is associated with an increased risk of cardiovascular disease [14]. Several factors contribute to the development of IR, including visceral fat accumulation [15], chronic low-grade inflammation [16], and alterations in adipokine secretion [17]. Unlike subcutaneous fat, visceral fat exhibits higher lipolytic activity and releases free fatty acids into the portal system, negatively affecting liver function and promoting IR [18]. Additionally, visceral adipose tissue secretes proinflammatory cytokines that interfere with insulin signaling [19].

Although individuals with metabolically healthy obesity (MHO) exhibit a more favorable metabolic profile compared to those with non-metabolically healthy obesity (NMHO), evidence suggests that this condition may be transient [20]. Various studies have indicated that MHO is not an entirely benign phenotype, as many individuals classified within this category may transition to a metabolically unhealthy state over time. The dynamic nature of MHO, which differentiates between individuals with a stable profile and those transitioning to NMHO, could explain the discrepancies observed in the literature. Additionally, research has shown that individuals with MHO have a higher risk of developing metabolic abnormalities over time, such as insulin resistance, dyslipidemia, and hypertension, increasing their vulnerability to cardiovascular and metabolic diseases [21,22]. Therefore, longitudinal follow-up is essential to identify individuals at greater risk of progression to a less favorable state and to design appropriate intervention strategies.

Epigenetic studies using biomarkers indicate that a significant proportion of MHO individuals develop IR and other metabolic complications over time [23]. Findings from the CORDIOPREV study, with a 5-year follow-up, revealed that 71.8% of people with MHO moved into the NMHO category [24]. The transition from an MHO phenotype to a metabolically unhealthy state may be influenced by factors such as aging [25], additional weight gain [26], physical inactivity [27], and genetic predisposition [28]. Furthermore, the ability of subcutaneous adipose tissue to expand and store excess energy without inducing inflammation or fibrosis appears to be a crucial determinant in maintaining metabolic health in obese individuals [29].

The early identification of IR in MHO individuals is essential for implementing preventive strategies to avoid progression toward NMHO states. The Homeostasis Model

Assessment (HOMA) index is a widely used tool for estimating IR in clinical and epidemiological studies [30]. Research in pediatric populations has demonstrated that the HOMA index is useful in distinguishing between metabolically healthy and unhealthy obesity, suggesting its applicability across different age groups [31].

In addition to IR assessment, it is important to consider other clinical and biochemical markers, such as adiponectin levels [32], C-reactive protein [33], and lipid profiles [34], for a more comprehensive characterization of the metabolic status of MHO individuals. Adiponectin, in particular, has been associated with increased insulin sensitivity [35] and a lower cardiovascular risk [36], with higher levels observed in MHO individuals compared to their NMHO counterparts.

Recognizing the metabolic heterogeneity among obese individuals has significant implications for clinical practice. While MHO individuals have a lower immediate risk of metabolic complications, they should not be considered risk free. Regular monitoring of metabolic parameters and the promotion of healthy lifestyle habits, including a balanced diet and regular physical activity, are essential for maintaining metabolic health and preventing the onset of IR and other comorbidities.

Interventions aimed at improving adipose tissue function, such as strategies to enhance the storage capacity of subcutaneous adipose tissue and reduce inflammation, may be beneficial in preventing the transition from an MHO phenotype to a NMHO state. Additionally, identifying genetic and molecular markers that predict susceptibility to developing IR in MHO individuals could facilitate the implementation of personalized interventions.

The objective of this study is to assess the level of IR risk in a cohort of workers classified as MHO.

## 2. Methods

### 2.1. Study Design and Participants

A cross-sectional descriptive analysis was conducted using data from occupational medical examinations performed on 68,884 obese Spanish workers (45,498 men and 23,386 women) across the primary, secondary, and tertiary sectors between January 2019 and June 2020.

Inclusion Criteria:

- Obesity, defined as a body mass index (BMI) $\geq 30$ kg/m$^2$.
- Age between 18 and 69 years.
- Employment at one of the participating companies.
- Voluntary participation in the study.

Exclusion Criteria:

- Individuals younger than 18 or older than 69 years.
- No employment contract with any participating company.
- Did not provide informed consent to participate in the study.
- Did not authorize the use of their data for epidemiological purposes.
- Missing variables necessary for calculations.
- Body mass index (BMI) $\leq 30$ kg/m$^2$.

The participant flowchart is presented in Figure 1.

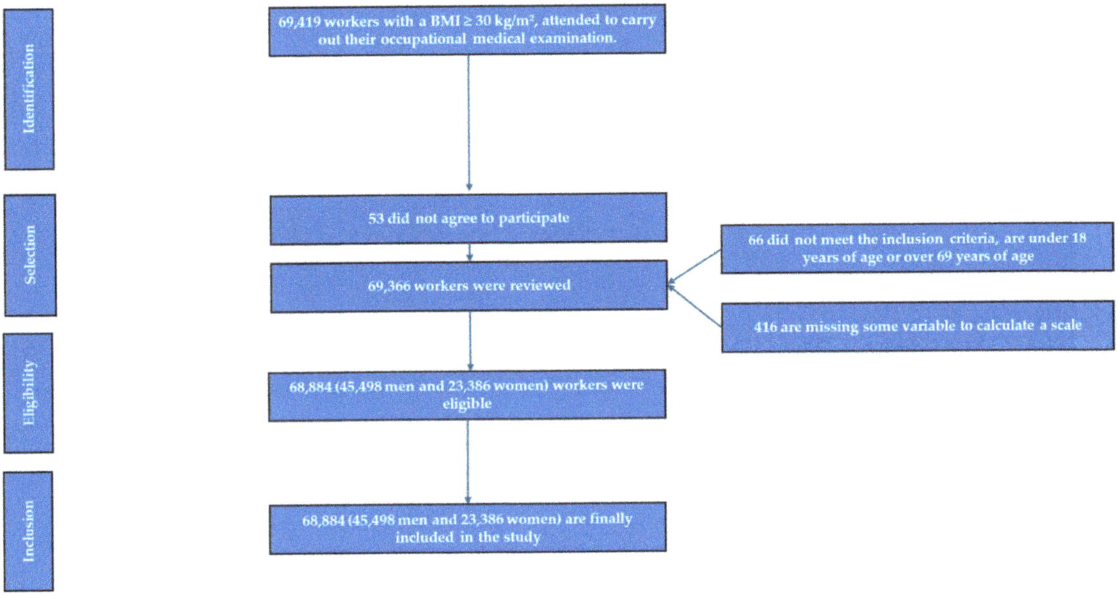


**Figure 1.** Flowchart of the participants in the study.

### 2.2. Variable Assessment

After standardizing measurement techniques, the study's medical and nursing personnel conducted clinical, analytical, and anthropometric assessments, including waist circumference, weight, and height.

Body weight and height were measured using a SECA 700 scale (SECA, Chino, CA, USA) and a SECA 220 stadiometer (SECA, Chino, CA, USA). Participants were barefoot and wearing underwear, following ISAK guidelines for anthropometric assessments [37]. Waist circumference was assessed with a SECA measuring tape (SECA, Chino, CA, USA), ensuring proper positioning: participants stood upright, with feet together and abdomen relaxed. The tape was placed parallel to the floor at the level of the lowest floating rib [38].

Blood pressure was recorded using a calibrated OMRON M3 automatic sphygmomanometer (OMRON, Osaka, Japan) while participants remained seated after a minimum rest period of 10 min. Three consecutive measurements were taken at 60 s intervals, and the final recorded value corresponded to the average of these readings.

### 2.3. Biochemical Analyses

Following a fasting period of at least 12 h, biochemical parameters were assessed. Concentrations of total cholesterol, glucose, and triglycerides were determined through automated enzymatic techniques. High-density lipoprotein cholesterol (HDL-c) levels were obtained using dextran sulfate-$MgCl_2$ precipitation methods. Low-density lipoprotein cholesterol (LDL-c) was indirectly estimated using the Friedewald equation [39], expressed in mg/dL:

$$\text{LDL-c} = \text{Total Cholesterol} - \text{HDL-c} + \text{Triglycerides}/5$$

Obesity was defined as a body mass index (BMI) $\geq 30$ kg/m$^2$.

### 2.4. Definition of Metabolically Healthy Obesity (MHO)

To classify individuals as metabolically healthy obese (MHO), the criteria established by the National Cholesterol Education Program Adult Treatment Panel III (NCEP-ATPIII) for metabolic syndrome (MS) were applied [40]. These criteria included the presence of at least one of the following metabolic risk factors:

- Waist circumference: ≥88 cm in women and ≥102 cm in men.
- Triglyceride levels: ≥150 mg/dL or undergoing lipid-lowering therapy.
- HDL cholesterol levels: <50 mg/dL in women or <40 mg/dL in men.
- Fasting glucose levels: ≥100 mg/dL or receiving glucose-lowering treatment.
- Blood pressure status: Systolic blood pressure (SBP) ≥ 130 mmHg and/or diastolic blood pressure (DBP) ≥ 85 mmHg, or the use of antihypertensive therapy.

Participants were subsequently categorized into three groups based on the number of metabolic syndrome components present:

- Group A: No metabolic syndrome factors.
- Group B: One metabolic syndrome factor.
- Group C: Up to two metabolic syndrome factors.

### 2.5. Demographic and Socioeconomic Variables

- Sex was recorded as a binary variable (male or female).
- Age was determined by subtracting the date of birth from the date of the medical ex-amination.
- Educational attainment was categorized into three levels: Primary education, High school education, and University education.
- Socioeconomic status was classified according to the Spanish Society of Epidemiolo-gy criteria, based on the 2011 National Occupational Classification (CNO-11) [41], and categorized as follows:
    - Social Class I: Executives, university-educated professionals, athletes, and artists.
    - Social Class II: Intermediate professionals and skilled self-employed workers.
    - Social Class III: Low-skilled workers.

Lifestyle and Behavioral Variables

- Participants were classified as smokers if they had consumed any form of tobacco at least once per day in the past 30 days or had ceased smoking within the preceding 12 months.
- Adherence to the Mediterranean diet was evaluated using a 14-item questionnaire, with responses scored as 0 or 1 point per item. A total score ≥ 9 was indicative of high adherence [42].
- Physical activity levels were assessed using the International Physical Activity Questionnaire (IPAQ), a self reported instrument designed to quantify physical activity patterns over the previous 7 days [43].

### 2.6. Statistical Analysis

Descriptive statistics were employed to summarize categorical variables, expressed as frequencies and distributions, while the normality of continuous variables was assessed using the Kolmogorov–Smirnov test. Means and standard deviations were calculated for quantitative variables. Bivariate analyses included a Student's t-test for mean comparisons and chi square tests for proportion analysis. To examine factors associated with metabolically healthy obesity (MHO), a multinomial logistic regression model was applied, with model fit assessed using the Hosmer–Lemeshow test. Stratified analyses were conducted to control for potential confounders, but no significant effects were detected. All statistical procedures were executed using SPSS (version 29.0), with statistical significance set at $p < 0.05$.

### 2.7. Ethical Considerations

This study was conducted in accordance with ethical research standards, including compliance with the 2013 Declaration of Helsinki. The anonymity and confidentiality of participants were strictly safeguarded throughout the study. Ethical approval was granted by the Balearic Islands Research Ethics Committee (CEI-IB) under reference number IB 4383/20, approved on 26 November 2020. All participant data were coded, ensuring that only the principal investigator had access to personally identifiable information. The majority of researchers involved in the study adhered to Organic Law 3/2018 (December 5) on Personal Data Protection and Digital Rights, guaranteeing that participants retained the right to access, rectify, erase, and object to the processing of their data at any time.

## 3. Results

Table 1 presents the characteristics of the study participants, highlighting that anthropometric, clinical, and analytical variables show less favorable values in men. The predominant age group in this study falls between 30 and 49 years. Most workers belong to the lowest socioeconomic levels (social class III) and have only primary education. Physical activity levels and adherence to the Mediterranean diet are notably low. More than 31% of men and slightly more than one in four women are smokers.

**Table 1.** Characteristics of the participants.

| | **Men n = 45,498** | **Women n = 23,386** | |
|---|---|---|---|
| | Mean (SD) | Mean (SD) | *p*-Value |
| Age (years) | 42.9 (10.0) | 42.0 (10.4) | <0.001 |
| Height (cm) | 173.2 (7.1) | 160.0 (6.7) | <0.001 |
| Weight (kg) | 99.7 (12.4) | 87.5 (12.3) | <0.001 |
| Waist (cm) | 96.7 (8.9) | 83.3 (8.8) | <0.001 |
| Hip (cm) | 108.6 (7.9) | 109.5 (9.3) | <0.001 |
| Systolic BP (mmHg) | 131.8 (16.2) | 124.0 (15.9) | <0.001 |
| Diastolic BP (mmHg) | 81.0 (10.7) | 76.9 (11.0) | <0.001 |
| Total cholesterol (mg/dL) | 204.1 (38.8) | 200.3 (37.4) | <0.001 |
| HDL-cholesterol (mg/dL) | 48.3 (7.0) | 51.2 (7.1) | <0.001 |
| LDL-cholesterol (mg/dL) | 124.5 (37.5) | 127.1 (37.0) | <0.001 |
| Triglycerides (mg/dL) | 158.6 (108.4) | 110.5 (55.8) | <0.001 |
| Glucose (mg/dL) | 92.3 (14.0) | 89.0 (13.4) | <0.001 |
| | % | % | *p*-Value |
| <30 years | 10.0 | 13.5 | <0.001 |
| 30–39 years | 28.3 | 28.2 | |
| 40–49 years | 34.5 | 32.3 | |
| 50–59 years | 22.6 | 21.9 | |
| 60–69 years | 4.6 | 4.3 | |
| Elementary school | 63.7 | 64.9 | <0.001 |
| High school | 32.3 | 30.6 | |
| University | 4.0 | 4.5 | |
| Social class I | 4.6 | 4.2 | <0.001 |
| Social class II | 15.7 | 21.4 | |
| Social class III | 79.7 | 74.4 | |
| No physical activity | 96.5 | 95.3 | <0.001 |
| Physical activity | 3.5 | 4.7 | |
| No Mediterranean diet | 91.8 | 85.1 | <0.001 |
| Mediterranean diet | 8.2 | 14.9 | |
| Non-smokers | 68.3 | 74.0 | <0.001 |
| Smokers | 31.7 | 26.0 | |

BP blood pressure. HDL High density lipoprotein. LDL Low density lipoprotein. SD Standard deviation.

In all cases, the differences observed between men and women are statistically significant ($p < 0.001$).

In Table 2, we present the mean values of the scales used to estimate the risk of developing insulin resistance or prediabetes. Meanwhile, Table 3 provides the prevalence of elevated values for these same scales, comparing these values between the MHO) and NMHO groups. In both cases, the same trend is observed, namely, higher values in the NMHO group. The differences observed across all scales consistently show statistical significance ($p < 0.001$).

**Table 2.** Mean values of different insulin resistance risk scales in metabolically healthy and unhealthy obese to sex.

| | **n = 8764** | **n = 36,734** | | **n = 24,264** | **n = 21,234** | | **n = 34,660** | **n = 10,838** | |
|---|---|---|---|---|---|---|---|---|---|
| | **MHO (A)** | **NMHO (A)** | | **MHO (B)** | **NMHO (B)** | | **MHO (C)** | **NMHO (C)** | |
| Men | Mean (SD) | Mean (SD) | *p*-Value | Mean (SD) | Mean (SD) | *p*-Value | Mean (SD) | Mean (SD) | *p*-Value |
| TyG index | 8.3 (0.3) | 8.9 (0.6) | <0.001 | 8.4 (0.4) | 9.0 (0.6) | <0.001 | 8.5 (0.5) | 9.1 (0.6) | <0.001 |
| TyG-BMI | 264.7 (19.6) | 297.6 (38.2) | <0.001 | 270.9 (23.3) | 303.5 (38.6) | <0.001 | 278.7 (27.1) | 313.0 (40.0) | <0.001 |
| TyG-waist | 774.5 (52.8) | 880.1(105.1) | <0.001 | 794.9 (65.5) | 898.6(103.7) | <0.001 | 822.0 (78.8) | 926.6(103.5) | <0.001 |
| TyG-WtHR | 4.5 (0.3) | 5.1 (0.6) | <0.001 | 4.6 (0.4) | 5.2 (0.6) | <0.001 | 4.7 (0.4) | 5.3 (0.6) | <0.001 |
| METS-IR | 45.6 (3.4) | 52.6 (7.0) | <0.001 | 47.0 (4.1) | 53.8 (7.0) | <0.001 | 48.7 (4.8) | 55.8 (7.2) | <0.001 |
| SPISE-IR | 2.1 (0.2) | 2.5 (0.5) | <0.001 | 2.1 (0.3) | 2.6 (0.5) | <0.001 | 2.2 (0.3) | 2.7 (0.5) | <0.001 |
| PRISQ | 17.4 (6.8) | 26.8 (8.4) | <0.001 | 20.4 (7.7) | 28.1 (8.0) | <0.001 | 22.7 (8.0) | 29.9 (7.6) | <0.001 |
| Women | n = 6146 | n = 17,240 | | n = 14,446 | n = 8938 | | n = 19,976 | n = 3410 | |
| TyG index | 8.1 (0.4) | 8.5 (0.5) | <0.001 | 8.2 (0.4) | 8.6 (0.5) | <0.001 | 8.3 (0.4) | 8.7 (0.5) | <0.001 |
| TyG-BMI | 257.2 (15.5) | 293.1 (40.6) | <0.001 | 267.3 (25.2) | 300.0 (41.6) | <0.001 | 276.4 (31.3) | 311.2 (43.3) | <0.001 |
| TyG-waist | 659.4 (47.0) | 775.6 (97.2) | <0.001 | 702.6 (75.2) | 793.8 (95.6) | <0.001 | 730.9 (84.3) | 820.5 (95.5) | <0.001 |
| TyG-WtHR | 4.2 (0.3) | 4.8 (0.6) | <0.001 | 4.4 (0.4) | 4.9 (0.6) | <0.001 | 4.6 (0.5) | 5.1 (0.6) | <0.001 |
| METS-IR | 43.2 (2.2) | 50.4 (6.9) | <0.001 | 45.4 (4.4) | 51.7 (7.0) | <0.001 | 47.3 (5.2) | 53.6 (7.3) | <0.001 |
| SPISE-IR | 1.9 (0.2) | 2.4 (0.5) | <0.001 | 2.1 (0.3) | 2.4 (0.5) | <0.001 | 2.2 (0.4) | 2.6 (0.5) | <0.001 |
| PRISQ | 15.1 (6.5) | 23.6 (8.3) | <0.001 | 17.5 (7.0) | 25.3 (8.0) | <0.001 | 19.9 (7.6) | 27.6 (7.7) | <0.001 |

TyG Triglyceride glucose index. BMI Body mass index. WtHR Waist to height ratio. METS-IR Metabolic score for insulin resistance. SPISE-IR Single-point insulin sensitivity estimator-insulin resistance. MHO Metabolically healthy obese. NMHO Non-Metabolically healthy obese. (A) 0 factors of metabolic syndrome. (B) <2 factors of metabolic syndrome (C) <3 factors of metabolic syndrome.

**Table 3.** Prevalence of high values of different insulin resistance risk scales in metabolically healthy and unhealthy obese to sex.

| | **n = 8764** | **n = 36,734** | | **n = 24,264** | **n = 21,234** | | **n = 34,660** | **n = 10,838** | |
|---|---|---|---|---|---|---|---|---|---|
| | **MHO (A)** | **NMHO (A)** | | **MHO (B)** | **NMHO (B)** | | **MHO (C)** | **NMHO (C)** | |
| Men | % | % | *p*-Value | % | % | *p*-Value | % | % | *p*-Value |
| TyG index high | 3.1 | 52.2 | <0.001 | 11.7 | 61.0 | <0.001 | 24.4 | 74.6 | <0.001 |
| METS-IR high | 9.4 | 58.9 | <0.001 | 18.3 | 67.8 | <0.001 | 32.1 | 80.3 | <0.001 |
| SPISE-IR high | 21.5 | 71.3 | <0.001 | 33.8 | 79.2 | <0.001 | 48.1 | 88.9 | <0.001 |
| PRISQ high | 5.3 | 51.8 | <0.001 | 19.9 | 58.1 | <0.001 | 30.7 | 67.6 | <0.001 |
| Women | n = 6146 | n = 17,240 | | n = 14,446 | n = 8938 | | n = 19,976 | n = 3410 | |
| TyG index high | 5.0 | 31.2 | <0.001 | 7.9 | 38.1 | <0.001 | 13.4 | 52.8 | <0.001 |
| METS-IR high | 0.3 | 42.2 | <0.001 | 11.0 | 50.7 | <0.001 | 22.9 | 63.1 | <0.001 |
| SPISE-IR high | 5.9 | 55.8 | <0.001 | 22.2 | 64.5 | <0.001 | 35.8 | 76.3 | <0.001 |
| PRISQ high | 2.7 | 25.7 | <0.001 | 5.1 | 31.8 | <0.001 | 10.3 | 44.4 | <0.001 |

TyG Triglyceride glucose index. METS-IR Metabolic score for insulin resistance. SPISE-IR Single-point insulin sensitivity estimator for insulin resistance. PRISQ Prediabetes Risk Score in Qatar. MHO Metabolically healthy obese. NMHO Non-Metabolically healthy obese. (A) 0 factors of metabolic syndrome. (B) <2 factors of metabolic syndrome (C) <3 factors of metabolic syndrome.

Table 4 presents the findings of the multinomial logistic regression analysis, demonstrating that all independent variables incorporated into the model—including sex, age, educational attainment, social class, smoking status, physical activity levels, adherence to the Mediterranean diet, and classification as either MHO or NMHO (based on the three established criteria)—exhibit significant associations with elevated scores on the insulin resistance and prediabetes risk scales. Among these factors, the most pronounced associations, as indicated by odds ratios (ORs), are observed for physical activity, adherence to the Mediterranean diet, and metabolic classification as MHO or NMHO.

**Table 4.** Multinomial logistic regression.

| | TyG Index High | SPISE-IR High | METS-IR High | PRISQ High |
|---|---|---|---|---|
| | OR (95% CI) | OR (95% CI) | OR (95% CI) | OR (95% CI) |
| Female | 1 | 1 | 1 | 1 |
| Male | 2.25 (2.14–2.35) | 1.22 (1.18–1.26) | 1.33 (1.26–1.40) | 1.36 (1.28–1.45) |
| <30 years | 1 | 1 | 1 | 1 |
| 30–39 years | 1.06 (1.03–1.09) | 1.09 (1.06–1.13) | 1.16 (1.09–1.23) | 1.10 (1.06–1.14) |
| 40–49 years | 1.11 (1.07–1.15) | 1.29 (1.20–1.38) | 1.35 (1.28–1.42) | 1.21 (1.16–1.26) |
| 50–59 years | 1.24 (1.12–1.37) | 1.59 (1.43–1.75) | 1.68 (1.50–1.86) | 1.85 (1.61–2.19) |
| 60–69 years | 1.61 (1.43–1.81) | 2.08 (1.80–2.36) | 1.99 (1.80–2.19) | 2.11 (1.88–2.34) |
| University | 1 | 1 | 1 | 1 |
| High school | 1.09 (1.06–1.12) | 1.12 (1.06–1.18) | 1.08 (1.04–1.12) | 1.07 (1.04–1.10) |
| Elementary school | 1.20 (1.13–1.27) | 1.28 (1.16–1.40) | 1.25 (1.18–1.32) | 1.23 (1.15–1.31) |
| Social class I | 1 | 1 | 1 | 1 |
| Social class II | 1.05 (1.02–1.08) | 1.21 (1.15–1.27) | 1.06 (1.03–1.10) | 1.16 (1.12–1.20) |
| Social class III | 1.29 (1.20–1.38) | 1.53 (1.37–1.70) | 1.33 (1.24–1.42) | 1.41 (1.31–1.51) |
| Physical activity | 1 | 1 | 1 | 1 |
| No physical activity | 6.34 (5.98–6.70) | 5.29 (4.96–5.62) | 6.78 (6.30–7.26) | 3.88 (3.59–4.18) |
| Mediterranean diet | 1 | 1 | 1 | 1 |
| No Mediterranean diet | 5.35 (4.99–5.71) | 3.40 (3.05–3.75) | 5.10 (4.70–5.51) | 2.90 (2.49–3.31) |
| Non-smokers | 1 | 1 | 1 | 1 |
| Smokers | 1.06 (1.03–1.10) | 1.16 (1.11–1.20) | 1.14 (1.09–1.18) | 1.03 (1.00–1.07) |
| MHO (A) | 1 | 1 | 1 | 1 |
| NMHO (A) | 4.67 (4.25–5.12) | 2.12 (2.02–2.21) | 2.05 (1.94–2.17) | 2.21 (2.07–2.36) |
| MHO (B) | 1 | 1 | 1 | 1 |
| NMHO (B) | 5.52 (5.27–5.79) | 2.98 (2.86–3.11) | 2.62 (2.51–2.74) | 2.36 (2.18–2.54) |
| MHO (C) | 1 | 1 | 1 | 1 |
| NMHO (C) | 8.79 (8.24–9.37) | 8.81 (8.10–9.58) | 4.25 (4.03–4.47) | 7.60 (6.59–8.77) |

TyG Triglyceride glucose index. METS-IR Metabolic score for insulin resistance. SPISE-IR Single-point insulin sensitivity estimator for insulin resistance. PRISQ Prediabetes Risk Score in Qatar. MHO Metabolically healthy obese. NMHO Non-Metabolically healthy obese. (A) 0 factors of metabolic syndrome. (B) <2 factors of metabolic syndrome (C) <3 factors of metabolic syndrome. OR Odds ratio.

## 4. Discussion

The findings of this study provide relevant evidence on the association between the risk of insulin resistance (IR) and prediabetes in workers classified as MHO. Although the MHO phenotype has been considered a condition with a lower metabolic risk, the results support the idea that individuals with MHO are not exempt from developing metabolic disorders.

The cross-sectional design prevents the establishment of causal relationships, as data are collected at a single time point, making it difficult to distinguish between causality and correlation. Additionally, selection bias may arise if the sample does not adequately represent the population. However, in our case, we consider that the large sample size reduces this bias.

One of the most significant findings is that, despite presenting a more favorable metabolic profile compared to NMHO individuals, workers with MHO also show signs of metabolic deterioration, as evidenced by the values of IR risk scales. In particular, physical activity [44–46] and adherence to the Mediterranean diet [47–49] have been identified as key protective factors against IR, highlighting the importance of promoting healthy lifestyle habits in this population.

Adipose tissue distribution appears to play a crucial role in the transition from the MHO phenotype to a NMHO state [50]. Previous studies have demonstrated that preferential fat storage in subcutaneous adipose tissue, rather than visceral adipose tissue, is associated with a lower metabolic risk [51]. However, over time, the capacity of subcutaneous adipose tissue to store excess energy is exceeded, leading to increased lipotoxicity and systemic inflammation, both of which are key factors in the development of IR [52].

Another aspect to consider is the influence of sociodemographic and lifestyle factors on the metabolic evolution of MHO individuals. In this study, age, educational level, and social class were found to be associated with a higher risk of IR and prediabetes [53–55], indicating that social inequalities may play a significant role in the progression of MHO to a pathological state. These findings align with previous research suggesting that limited access to healthy foods [56], reduced opportunities for physical activity [57], and chronic stress [58] contribute to metabolic deterioration in vulnerable populations.

It would be of great interest to further explore the relationship between metabolic health and the organizational level of workers within each occupational category, considering classifications such as directors, managers, technicians, officers, and laborers. This analysis would help identify whether specific patterns exist in the distribution of healthy lifestyle habits according to occupational hierarchy and determine whether certain organizational levels present a higher metabolic risk.

Additionally, it would be relevant to describe the predominant employment profiles, differentiating between manual labor, sedentary work, and shift work. Each of these occupational types involves different physical demands and stress levels, which could influence the prevalence of insulin resistance and other metabolic disorders.

This approach would provide a better understanding of how workplace characteristics impact workers' health, including factors such as available time for physical activity, access to healthy nutrition, and exposure to stressors. The interaction between occupational type, job-related physical demands, lifestyle habits, and access to health resources could offer valuable insights for designing workplace health promotion and prevention strategies.

Therefore, this analysis represents a key aspect to consider in future research on occupational health and the risk of developing insulin resistance.

From a clinical perspective, these results highlight the need for periodic monitoring of MHO individuals to identify early signs of transition toward IR and other metabolic complications such as prediabetes. The use of tools such as the Homeostatic Model Assessment (HOMA) index for evaluating insulin resistance [59], along with biomarkers such as adiponectin [60] and C-reactive protein [61], could allow for more precise stratification of metabolic risk in this population. Combining these markers with imaging techniques, such as magnetic resonance imaging (MRI) [62] or computed tomography (CT) [63], could provide a more detailed assessment of the metabolic status of MHO individuals. However, these data are not available in our study and should be considered in future research.

Physical activity plays a crucial role in preventing insulin resistance and the development of prediabetes, as evidenced by the findings from the multinomial logistic regression analysis. The results show significant associations between high scores on insulin resistance scales and the risk of prediabetes, with physical activity acting as a protective factor. This is reflected in the Odds Ratio values, which range from 3.88 to 6.78, indicating that individuals with lower physical activity levels have a significantly higher probability of developing insulin resistance compared to those who engage in regular exercise.

This protective effect can be explained by several physiological mechanisms. Physical activity enhances insulin sensitivity by increasing glucose uptake in skeletal muscles, thereby reducing blood glucose levels. Additionally, exercise promotes a reduction in visceral adiposity, which is closely linked to chronic inflammation and metabolic dysfunction. It also influences the regulation of adipokines and inflammatory cytokines, modulating metabolic responses and lowering the risk of developing insulin resistance [64].

The findings of this study reinforce the importance of promoting physical activity as a key strategy for preventing metabolic diseases. Including specific recommendations on exercise frequency, intensity, and type could help develop more effective interventions in at-risk populations [65]. Since physical activity is a modifiable factor, its promotion in workplaces, educational settings, and community programs could be an effective strategy to reduce the burden of type 2 diabetes and other related metabolic diseases. These findings highlight the need for further research in this area to optimize prevention strategies.

The Mediterranean diet is a fundamental pillar in preventing metabolic disorders, particularly insulin resistance. The results from the multinomial logistic regression analysis indicate that lack of adherence to this dietary pattern significantly increases the risk of developing insulin resistance, with Odds Ratio values ranging from 2.90 to 5.35. This suggests that individuals who do not follow the Mediterranean diet have nearly three to more than five times the likelihood of developing insulin resistance compared to those who adhere to it.

The metabolic benefits of the Mediterranean diet can be attributed to its composition, which is rich in monounsaturated fatty acids from olive oil, a high intake of fruits, vegetables, legumes, and nuts, and a moderate consumption of fish and dairy products. These foods contain bioactive compounds that reduce systemic inflammation, oxidative stress, and improve insulin sensitivity. Additionally, dietary fiber from fruits, vegetables, and whole grains modulates the glycemic response and supports the gut microbiome balance, contributing to better metabolic regulation [66].

This study reinforces the importance of promoting the Mediterranean diet as a key strategy in preventing insulin resistance and related metabolic disorders such as type 2 diabetes and metabolic syndrome. Nutritional education and public health policies that encourage adherence to this dietary pattern could be essential in reducing the incidence of these conditions. Furthermore, personalized interventions could be designed to improve Mediterranean diet adherence, particularly in populations with high-risk factors. These results underscore the need for continued research on the relationship between nutrition and metabolic health.

Smoking is established as a modifiable risk factor in the development of insulin resistance, as evidenced by the results of the multinomial logistic regression analysis. Our analysis shows an increased risk of insulin resistance ranging from 3% to 16% in smokers compared to non-smokers, highlighting the importance of addressing this habit in the prevention of metabolic disorders.

The pathophysiological mechanisms underlying this relationship include oxidative stress and chronic inflammation induced by toxic tobacco components, which impair endothelial function and disrupt insulin signaling [67]. Additionally, smoking is associated with an unfavorable distribution of body fat, promoting the accumulation of visceral fat—a key factor in insulin resistance [68].

Since smoking is a modifiable risk factor, its control should be a priority in public health strategies. Implementing smoking cessation programs and raising awareness of its metabolic effects could significantly reduce the risk of developing insulin resistance and associated metabolic diseases.

Furthermore, it is essential to design intervention strategies aimed at improving the metabolic health of MHO individuals. Interventions that promote physical activity maintenance, the adoption of a healthy diet, and stress reduction could play a crucial role in preventing the development of IR [69,70]. In this regard, implementing health promotion programs in the workplace could be an effective strategy for improving workers' wellbeing and preventing the progression of MHO to a pathological state [71]. Strategies that include personalized nutritional counseling, tailored physical training, and stress management programs could be particularly beneficial for this population group.

The role of genetics and epigenetics in the evolution of MHO individuals is another factor that warrants special attention [72]. Recent studies have demonstrated that certain genetic variants may predispose individuals to transition to an NMHO state [28]. Additionally, epigenetic regulation induced by environmental factors such as diet and physical exercise can modulate the expression of genes related to inflammation [73], glucose metabolism, and insulin sensitivity [74]. Research in this field could open new avenues for the development of personalized therapies aimed at preventing the progression of IR in these individuals.

It is important to note that variability in the diagnostic criteria for the MHO phenotype poses a challenge for comparability across studies. Different studies have used varying thresholds to define insulin resistance and other metabolic risk factors, which may influence the estimated prevalence of this phenotype and the interpretations of its clinical impact [75,76]. Standardizing these criteria and incorporating longitudinal analyses would facilitate a better understanding of the evolution of MHO individuals and the factors contributing to their transition to a metabolically unhealthy state.

Another key aspect is the impact of public health policies on the prevention and management of the MHO phenotype. Government initiatives aimed at promoting healthy lifestyles, improving access to nutritious foods, and reducing work-related stress and bur-dens among workers could play a crucial role in reducing the incidence of IR in this pop-ulation [77,78]. Collaboration between the health, education, and labor sectors could yield more effective strategies for promoting long-term metabolic health.

Among the essential strategies to improve employee health, several concrete actions can be implemented in the workplace. First, adequate health education training for all workers is fundamental to promoting the adoption of healthy habits and preventing chronic diseases. The promotion of healthy lifestyles should be supported by awareness programs tailored to the needs of each occupational group.

Second, the implementation of workplace nutrition policies is key to improving employees' dietary habits. This includes offering healthy meal options in workplace cafeterias and eliminating vending machines that promote the consumption of ultra-processed foods. Another essential measure is ensuring work schedules that allow employees sufficient time to eat properly, preventing rushed or unbalanced meals due to a lack of breaks. Additionally, the installation of fitness areas in the workplace would encourage regular physical activity, benefiting cardiovascular health and overall well-being.

Finally, companies can develop physical exercise and stress management programs, such as mindfulness, yoga, and relaxation techniques. These strategies would not only improve individual health and well-being but could also enhance productivity and company profitability by reducing absenteeism and improving employee performance.

*Strengths and Limitations*

A key strength of this study is its large sample size, comprising nearly 69,000 obese workers, making it one of the most extensive investigations of MHO conducted globally. Another notable advantage is the wide range of analyzed variables, encompassing both sociodemographic and lifestyle-related factors, and their relationship with MHO. Furthermore, the use of validated questionnaires to assess physical activity levels and adherence to the Mediterranean diet enhances the study's reliability, offering a cost-effective and practical approach for evaluation and longitudinal monitoring.

However, this study is subject to certain limitations. One of the primary constraints is its cross-sectional design, which precludes the ability to establish causal relationships.

Additionally, the exclusion of unemployed individuals, retirees, and those under 18 or over 69 years of age limits the generalizability of the findings to the broader population. Nevertheless, the large sample size is expected to mitigate this limitation to some extent. Similarly, as the study was conducted exclusively within a Spanish population, the findings may not be directly applicable to other populations, necessitating caution in extrapolating the results.

Not stratifying by hierarchical level within each occupation limits the analysis of patterns according to job hierarchy and specific sectors. Understanding how the work environment, physical demands, and access to health resources influence lifestyle habits is essential for designing preventive strategies and guiding future research in occupational health.

The lack of biomarkers is another limitation of our work, as they would be very useful in allowing for more precise metabolic risk stratification in this population.

Another potential limitation stems from the use of self-administered questionnaires, which are inherently susceptible to recall bias and social desirability bias. Future research should consider integrating objective validation methods to enhance data accuracy. Additionally, certain confounding factors, such as comorbidities and pharmacological treatments, were not accounted for due to data unavailability, which may have influenced the outcomes.

## 5. Conclusions

The results of this study reinforce the evidence that the MHO phenotype should not be considered a stable or benign condition, but rather a transitory state that may evolve into metabolic dysfunction over time. Early identification of IR risk and the implementation of prevention strategies based on the promotion of healthy lifestyles are essential to minimize the complications associated with obesity in this population. Adopting a comprehensive approach that combines clinical assessments, advanced biomarkers, genetic and epigenetic studies, and personalized intervention strategies could be key to improving long-term metabolic outcomes in MHO individuals.

**Author Contributions:** M.G.S.: Conceptualization, investigation, original manuscript writing. P.J.T.L.: Validation, statistical analysis. Á.A.L.-G.: Methodology, manuscript review. H.P.: Data collection and curation. E.M.-A.R.: Methodology, original manuscript writing. J.I.R.-M.: Conceptualization, manuscript review. All authors have read and agreed to the published version of the manuscript.

**Funding:** This research received no external funding.

**Institutional Review Board Statement:** This study was conducted in strict accordance with both national and international ethical standards for health-related research, as stipulated by the Declaration of Helsinki. Specific measures were implemented to protect participant anonymity and maintain the confidentiality of all data collected. Ethical approval was obtained from the Ethics and Research Committee of the Balearic Islands (CEI-IB) under reference number IB 4383/20, with approval granted on 26 November 2020. Participation in the study was entirely voluntary. All participants were informed about the study's objectives and procedures and provided written informed consent. To ensure confidentiality, all data were anonymized through the assignment of unique codes, which were accessible only to the Project coordinator. No personally identifiable information will be disclosed in published reports or shared by the research team. Participants were fully informed of their rights to access, modify, delete, or oppose the processing of their data, in alignment with ethical principles. Moreover, the research team adhered to the provisions of Organic Law 3/2018 of 5 December concerning the protection of personal data and the guarantee of digital rights.

**Informed Consent Statement:** Informed consent was obtained from all subjects involved in the study.

**Data Availability Statement:** Data are not available due to ethical or privacy restrictions. This study's data are stored in a database that complies with all security measures at the ADEMA-Escuela Universitaria. The Data Protection Delegate is Ángel Arturo López González.

**Conflicts of Interest:** The authors declare no conflicts of interest.

## References


1. Naghizadeh, M.; Maskouni, S.J.; Mortazavi, Z.; Ahmadi, M.; Shokri, S. The Impact of Fast Food Consumption on the Development of General and Central Obesity. *Acad. J. Health Sci.* **2024**, *39*, 44–48. [CrossRef]
2. Suren Garg, S.; Kushwaha, K.; Dubey, R.; Gupta, J. Association between obesity, inflammation and insulin resistance: Insights into signaling pathways and therapeutic interventions. *Diabetes Res. Clin. Pract.* **2023**, *200*, 110691. [CrossRef] [PubMed]
3. Blüher, M. Metabolically Healthy Obesity. *Endocr Rev.* **2020**, *41*, bnaa004. [CrossRef] [PubMed] [PubMed Central]
4. Petersen, M.C.; Smith, G.I.; Palacios, H.H.; Farabi, S.S.; Yoshino, M.; Yoshino, J.; Cho, K.; Davila-Roman, V.G.; Shankaran, M.; Barve, R.A.; et al. Cardiometabolic characteristics of people with metabolically healthy and unhealthy obesity. *Cell Metab.* **2024**, *36*, 745–761.e5. [CrossRef] [PubMed] [PubMed Central]
5. Griera Borrás, J.L.; Contreras Gilbert, J. Are there healthy obese? *Endocrinol. Nutr.* **2014**, *61*, 47–51. [CrossRef] [PubMed]
6. Tsatsoulis, A.; Paschou, S.A. Metabolically Healthy Obesity: Criteria, Epidemiology, Controversies, and Consequences. *Curr. Obes. Rep.* **2020**, *9*, 109–120. [CrossRef] [PubMed]
7. Barrea, L.; Muscogiuri, G.; Pugliese, G.; de Alteriis, G.; Colao, A.; Savastano, S. Metabolically Healthy Obesity (MHO) vs. Metabolically Unhealthy Obesity (MUO) Phenotypes in PCOS: Association with Endocrine-Metabolic Profile, Adherence to the Mediterranean Diet, and Body Composition. *Nutrients* **2021**, *13*, 3925. [CrossRef]
8. Gómez-Zorita, S.; Queralt, M.; Vicente, M.A.; González, M.; Portillo, M.P. Metabolically healthy obesity and metabolically obese normal weight: A review. *J. Physiol. Biochem.* **2021**, *77*, 175–189. [CrossRef] [PubMed]
9. Su, Z.; Efremov, L.; Mikolajczyk, R. Differences in the levels of inflammatory markers between metabolically healthy obese and other obesity phenotypes in adults: A systematic review and meta-analysis. *Nutr. Metab. Cardiovasc. Dis.* **2024**, *34*, 251–269. [CrossRef]
10. Kang, Y.M.; Jung, C.H.; Cho, Y.K.; Jang, J.E.; Hwang, J.Y.; Kim, E.H.; Lee, W.J.; Park, J.-Y.; Kim, H.-K. Visceral adiposity index predicts the conversion of metabolically healthy obesity to an unhealthy phenotype. *PLoS ONE* **2017**, *12*, e0179635. [CrossRef]
11. Wang, J.-S.; Xia, P.-F.; Ma, M.-N.; Li, Y.; Geng, T.-T.; Zhang, Y.-B.; Tu, Z.-Z.; Jiang, L.; Zhou, L.-R.; Zhang, B.-F.; et al. Trends in the Prevalence of Metabolically Healthy Obesity Among US Adults, 1999–2018. *JAMA Netw. Open* **2023**, *6*, e232145. [CrossRef]
12. Sastre-Alzamora, T.; Tomás-Gil, P.; Paublini, H.; Pallarés, L.; Ramírez-Manent, J.I.; López-González, A.A. Relationship between heart age and insulin resistance risk scales in 139634 Spanish workers. *Acad. J. Health Sci.* **2024**, *39*, 16–22. [CrossRef]
13. Lee, S.H.; Park, S.Y.; Choi, C.S. Insulin Resistance: From Mechanisms to Therapeutic Strategies. *Diabetes Metab. J.* **2022**, *46*, 15–37. [CrossRef]
14. Kosmas, C.E.; Bousvarou, M.D.; Kostara, C.E.; Papakonstantinou, E.J.; Salamou, E.; Guzman, E. Insulin resistance and cardiovascular disease. *J. Int. Med. Res.* **2023**, *51*, 3000605231164548. [CrossRef]
15. He, M.; Wang, J.; Liang, Q.; Li, M.; Guo, H.; Wang, Y.; Deji, C.; Sui, J.; Wang, Y.-W.; Liu, Y.; et al. Time-restricted eating with or without low-carbohydrate diet reduces visceral fat and improves metabolic syndrome: A randomized trial. *Cell Rep. Med.* **2022**, *3*, 100777. [CrossRef]
16. Li, H.; Meng, Y.; He, S.; Tan, X.; Zhang, Y.; Zhang, X.; Wang, L.; Zheng, W. Macrophages, Chronic Inflammation, and Insulin Resistance. *Cells* **2022**, *11*, 3001. [CrossRef]
17. Al-Mansoori, L.; Al-Jaber, H.; Prince, M.S.; Elrayess, M.A. Role of Inflammatory Cytokines, Growth Factors and Adipokines in Adipogenesis and Insulin Resistance. *Inflammation* **2022**, *45*, 31–44. [CrossRef]
18. Tanase, D.M.; Gosav, E.M.; Costea, C.F.; Ciocoiu, M.; Lacatusu, C.M.; Maranduca, M.A.; Ouatu, A.; Floria, M. The Intricate Relationship between Type 2 Diabetes Mellitus (T2DM), Insulin Resistance (IR), and Nonalcoholic Fatty Liver Disease (NAFLD). *J. Diabetes Res.* **2020**, *2020*, 3920196. [CrossRef]
19. Kolb, H. Obese visceral fat tissue inflammation: From protective to detrimental? *BMC Med.* **2022**, *20*, 494. [CrossRef]
20. Schulze, M.B.; Stefan, N. Metabolically healthy obesity: From epidemiology and mechanisms to clinical implications. *Nat. Rev. Endocrinol.* **2024**, *20*, 633–646. [CrossRef]
21. Abiri, B.; Koohi, F.; Ebadinejad, A.; Valizadeh, M.; Hosseinpanah, F. Transition from metabolically healthy to unhealthy overweight/obesity and risk of cardiovascular disease incidence: A systematic review and meta-analysis. *Nutr. Metab. Cardiovasc. Dis.* **2022**, *32*, 2041–2051. [CrossRef] [PubMed]
22. Song, Z.; Gao, M.; Lv, J.; Yu, C.; Guo, Y.; Bian, Z.; Wei, Y.; Yang, L.; Du, H.; Chen, Y.; et al. Metabolically healthy obesity, transition to unhealthy phenotypes, and type 2 diabetes in 0.5 million Chinese adults: The China Kadoorie Biobank. *Eur. J. Endocrinol.* **2022**, *186*, 233–244. [CrossRef] [PubMed] [PubMed Central]
23. Gutiérrez-Repiso, C.; Linares-Pineda, T.M.; Gonzalez-Jimenez, A.; Aguilar-Lineros, F.; Valdés, S.; Soriguer, F.; Rojo-Martínez, G.; Ti-nahones, F.J.; Morcillo, S. Epigenetic Biomarkers of Transition from Metabolically Healthy Obesity to Metabolically Unhealthy Obesity Phenotype: A Prospective Study. *Int. J. Mol. Sci.* **2021**, *22*, 10417. [CrossRef]
24. Martin-Piedra, L.; Alcala-Diaz, J.F.; Gutierrez-Mariscal, F.M.; de Larriva, A.P.A.; Romero-Cabrera, J.L.; Torres-Peña, J.D.; Caballero-Villarraso, J.; Luque, R.M.; Perez-Martinez, P.; Lopez-Miranda, J.; et al. Evolution of Metabolic Phenotypes of Obesity in Coronary Patients after 5 Years of Dietary Intervention: From the CORDI-OPREV Study. *Nutrients* **2021**, *13*, 1016. [CrossRef]

25. Colleluori, G.; Villareal, D.T. Aging, obesity, sarcopenia and the effect of diet and exercise intervention. *Exp. Gerontol.* **2021**, *155*, 111561. [CrossRef]
26. Chaput, J.-P.; McHill, A.W.; Cox, R.C.; Broussard, J.L.; Dutil, C.; da Costa, B.G.G.; Sampasa-Kanyinga, H.; Wright, K.P. The role of insufficient sleep and circadian misa-lignment in obesity. *Nat. Rev. Endocrinol.* **2023**, *19*, 82–97. [CrossRef]
27. Murlasits, Z.; Kupai, K.; Kneffel, Z. Role of physical activity and cardiorespiratory fitness in metabolically healthy obesity: A nar-rative review. *BMJ Open Sport. Exerc. Med.* **2022**, *8*, e001458. [CrossRef]
28. Ojalehto Lindfors, E.; De Oliveira, T.L.; Reynolds, C.A.; Zhan, Y.; Dahl Aslan, A.K.; Jylhävä, J.; Sjölander, A.; Karlsson, I.K. Genetic influences, lifestyle and psychosocial aspects in relation to metabolically healthy obesity and conversion to a metabolically unhealthy state. *Diabetes Obes. Metab.* **2025**, *27*, 207–214. [CrossRef]
29. Stefan, N. Causes, consequences, and treatment of metabolically unhealthy fat distribution. *Lancet Diabetes Endocrinol.* **2020**, *8*, 616–627. [CrossRef]
30. Tutunchi, H.; Naeini, F.; Ebrahimi-Mameghani, M.; Najafipour, F.; Mobasseri, M.; Ostadrahimi, A. Metabolically healthy and unhealthy obesity and the progression of liver fibrosis: A cross-sectional study. *Clin. Res. Hepatol. Gastroenterol.* **2021**, *45*, 101754. [CrossRef]
31. Cho, A.Y.; Roh, J.G.; Shim, Y.S.; Lee, H.S.; Hwang, J.S. Biochemical predictors of metabolically unhealthy obesity in children and ado-lescents. *J. Pediatr. Endocrinol. Metab.* **2021**, *35*, 97–103. [CrossRef]
32. Aisike, G.; Kuerbanjiang, M.; Muheyati, D.; Zaibibuli, K.; Lv, M.X.; Han, J. Correlation analysis of obesity phenotypes with leptin and adiponectin. *Sci. Rep.* **2023**, *13*, 17718. [CrossRef]
33. Xu, R.; Shen, P.; Wu, C.; Wan, Y.; Fan, Z.; Gao, X. BMI, high-sensitivity C-reactive protein and the conversion from metabolically healthy to unhealthy phenotype in Chinese adults: A cohort study. *Public. Health Nutr.* **2021**, *24*, 4124–4131. [CrossRef]
34. Ler, P.; Ojalehto, E.; Zhan, Y.; Finkel, D.; Dahl Aslan, A.K.; Karlsson, I.K. Conversions between metabolically unhealthy and healthy obesity from midlife to late-life. *Int. J. Obes.* **2024**, *48*, 433–436. [CrossRef]
35. Jéru, I.; Fellahi, S.; Capeau, J.; Bastard, J.P.; Vigouroux, C.; Pour le groupe de travail RIHN Adipokinesb. Leptine, adiponectine, syndromes lipodystrophiques et d'insulino-résistance sévère. *Ann. Biol. Clin.* **2020**, *78*, 261–264. (In French) [CrossRef]
36. Li, S.; Han, X.; Song, J.; Dong, M.; Xie, T. Mechanism of Action and Risk Prediction of Adiponectin in Cardiovascular Diseases. *Front. Biosci. (Landmark Ed.)* **2024**, *29*, 286. [CrossRef]
37. Petri, C.; Campa, F.; Holway, F.; Pengue, L.; Arrones, L.S. ISAK-Based Anthropometric Standards for Elite Male and Female Soccer Players. *Sports* **2024**, *12*, 69. [CrossRef]
38. Ramírez-Manent, J.I.; Tomás-Gil, P.; Coll-Villalonga, J.L.; Marti-Lliteras, P.; López-González, A.A.; Paublini, H. Influence of socio-demographic variables and tobacco consumption on the prevalence of atherogenic dyslipidemia and lipid triad in 418.343 spanish workers. *Acad. J. Health Sci.* **2023**, *38*, 84–89. [CrossRef]
39. Friedewald, W.T.; Levy, R.I.; Fredrickson, D.S. Estimation of the concentration of low-density lipoprotein cholesterol in plasma, without use of the preparative ultracentrifuge. *Clin. Chem.* **1972**, *18*, 499–502. [CrossRef]
40. Sastre-Alzamora, T.; Tomás-Gil, P.; Paublini, H.; Pallarés, L.; Ramírez-Manent, J.I.; López-González, A.A. Relationship between heart age and cardiometabolic risk scales in 139634 Spanish workers. *Acad. J. Health Sci.* **2024**, *39*, 141–148. [CrossRef]
41. Domingo-Salvany, A.; Bacigalupe, A.; Carrasco, J.M.; Espelt, A.; Ferrando, J.; Borrell, C. del Grupo de Determinantes Sociales de Sociedad Española de Epidemiología. Propuestas de clase social neoweberiana y neomarxista a partir de la Clasificación Nacional de Ocupaciones 2011 [Proposals for social class classification based on the Spanish National Classification of Occupations 2011 using neo-Weberian and neo-Marxist approaches]. *Gac. Sanit.* **2013**, *27*, 263–272.
42. Mestre-Font, M.; Busquets-Cortés, C.; Ramírez-Manent, J.I.; Tomás-Gil, P.; Paublini, H.; López-González, A.A. Influence of socio-demographic variables and healthy habits on the values of type 2 diabetes risk scales. *Acad. J. Health Sci.* **2024**, *39*, 99–106. [CrossRef]
43. Lee, P.H.; Macfarlane, D.J.; Lam, T.H.; Stewart, S.M. Validity of the International Physical Activity Questionnaire Short Form (IPAQ-SF): A systematic review. *Int. J. Behav. Nutr. Phys. Act.* **2011**, *8*, 115. [CrossRef]
44. Gallardo-Alfaro, L.; Bibiloni, M.d.M.; Mascaró, C.M.; Montemayor, S.; Ruiz-Canela, M.; Salas-Salvadó, J.; Corella, D.; Fitó, M.; Romaguera, D.; Vioque, J.; et al. Leisure-Time Physical Activity, Sedentary Behaviour and Diet Quality are Associated with Metabolic Syndrome Severity: The PREDIMED-Plus Study. *Nutrients.* **2020**, *12*, 1013. [CrossRef] [PubMed] [PubMed Central]
45. García-Hermoso, A.; López-Gil, J.F.; Izquierdo, M.; Ramírez-Vélez, R.; Ezzatvar, Y. Exercise and Insulin Resistance Markers in Children and Adolescents With Excess Weight: A Systematic Review and Network Meta-Analysis. *JAMA Pediatr.* **2023**, *177*, 1276–1284, Erratum in: *JAMA Pediatr.* **2023**, *177*, 1362. https://doi.org/10.1001/jamapediatrics.2023.5135. [CrossRef] [PubMed] [PubMed Central]
46. Fowler, J.R.; Tucker, L.A.; Bailey, B.W.; LeCheminant, J.D. Physical Activity and Insulin Resistance in 6,500 NHANES Adults: The Role of Abdominal Obesity. *J. Obes.* **2020**, *2020*, 3848256. [CrossRef] [PubMed] [PubMed Central]

47. Mirabelli, M.; Chiefari, E.; Arcidiacono, B.; Corigliano, D.M.; Brunetti, F.S.; Maggisano, V.; Russo, D.; Foti, D.P.; Brunetti, A. Mediterranean Diet Nutrients to Turn the Tide against Insulin Resistance and Related Diseases. *Nutrients* **2020**, *12*, 1066. [CrossRef] [PubMed] [PubMed Central]
48. Guasch-Ferré, M.; Willett, W.C. The Mediterranean diet and health: A comprehensive overview. *J. Intern. Med.* **2021**, *290*, 549–566. [CrossRef] [PubMed]
49. Pavlidou, E.; Papadopoulou, S.K.; Fasoulas, A.; Papaliagkas, V.; Alexatou, O.; Chatzidimitriou, M.; Mentzelou, M.; Giaginis, C. Diabesity and Dietary Inter-ventions: Evaluating the Impact of Mediterranean Diet and Other Types of Diets on Obesity and Type 2 Diabetes Management. *Nutrients* **2023**, *16*, 34. [CrossRef] [PubMed] [PubMed Central]
50. Camhi, S.M.; Katzmarzyk, P.T. Differences in body composition between metabolically healthy obese and metabolically abnormal obese adults. *Int. J. Obes.* **2014**, *38*, 1142–1145. [CrossRef] [PubMed] [PubMed Central]
51. Hwang, Y.-C.; Hayashi, T.; Fujimoto, W.Y.; Kahn, S.E.; Leonetti, D.L.; McNeely, M.J.; Boyko, E.J. Visceral abdominal fat accumulation predicts the conversion of metabolically healthy obese subjects to an unhealthy phenotype. *Int. J. Obes.* **2015**, *39*, 1365–1370. [CrossRef] [PubMed] [PubMed Central]
52. Adeva-Andany, M.M.; Domínguez-Montero, A.; Adeva-Contreras, L.; Fernández-Fernández, C.; Carneiro-Freire, N.; González-Lucán, M. Body Fat Distribution Contributes to Defining the Relationship between Insulin Resistance and Obesity in Human Diseases. *Curr. Diabetes Rev.* **2024**, *20*, e160823219824. [CrossRef] [PubMed]
53. Cai, S.; Dang, J.; Zhong, P.; Ma, N.; Liu, Y.; Shi, D.; Zou, Z.; Dong, Y.; Ma, J.; Song, Y. Sex differences in metabolically healthy and metabolically unhealthy obesity among Chinese children and adolescents. *Front. Endocrinol.* **2022**, *13*, 980332, Erratum in: *Front. Endocrinol.* **2022**, *13*, 1074024. https://doi.org/10.3389/fendo.2022.1074024. [CrossRef] [PubMed] [PubMed Central]
54. Kim, H.Y.; Kim, J.H. Temporal trends in the prevalence of metabolically healthy overweight and obesity in Korean youth: Data from the Korea National Health and Nutrition Examination Survey 2011–2019. *Ann. Pediatr. Endocrinol. Metab.* **2022**, *27*, 134–141. [CrossRef] [PubMed] [PubMed Central]
55. Aguiló Juanola, M.C.; López-González, A.A.; Tomás-Gil, P.; Paublini, H.; Tárraga-López, P.J.; Ramírez-Manent, J.I. Influence of tobacco consumption on the values of different insulin resistance risk scales and non-alcoholic fatty liver disease and hepatic fibrosis scales in 418,343 spanish people. *Acad. J. Health Sci.* **2024**, *39*, 9–15. [CrossRef]
56. Cano-Ibañez, N.; Gea, A.; Ruiz-Canela, M.; Corella, D.; Salas-Salvadó, J.; Schröder, H.; Navarrete-Muñoz, E.M.; Romaguera, D.; Martínez, J.A.; Barón-López, F.J.; et al. Diet quality and nutrient density in subjects with metabolic syndrome: Influence of socioeconomic status and lifestyle factors. A cross-sectional assessment in the PRED-IMED-Plus study. *Clin. Nutr.* **2020**, *39*, 1161–1173. [CrossRef] [PubMed]
57. Paudel, S.; Ahmadi, M.; Phongsavan, P.; Hamer, M.; Stamatakis, E. Do associations of physical activity and sedentary behaviour with cardiovascular disease and mortality differ across socioeconomic groups? A prospective analysis of device-measured and self-reported UK Biobank data. *Br. J. Sports Med.* **2023**, *57*, 921–929. [CrossRef] [PubMed] [PubMed Central]
58. Li, G.; Ma, Z.; Lu, Y.; Jiang, Y.; Zhao, H.; Sun, M.; Wang, Y.; He, Q.; Feng, Z.; Li, T.; et al. Associations of socioeconomic status and chronic stress with incident atrial fibrillation among older adults: A prospective cohort study from the UK biobank. *Int. J. Cardiol.* **2025**, *418*, 132633. [CrossRef] [PubMed]
59. Tahapary, D.L.; Pratisthita, L.B.; Fitri, N.A.; Marcella, C.; Wafa, S.; Kurniawan, F.; Rizka, A.; Tarigan, T.J.E.; Harbuwono, D.S.; Purnamasari, D.; et al. Challenges in the diagnosis of insulin resistance: Focusing on the role of HOMA-IR and Tryglyceride/glucose index. *Diabetes Metab. Syndr.* **2022**, *16*, 102581. [CrossRef] [PubMed]
60. Khoramipour, K.; Chamari, K.; Hekmatikar, A.A.; Ziyaiyan, A.; Taherkhani, S.; Elguindy, N.M.; Bragazzi, N.L. Adiponectin: Structure, Physio-logical Functions, Role in Diseases, and Effects of Nutrition. *Nutrients* **2021**, *13*, 1180. [CrossRef] [PubMed] [PubMed Central]
61. Cui, C.; Liu, L.; Qi, Y.; Han, N.; Xu, H.; Wang, Z.; Shang, X.; Han, T.; Zha, Y.; Wei, X.; et al. Joint association of TyG index and high sensitivity C-reactive protein with cardiovascular disease: A national cohort study. *Cardiovasc. Diabetol.* **2024**, *23*, 156. [CrossRef] [PubMed] [PubMed Central]
62. Rodriguez-Garcia, E.; Ruiz-Nava, J.; Santamaria-Fernandez, S.; Fernandez-Garcia, J.C.; Vargas-Candela, A.; Yahyaoui, R.; Tinahones, F.J.; Bernal-Lopez, M.R.; Gomez-Huelgas, R. Impli-cations of the Mediterranean diet and physical exercise on the lipid profile of metabolically healthy obese women as measured by nuclear magnetic resonance spectroscopy (1H NMR). *Chem. Phys. Lipids.* **2018**, *213*, 68–75. [CrossRef] [PubMed]
63. Oh, E.; Cho, N.J.; Kang, H.; Kim, S.H.; Park, H.K.; Kwon, S.H. Computed tomography evaluation of skeletal muscle quality and quantity in people with morbid obesity with and without metabolic abnormality. *PLoS ONE* **2023**, *18*, e0296073. [CrossRef] [PubMed] [PubMed Central]
64. Kolahdouzi, S.; Baghadam, M.; Kani-Golzar, F.A.; Saeidi, A.; Jabbour, G.; Ayadi, A.; De Sousa, M.; Zouita, A.; Abderrahmane, A.B.; Zouhal, H. Progressive circuit resistance training improves inflammatory biomarkers and insulin resistance in obese men. *Physiol. Behav.* **2019**, *205*, 15–21. [CrossRef] [PubMed]

65. Wang, X.; Fan, M.; Meng, Q.; Wu, H.; Wang, Q.; Liu, T. Comparative study on the function of high-intensity intermittent exercise and continuous aerobic exerciseon obese children. *Acad. J. Health Sci.* **2024**, *39*, 40–49. [CrossRef]
66. Celada Roldana, C.; López Díez, J.; Cerezuela, M.A.; Rider, F.; Tárraga Marcos, A.; Tárraga López, P.J.; López González, A.A.; Ramírez Manent, J.I. Cardiovascular effects of a nutritional educational intervention in diabetic patients with poor control. *Acad. J. Health Sci.* **2023**, *38*, 57–65. [CrossRef]
67. Mukharjee, S.; Bank, S.; Maiti, S. Chronic Tobacco Exposure by Smoking Develops Insulin Resistance. *Endocr. Metab. Immune Disord. Drug Targets* **2020**, *20*, 869–877. [CrossRef] [PubMed]
68. Maddatu, J.; Anderson-Baucum, E.; Evans-Molina, C. Smoking and the risk of type 2 diabetes. *Transl Res.* **2017**, *184*, 101–107. [CrossRef] [PubMed] [PubMed Central]
69. Watanabe, K.; Wilmanski, T.; Diener, C.; Earls, J.C.; Zimmer, A.; Lincoln, B.; Hadlock, J.J.; Lovejoy, J.C.; Gibbons, S.M.; Magis, A.T.; et al. Multiomic signatures of body mass index identify heterogeneous health phenotypes and responses to a lifestyle intervention. *Nat. Med.* **2023**, *29*, 996–1008. [CrossRef] [PubMed] [PubMed Central]
70. Torres García, J.C.; Tárraga López, P.J.; Ramírez Gallegos, I.; Tarraga Marcos, A.; López González, A.A.; Manent, J.I.R. Relación entre actividad Física y Riesgo Cardiovascular: Una revisión sistemática. *Acad. J. Health Sci.* **2024**, *39*, 26–40. [CrossRef]
71. Papakonstantinou, E.; Oikonomou, C.; Nychas, G.; Dimitriadis, G.D. Effects of Diet, Lifestyle, Chrononutrition and Alternative Dietary Interventions on Postprandial Glycemia and Insulin Resistance. *Nutrients* **2022**, *14*, 823. [CrossRef] [PubMed] [PubMed Central]
72. Trang, K.; Grant, S.F.A. Genetics and epigenetics in the obesity phenotyping scenario. *Rev. Endocr. Metab. Disord.* **2023**, *24*, 775–793. [CrossRef] [PubMed] [PubMed Central]
73. Gasmi, A.; Noor, S.; Menzel, A.; Doşa, A.; Pivina, L.; Bjørklund, G. Obesity and Insulin Resistance: Associations with Chronic In-flammation, Genetic and Epigenetic Factors. *Curr. Med. Chem.* **2021**, *28*, 800–826. [CrossRef] [PubMed]
74. Ling, C. Epigenetic regulation of insulin action and secretion—Role in the pathogenesis of type 2 diabetes. *J. Intern. Med.* **2020**, *288*, 158–167. [CrossRef] [PubMed]
75. Zembic, A.; Eckel, N.; Stefan, N.; Baudry, J.; Schulze, M.B. An Empirically Derived Definition of Metabolically Healthy Obesity Based on Risk of Cardiovascular and Total Mortality. *JAMA Netw. Open* **2021**, *4*, e218505. [CrossRef] [PubMed] [PubMed Central]
76. WWang, W.-Q.; Wei, B.; Song, Y.-P.; Guo, H.; Zhang, X.-H.; Wang, X.-P.; Yan, Y.-Z.; Ma, J.-L.; Wang, K.; Keerman, M.; et al. Metabolically healthy obesity and unhealthy normal weight rural adults in Xinjiang: Prevalence and the associated factors. *BMC Public Health* **2021**, *21*, 1940. [CrossRef] [PubMed] [PubMed Central]
77. García-Perea, A.; Fernández-Cruz, E.; de la O-Pascual, V.; Gonzalez-Zorzano, E.; Moreno-Aliaga, M.J.; Tur, J.A.; Martinez, J.A. Nutritional and Lifestyle Features in a Mediterranean Cohort: An Epidemiological Instrument for Categorizing Metabotypes Based on a Computational Algorithm. *Medicina* **2024**, *60*, 610. [CrossRef] [PubMed] [PubMed Central]
78. Safaei, M.; Sundararajan, E.A.; Driss, M.; Boulila, W.; Shapi'i, A. A systematic literature review on obesity: Understanding the causes & consequences of obesity and reviewing various machine learning approaches used to predict obesity. *Comput. Biol. Med.* **2021**, *136*, 104754. [CrossRef] [PubMed]

nutrients

MDPI

*Article*

# Metabolic Syndrome in the Amazon: Customizing Diagnostic Methods for Urban Communities

**José M. Alcaide-Leyva [1,2], Manuel Romero-Saldaña [1,2,*], María García-Rodríguez [3], Rafael Molina-Luque [1,2], María del Rocío Jiménez-Mérida [1,2] and Guillermo Molina-Recio [1,2]**

1 Department of Nursing, Pharmacology and Physiotherapy, Faculty of Medicine and Nursing, University of Cordoba, 14014 Cordoba, Spain; jmalcaide@uco.es (J.M.A.-L.); p72molur@uco.es (R.M.-L.); en1moreg@uco.es (G.M.-R.)

2 Associated Research Group GA16 Lifestyles, Technology and Health, Maimonides Institute for Biomedical Research of Cordoba (IMIBIC), 14014 Cordoba, Spain

3 Department of Nursing and Nutrition, Faculty of Biomedical and Health Sciences, Universidad Europea de Madrid, Calle Tajo S/N, 28670 Madrid, Spain

* Correspondence: z92rosam@uco.es

**Abstract: Background/Objectives**: Metabolic syndrome is a significant public health issue, particularly in urbanizing regions like the Peruvian Amazon, where lifestyle changes have increased the prevalence of metabolic disorders. This study aimed to develop and validate a simple, cost-effective diagnostic model for early detection of metabolic syndrome in the urban population of San Juan Bautista, Iquitos. **Methods**: A cross-sectional study was conducted with 251 adults aged over 18 years. Data collection included anthropometric measurements, body composition analysis, and biochemical assessments. Logistic regression analyses identified key predictors of metabolic syndrome, and clinical decision trees were developed to enhance diagnostic accuracy. **Results**: The prevalence of metabolic syndrome was 47.9%. Systolic blood pressure, triglycerides, and very-low-density lipoprotein cholesterol were the strongest predictors. The most effective diagnostic model, combining very-low-density lipoprotein cholesterol and systolic blood pressure, achieved a sensitivity of 91.6% and a specificity of 78.5%, demonstrating high diagnostic accuracy. **Conclusions**: The proposed model offers a practical, low-cost tool for early detection of metabolic syndrome in resource-limited urban settings. However, its findings are limited by the small sample size and the lack of external validation, requiring further studies to confirm its generalizability and applicability to other populations. Its implementation in primary healthcare could facilitate timely interventions, reducing the risk of chronic diseases in vulnerable populations.

**Keywords:** metabolic syndrome; diagnostic model; urban Amazonian population; clinical decision tree; public health; early detection

## 1. Introduction

### *1.1. Metabolic Syndrome: Definition and Global Relevance*

Metabolic syndrome (MetS) is a set of metabolic disturbances that significantly increase the risk of developing chronic non-communicable diseases (NCDs), such as type 2 diabetes mellitus (T2D) and cardiovascular disease (CVD). The main criteria defining MetS include abdominal obesity, hyperglycaemia, high blood pressure (HBP), hypertriglyceridaemia and reduced high-density lipoprotein (HDL) levels [1,2]. This set of interrelated risk factors significantly increases the likelihood of severe complications, doubling the risk of cardiovascular events and increasing the risk of developing T2D by fivefold [3,4]. Globally, MetS affects approximately 25% of the adult population, and its prevalence has been increasing in recent decades due to various environmental and lifestyle factors, especially in urban settings where diet and physical activity levels have changed dramatically [5,6].

Accelerated urbanisation and the Nutritional Transition are among the main factors contributing to the increase of METS. In many regions of the world, dietary habits have shifted towards increased consumption of ultra-processed and high-calorie foods rich in saturated fats, sugars and salt, while consumption of fresh and nutritious foods has declined [7]. At the same time, changing lifestyles have reduced physical activity levels due to the increasing adoption of sedentary jobs and the use of technologies that facilitate transport and reduce the need for physical exertion. This context has significantly increased the prevalence of obesity and other risk factors contributing to MetS in urban populations from diverse cultural and economic backgrounds [8].

### 1.2. Prevalence and Risk Factors for MetS in Peru and Latin America

In Latin America, MetS is an increasingly relevant public health problem, with a steadily growing prevalence. Factors such as urbanisation, an increasing per capita income and the globalisation of dietary patterns have transformed the diet and lifestyle of Latin American populations, placing them at high risk of metabolic diseases [9]. In Peru, the prevalence of MetS reaches 31% in adults, reflecting the severity of this problem nationwide. Moreover, prevalence is particularly high in urban areas compared to rural areas, indicating a direct relationship between urbanisation and the increase in risk factors associated with MetS, such as overweight, abdominal obesity and dyslipidaemia [10]. This phenomenon is attributed to changes in lifestyle habits, with increasing access to ultra-processed foods and a decrease in physical activity levels that characterises urban areas of the country [11,12].

### 1.3. MetS in the Peruvian Amazon and the Impact of Urbanisation

The Peruvian Amazon faces unique public health challenges, and MetS is one of the emerging problems in this region. The 'double burden' of malnutrition is a distinctive feature of the Peruvian Amazon, where undernutrition and an increased prevalence of overweight and obesity coexist. This complex situation is driven by a nutritional transition in a region that has historically been dependent on local, nutrient-rich foods, but which in recent decades has experienced an increase in the availability of processed and high-calorie foods. This dietary change, coupled with increasingly sedentary urban lifestyles, has increased the burden of chronic non-communicable diseases, of which MetS is central [13,14].

Iquitos, the largest city in the Peruvian Amazon and capital of the department of Loreto, presents a particular context in this sense. Being unconnected by road to the rest of the country and dependent on river and air routes, Iquitos faces a series of limitations that complicate access to health services and to a varied and high-quality nutritional diet. These conditions exacerbate the vulnerability of the Iquitos population to MetS and other metabolic diseases, as dietary options are often limited and geographic barriers hinder the implementation of effective public health policies [15].

### 1.4. San Juan Bautista: Characterisation of an Urban Amazonian District

Within Iquitos, the district of San Juan Bautista is one of the areas that best represents the challenges of urbanisation in the Peruvian Amazon. With a mainly urban population, San Juan Bautista has witnessed a change in the lifestyle and dietary habits of its inhabitants, which has significantly increased the risk factors for MetS in this community. Data indicate that abdominal obesity and dyslipidaemia are increasingly common in the district, affecting even individuals with a body mass index (BMI) considered normal by international standards [16,17]. These findings highlight the need to develop tailored diagnostic models that take into account the anthropometric and metabolic particularities of the Peruvian Amazonian population, where risk thresholds established for other populations may not adequately reflect the risk profile of this population [10,18].

### *1.5. The Harmonised MetS Diagnostic Model and Its Application in Specific Populations*

To respond to variations in risk profiles between different ethnicities and regions, the harmonised model for the diagnosis of MetS, promoted by the International Diabetes Federation (IDF), has become an international standard for the identification of at-risk individuals. This model establishes specific cut-off points for key risk factors, such as waist circumference, adapting these values to reflect variations in body composition and metabolic susceptibility among different groups [19]. However, studies have highlighted that the application of this model in Latin American and Amazonian populations requires local adjustments, as these communities have particular susceptibility to MetS and its comorbidities, which may not be adequately captured in the standard criteria of the harmonised model [20,21]. Adapting international models to local contexts presents several challenges. First, the cut-off points for anthropometric and metabolic variables often do not reflect the unique characteristics of populations in regions such as the Peruvian Amazon, where body composition and genetic predispositions differ significantly from those in Western populations [20,22]. Second, cultural and socioeconomic factors, such as dietary patterns, access to healthcare, and levels of physical activity, vary greatly and influence the prevalence and risk factors of MetS [17,23]. Finally, the availability of resources and diagnostic tools in low-resource settings can limit the feasibility of implementing standardised criteria [13]. For instance, while the IDF model provides a global framework, its practical application in vulnerable communities like San Juan Bautista requires tailoring to account for these local realities. These challenges underscore the need for models that are both scientifically robust and contextually appropriate

In the case of the Peruvian Amazon, previous studies have shown that variables such as waist-to-height ratio (WHtR) and waist circumference (WC) are useful diagnostic tools in low-resource settings, as they allow for practical and accessible risk assessment without the need for advanced technology [24]. These anthropometric measures, adapted to specific cut-off points for the Amazonian population, facilitate early and affordable identification of estimated risk in urban settings such as San Juan Bautista, which is particularly important in areas where resources for diagnosis and treatment are limited.

Additionally, several diagnostic models validated in comparable populations provide further evidence supporting the use of tailored approaches in resource-limited contexts. For instance, the FINDRISC model has been shown to effectively predict cardiometabolic risk in low-resource environments through non-invasive measures [25]. Similarly, the Triglycerides and Glucose (TyG) index has demonstrated high diagnostic accuracy in Latin American populations by integrating simple biochemical parameters [26,27]. These models highlight the importance of adapting diagnostic tools to specific sociodemographic and cultural contexts, as they account for regional variations in metabolic and anthropometric profiles. Building upon this evidence, our study aims to develop a diagnostic model tailored specifically to the urban Amazonian population, addressing their unique characteristics and public health challenges.

## 2. Materials and Methods

The study population consisted of EsSalud (Social Health Insurance) workers at the health post in the district of San Juan Bautista in the city of Iquitos and the service users themselves.

Study sample

A non-probabilistic convenience sample was used in which an attempt was made to include as many subjects as possible based on the time and technical resources available. In the end, 251 subjects were included in the study.

### 2.1. Eligibility Criteria

Persons over 18 years of age who agreed to participate in the study and sign the informed consent form were included, and those with an inability to stand upright during anthropometry and bioimpedance were excluded.

- Study variables and measurementThe dependent variable of the study was the diagnosis of MetS according to the NCEP ATP III criteria [28]. These criteria establish the presence of STEM when three or more of the following risk factors are present: Obesity Central. CC $\geq$ 94 cm for males o $\geq$88 cm for females.
  - High blood pressure. SBP $\geq$ 130 mmHg and/or DBP $\geq$ 85 mmHg or antihypertensive treatment.
  - High triglycerides. TG $\geq$ 150 mg/dL or lipid-lowering treatment.
  - High blood glucose. FG $\geq$ 100 mg/dL or hypoglycaemic treatment.
  - Low HDL. HDL < 40 mg/dL in women or HDL < 50 mg/dL in men or pharmacological treatment to address it.
- The independent variables of the study were:
  - Sociodemographics: Age (years) and sex (male/female).
  - Anthropometric. Height (cm), weight (kg), BMI (kg/m$^2$), waist circumference (WC, cm), body fat percentage (FP%), muscle mass (MM, kg), basal metabolic rate (BMR, kcal), waist-to-height ratio (WHtR), A New Body Shape Index (ABSI) (113) and Body Adiposity Index (BAI) (114). In addition, the BMI was used to assess nutritional status according to the cut-off points established by the WHO (111) for underweight ($\leq$18.49), normal weight (18.5–24.99 kg/m$^2$), overweight (25.00–29.99 kg/m$^2$) and obesity ($\geq$30.00 kg/m$^2$). WHtR was categorised as healthy (Males (M): 0.43 to 0.52 and Females (F): 0.42 to 0.48); overweight (M: 0.53 to 0.57 and F: 0.49 to 0.53); elevated overweight (M: 0.58 to 0.62 and F: 0.54 to 0.57), and obese (M: $\geq$0.63 and F: $\geq$0.58) [29,30].
  - Laboratory tests. FG (mg/dL), HDL cholesterol (mg/dL), TG (mg/dL), VLDL cholesterol according to Friedewald's formula (mg/dL) [31].

### 2.2. Data Collection

For data collection, several teams were formed, composed of nurses, nutritionists and students previously trained in data collection. The students belonged to the final courses of Nursing, Nutrition and Medicine at the University of the Peruvian Amazon. Regarding measurements, height was taken using a Seca 213 portable stadiometer (Seca. Hamburg, Germany). Body composition and weight were measured with a Tanita BC-545N (Tanita Corp., Itabashini-Ku, Tokyo, Japan). Bioimpedance analysis was chosen for assessing body composition due to its practicality, portability, and cost-effectiveness in resource-limited settings such as San Juan Bautista. While BIA has limitations compared to gold-standard methods like dual-energy X-ray absorptiometry, it is widely validated in population-based studies. BIA provides reliable estimates of body fat percentage, muscle mass, and basal metabolic rate, making it a suitable and effective tool for large-scale community-based studies. CC was measured at the midpoint between the lower limit of the last rib and the iliac crest. Both variables were collected with a Lufki W606PM (Lufki, Missouri City, TX, USA) metal tape with an accuracy of 0.1 cm (118). Both circumferences were measured at the end of a regular exhalation in an upright position with arms suspended alongside the torso [32]. Blood pressure was measured using an OMRON M4 digital sphygmomanometer (OMRON Corporation Ltd., Tokyo, Japan) according to blood pressure measurement standards. Finally, biochemical variables were measured with a Cardiocheck (pts Diagnostics, Whitestown, IN, USA) and PTS Panels self-testing strips (pts Diagnostics, USA) [33].

### 2.3. Statistical Analysis

Quantitative variables were presented using the mean and standard deviation. Qualitative variables were expressed as absolute frequency and percentages.

To study the goodness of fit of the quantitative variables to the normal distribution, the Kolmogorov–Smirnov test with the Lilliefors correction was used, together with the analysis of their histograms and Q-Q and P-P plots.

For the comparison of means, Student's *t*-test or one-factor ANOVA was used when the parametricity criteria were met. In the latter case, post hoc contrasts were used using the Bonferroni test. In the absence of normality of the data, non-parametric tests (Mann–Whitney U and Kruskal–Wallis) were used. For hypothesis testing of qualitative variables, the chi-square test and Fisher's exact test were used.

On the other hand, binary logistic regressions were performed. In this analysis, crude and adjusted Odds Ratios (OR) were obtained. The Wald test was applied as a statistical contrast method to assess the significance of the coefficients in the logistic regression model. The goodness-of-fit of the model was assessed using the Hosmer–Lemeshow test. Finally, to assess the predictive ability of the model, we calculated the Cox–Snell and Nagelkerke tests, together with the coefficients of variance and determination.

### 2.4. Ethical Considerations

Participants were treated within the bioethical legislative framework of the Republic of Peru. The guidelines of the Declaration of Helsinki [34], which establishes the fundamental ethical principles for medical research, were strictly followed. All participants were informed personally, verbally and in writing, of the objectives of the research study. The researchers also informed them of the dangers and advantages of their participation in this project. All informed consents were signed and retained.

To ensure inclusivity and respect for the cultural and social characteristics of the local population, the study involved collaboration with local healthcare professionals, including physicians, nutritionists, and nurses, who were familiar with the community and its sociocultural dynamics. Their participation facilitated trust-building and effective communication with participants. Additionally, recruitment materials and consent forms were adapted to the local context, using culturally appropriate language and formats to ensure comprehension and meaningful participation. Efforts were also made to achieve gender balance and include participants across a wide age range to reflect the diversity of the population.

In addition, the provisions of Law No. 26842—Peru's General Health Law [35], which establishes the guiding principles of the health system in the country and addresses issues related to medical ethics and health research, were complied with. In the area of data protection, the regulations of the European Union's General Data Protection Regulation (GDPR) [36] were applied, guaranteeing the privacy and rights of participants. This ethical and legal approach, both at local and European levels, ensured the protection of the rights and welfare of the study participants. The research project of this Doctoral Thesis was approved by the Research Ethics Committee of Cordoba (act 348/reference 5610).

## 3. Results

### 3.1. Characteristics of the Sample

The sample consisted of 251 participants, whose sociodemographic and anthropometric characteristics are shown in Table 1.

**Table 1.** Sociodemographic and anthropometric characteristics.

| Variable | Total $n = 251$ | Women 164 (65.3%) | Men 87 (34.7%) | $p$ |
|---|---|---|---|---|
| **Age (years)** | 47.93 (SD 15.71) | 47.68 (SD15.68) | 48.39 (1SD3.96) | |
| | | **Anthropometry** | | |
| **WC (cm)** | 99.64 (SD9.65) | 96.53 (53 (8.2) | 105.49 (SD9.51) | <0.001 |
| | | **Level of WC** | | |
| **Low** | 7 (2.8%) | 3 (42.9%) | 4 (57.1%) | |
| **High** | 244 (97.2%) | 161 (66%) | 83 (34%) | NS |
| **Weight (kg)** | 73.83 (SD15.17) | 67.98 (SD11.92) | 71.57(SD6.48) | <0.001 |
| **Height (cm)** | 154.76 (SD1.54) | 1.51 (SD0.05) | 1.62 (SD0.06) | <0.001 |
| **WHtR** | 0.64 (SD0.07) | 0.63 (SD0.07) | 0.65 (SD0.05) | |
| | | **Level of WHtR** | | |
| **Low** | 5 (2) | 4 (80) | 1 (20%) | NS |
| **High** | 244 (98) | 158 (64.8) | 86 (35.2%) | |
| **BMI (kg/m²)** | 30.360 (SD4.86) | 29.83(SD 3.12) | 32 (SD4.44) | <0.001 |
| | | **Level of BMI** | | |
| **Underweight** | 2 (0.8%) | 2 (100%) | 0 | <0.001 |
| **Healthy weight** | 23.8 (9.2%) | 20 (87%) | 3 (13%) | |
| **Overweight** | 96 (38.2%) | 69 (71.1%) | 27 (28.1%) | |
| **Obesity** | 119 (47.4%) | 66 (55.5%) | 52 (44.5%) | |

Quantitative variables with mean and SD. Qualitative variables with absolute frequency and percentage; BMI: Body Mass Index; WC: Waist Circumference; WHtR: waist-to-height ratio. SD: Standar Desviation; NS: No Significant

The mean age of the participants was 47.93 ± 15.71 years, with a higher proportion of women. In terms of anthropometric characteristics, the mean WC was 99.64 ± 9.65 cm, which determined that the majority of participants had a WC considered high. Similarly, the mean WhtR was 0.64 ± 0.067, also above the values indicating good nutritional status, which meant that 97.2% of the sample had a high WhtR. Finally, BMI averaged 30.36 ± 4.86 kg/m$^2$, resulting in a high percentage of overweight and obese individuals.

Regarding the characteristics related to the data obtained from the bioimpedance and clinical variables (Table 2), a mean FP of 32.73 ±7.17% stood out, with 56.6% of the participants in the high level. Regarding the clinical variables, 80.5% of the participants had a high HDL-C and 41.4% a high TG. The mean AG was 103.42 ±41.79 mg/dL.

**Table 2.** Characteristics according to bioimpedance and clinical variables.

| Variable | Total | Women 164 (65.3%) | Men 87 (34.7%) | $p$ |
|---|---|---|---|---|
| | | **Bioimpedance variables** | | |
| **FP (%)** | 32.73 (SD7.17) | 35.21 (SD6.67) | 28.06 (SD5.61) | <0.001 |
| **MM (kg)** | 46.86 (SD 4.05) | 47.26 (SD5.53) | 52.39 (SD4.27) | <0.001 |
| **BMR (kcal)** | 1492.53 (SD296.48) | 1334.61 (SD162.31) | 1791.02 (SD260.85) | <0.001 |
| **MA (years)** | 51 (SD10.91) | 49 (SD10.8) | 54.8 (SD10.13) | <0.001 |

**Table 2.** *Cont.*

| Variable | Total | Women 164 (65.3%) | Men 87 (34.7%) | *p* |
|---|---|---|---|---|
| | | **Clinical variables** | | |
| **SBP (mmHg)** | 130.37 (DE 23.65) | 125.41 (SD 23.44) | 139.70 (SD 21.21) | <0.001 |
| **DBP (mmHg)** | 79.06 (DE 13.07) | 75.68 (SD 12.83) | 85.43 (SD 11.04) | <0.001 |
| **HDL-C: (mg/dL)** | 38.18 (DE 13.31) | 42.38 (SD 12.61) | 30.24 (SD 6.479) | <0.001 |
| | | **Level of HDL-C** | | |
| **Low** | 49 (19.5%) | 39 (79.6%) | 10 (20.4%) | <0.05 |
| **High** | 202 (80.5%) | 125 (61.9%) | 77 (38.1%) | |
| **TG (mg/dL)** | 152.12 (SD 69.5) | 134.01 (SD 124.01) | 170.44 (SD 76.17) | <0.001 |
| | | **TG level** | | |
| **Low** | 147 (58.6%) | 106 (72.1%) | 41 (27.9%) | <0.05 |
| **High** | 104 (41.4%) | 58 (55.8%) | 46 (44.2%) | |
| **FG (mg/dL)** | 103.42 (SD 41.79) | 102.63 (SD 39.42) | 104.91 (SD 46.13) | NS |
| **Low** | 169 (67.3%) | 112 (66.3%) | 57 (33.7%) | NS |
| **High** | 82 (32.7%) | 52 (63.4%) | 30 (36.6%) | |
| **VLDL** | 70.10 (SD 37.81) | 45.48(SD 14.29) | 82.45 (SD 39.87) | <0.001 |

Quantitative variables with mean and SD. Qualitative variables with absolute frequency and percentage; FP: fat percentage; MM: muscle mass; BMR: basal metabolism rate; MA: metabolic age; SST: systolic blood pressure; DBP: diastolic blood pressure; HDL-C: cholesterol; TG: triglycerides; FG: fasting glucose; VLDL: very low-density lipoprotein. SD: Standar Desviation; NS: No Significant.

### 3.2. Bivariate Analysis and Logistic Regression for MetS

Data concerning bivariate analysis and logistic regression for MetS are shown in Table 3. In relation to the presence of MetS, the diseased population showed a mean age seven years older than the healthy. In addition, men had a much higher prevalence than women, being 5.54 times more likely to develop this syndrome in the former group.

Regarding anthropometric variables, WC, weight and height were associated with a higher prevalence of MetS ($p < 0.001$). However, WHtR did not show this relationship. The FP was significantly related to MetS (crude OR = 1.22, 95%CI: 1.05–1.43, $p < 0.05$). Similarly, other bioimpedance parameters such as MM, BMR and MA were related to the presence of this condition. This association was also evident for all clinical variables. Finally, the adjusted model included SBP, DBP, TG, FG and VLDL.

**Table 3.** Bivariate analysis and crude and adjusted logistic regression for MS.

| Variable | No MS 84 (33.5%) | Yes MS 167 (66.5%) | Raw OR | *p* | Adjusted OR | *p* |
|---|---|---|---|---|---|---|
| **Age (years)** | 43.74 (14.4) | 50.04 (14.51) | 1.03 (1.01–1.05) | $p < 0.05$ | | NS |
| | | | **Sex** | | | |
| **Women** | 73 (86.9%) | 91 (54.5%) | 1 | | | |
| **Men** | 11 (13.1%) | 76 (45.5%) | 5.54 (2.74–11.19) | $p < 0.001$ | | NS |
| | | | **Anthropometry** | | | |
| **WC (cm)** | 96.31 (8.55) | 101.31 (9.76) | 1.06 (1.02–1.09) | $p < 0.001$ | | NS |
| | | | **Level of WC** | | | |
| **Low** | 5 (6%) | 2 (1.2%) | 1 | | | |
| **High** | 79 (94%) | 165 (98.8%) | 5.22 (0.99–27.5) | $p = 0.51$ | | NS |
| **Weight (kg)** | 86.91 (11.75) | 76.29(16.1) | 1.03 (1.01–1.05) | $p < 0.001$ | | NS |
| **Height (cm)** | 152 (6.2) | 155 (8.6) | 1.08 (1.02–1.14) | $p < 0.001$ | | NS |
| **WHtR** | 0.63 (0.05) | 0.64 (0.07) | 1.24 (0.77–2.01) | NS | | |

**Table 3.** *Cont.*

| Variable | No MS 84 (33.5%) | Yes MS 167 (66.5%) | Raw OR | *p* | Adjusted OR | *p* |
|---|---|---|---|---|---|---|
| | | | **Level of WHtR** | | | |
| **Low** | 3 (3.6%) | 2 (1.2%) | 1 | | | |
| **High** | 81 (96.4%) | 163 (98.8%) | 3.01 (0.49– 18.42) | NS | | |
| **BMI (kg/m²)** | 29.45 (4.19) | 30.81 (5.12) | 1.06 (1.001–1.12) | $p < 0.05$ | | NS |
| | | | **Level of BMI** | | | |
| **Underweight** | 1 (1.3%) | 1 (0.6%) | | | | NS |
| **Healthy weight** | 8 (10%) | 15 (9.4%) | | | | |
| **Overweight** | 40 (50%) | 56 (35%) | | | | |
| **Obesity** | 31 (38.8%) | 88 (55%) | | | | |
| **Variable** | MetS No 84 (33.5%) | MetS Yes 167 (66.5%) | Raw OR | *p* | Adjusted OR | *p* |
| | | | **Bioimpedance variables** | | | |
| **FP (%)** | 34.97 (7.94) | 31.61 (6.489) | 1.22 (1.05–1.43) | $p < 0.05$ | | NS |
| **MM (kg)** | 42.34 (6.96) | 49.03 (10.38) | 1.09 (1.05–1.12) | $p < 0.001$ | | NS |
| **BM (kcal)** | 1364 (189.73) | 1556.31 (319.31) | 1.003 (1.002–1.004) | $p < 0.001$ | | NS |
| **MA (years)** | 46.61 (10.18) | 53.19 (10.63) | 1.06 (1.03–1.09) | $p < 0.001$ | | NS |
| | | | **Clinical variables** | | | |
| **SBP (mmHg)** | 115.27 (17) | 137.96 (22.91) | 1.06 (1.04–108) | $p < 0.001$ | 1.08 (1.05–1.11) | $p < 0.001$ |
| **DBP (mmHg)** | 72.61 (8.66) | 82.3 (13.72) | 1.07 (1.04–1.11) | $p < 0.001$ | 1.23 (1.12–1.28) | $p < 0.001$ |
| **HDL-C: (mg/dL)** | 43.96 (12.54) | 35.26 (11.15) | 0.91 (0.89–0.95) | $p < 0.001$ | | NS |
| | | | **Level of HDL-C** | | | |
| **Low** | 52 (61.9%) | 150 (89.8%) | 1 | | | |
| **High** | 32 (38.1%) | 17 (10.2%) | 0.18 (0.09–0.35) | $p < 0.001$ | | NS |
| **TG (mg/dL)** | 98.7 (31.02) | 170.75 (71.04) | 1.03 (1.02–1.04) | $p < 0.001$ | 1.03 (1.02–1.04) | $p < 0.001$ |
| | | | **TG level** | | | |
| **Low** | 82 (97.6%) | 65 (38.9%) | 1 | | | |
| **High** | 2 (2.4%) | 102 (61.1%) | 64.38 (15.29–270.64) | $p < 0.001$ | | NS |
| **FG (mg/dL)** | 90.29 (19.74) | 110.02 (48) | 1.03 (1.01–1.05) | $p < 0.001$ | 1.02 (1.01–1.09) | $p < 0.001$ |
| | | | **Level of FG** | | | |
| **Low** | 80 (95.2%) | 89 (53.3%) | 1 | | | |
| **High** | 4 (4.8%) | 78 (46.7%) | 17.52 (6.13–50.04) | $p < 0.001$ | | NS |
| **VLDL** | 45.48 (14.29) | 82.48 (39.87) | 1.06 (1.043–1.08) | $p < 0.001$ | 1.04 (1.01–1.07) | $p < 0.001$ |

Quantitative variables with mean and SD. Qualitative variables with absolute frequency and percentage; BMI: Body Mass Index; WC: Waist Circumference; FP: fat percentage; MM: muscle mass; BM: basal metabolism; MA: metabolic age; SBP: systolic blood pressure; DBP: diastolic blood pressure; HDL-C: cholesterol; TG: triglycerides; FG: fasting glucose; VLDL: very low-density lipoprotein. NS: No Significant.

### 3.3. Development of the Clinical Decision Tree

Figure 1 shows the ROC curves for all variables included in the regression model fitted for MetS detection. Thus, the cut-off points that showed the best Youden index are shown (Table 4).

The variables were grouped logically by selecting those with the least complexity of application in the populations of the area studied. Three diagnostic models were then developed based on the cut-off points obtained. For this purpose, the SBP and DBP variables were transformed into dichotomous categorical variables that were used to develop the tree without forcing the first variable (Figure 2) and thus test the effectiveness of diagnosing MetS based on non-invasive clinical variables. In the second tree (Figure 3), the level of TG was categorised into a dichotomous variable. Once transformed, and together with the dichotomous SBP, a mixed model was designed with invasive (but easy to measure with portable devices) and non-invasive variables, without forcing the first variable. Finally, for the third model (Figure 4), the VLDL variable was dichotomised from the cut-off point calculated using the Youden index. In this case, the first discriminant variable was forced to be VLDL and, using the CHAID system, DBP was discarded and SBP was finally selected (Table 5).

**Table 4.** Comparison of diagnostic accuracy between variables.

| Variable | AUC | *p* | 95%IC | Cut-Off Point | Sensitivity | Specificity | J |
|---|---|---|---|---|---|---|---|
| TG | 0.83 | <0.001 | 0.78–0.88 | 149.5 | 0.611 | 0.976 | 0.587 |
| VLDL | 0.82 | <0.001 | 0.77–0.872 | 68.89 | 0.591 | 0.914 | 0.612 |
| SBP | 0.819 | <0.001 | 0.71–0.83 | 125.5 | 0.725 | 0.81 | 0.534 |
| DBP | 0.756 | <0.001 | 0.69–0.82 | 75.5 | 0.737 | 0.69 | 0.424 |

TG: Triglycerides; SBP: Systolic Blood Pressure; DBP: Diastolic Blood Pressure; VLDL: Very Low-Density Lipoprotein; AUC: Area Under the Curve; IC: Confidence Interval; J: Youden Index.

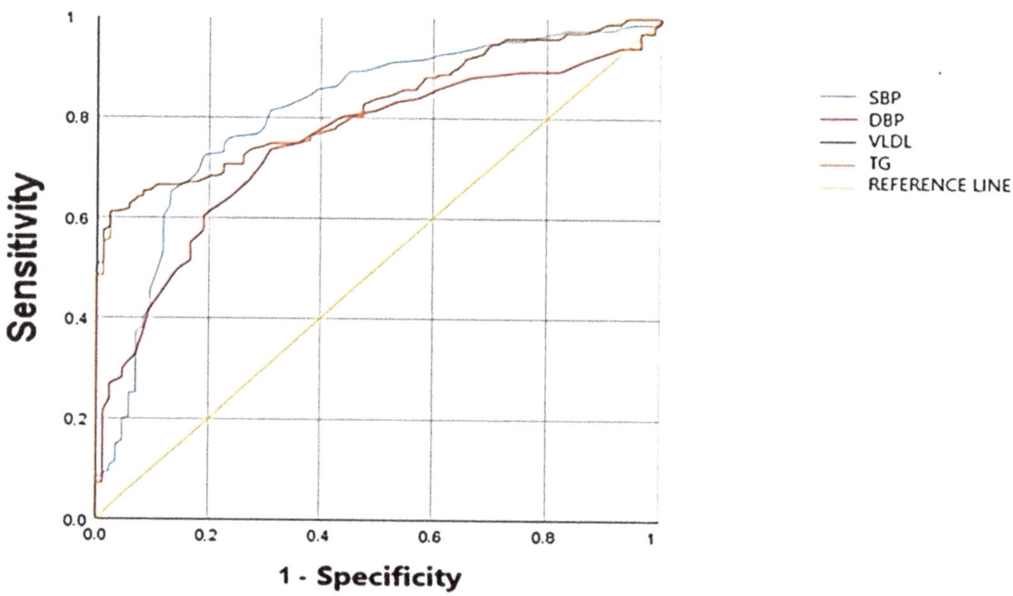


**Figure 1.** Area under the curve of the selected variables.

**Table 5.** Comparative diagnostic accuracy of clinical decision trees.

| | Sensitivity (%) | Specificity (%) | Validity Index (%) | PPV (%) | NVP (%) | Youden |
|---|---|---|---|---|---|---|
| Model 1 | 84.43 (78.63–90.23) | 65.48 (54.71–76.24) | 78.09 (72.77–83.40) | 83.94 (76.99–88.89) | 67.90 (57.12–79.69) | 0.5 (0.38–0.61) |
| Model 2 | 92.22 (87.85–96.58) | 61.90 (50.92–72.88) | 82.07 (77.13–87.02) | 82.80 (77.10–88.49) | 80 (69.51–90.49) | 0.54 (0.43–0.65) |
| Model 3 | 91.62 (87.11–96.12) | 78.57 (69.2–87.94) | 87.25 (82.93–91.58) | 89.47 (84.58–94.37) | 82.50 (73.55–91.45) | 0.7(0.6–0.8) |

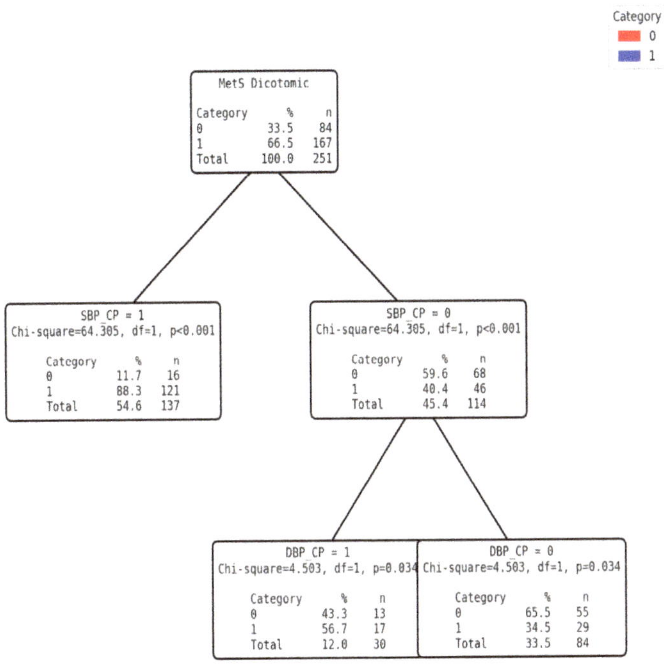


**Figure 2.** Clinical decision tree for MS based on SBP CP (SBP Cut-off point) and DBP CP (DBP Cut-off point).

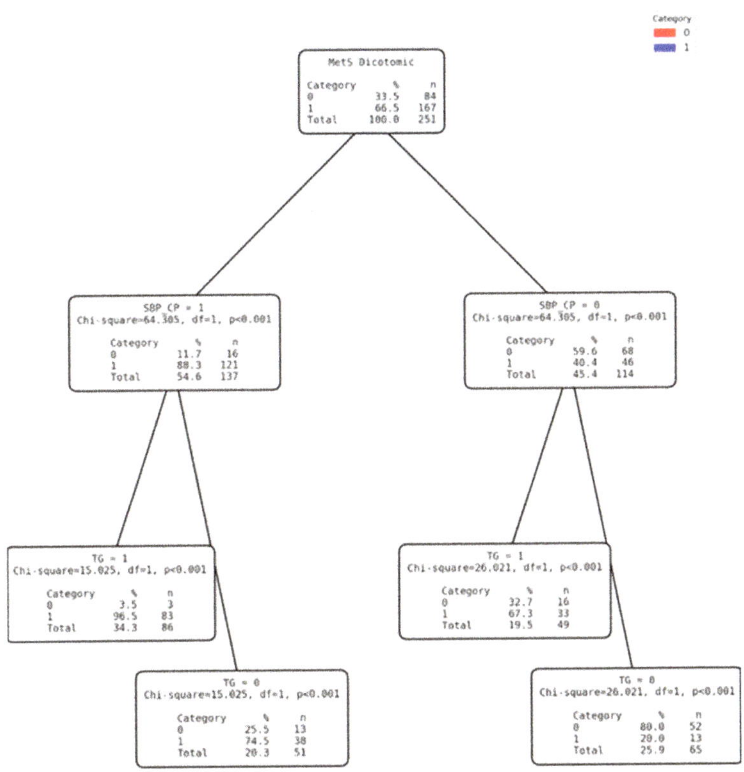


**Figure 3.** Clinical decision tree for MetS based on SBP CP(SBP Cut-off point) and TG.

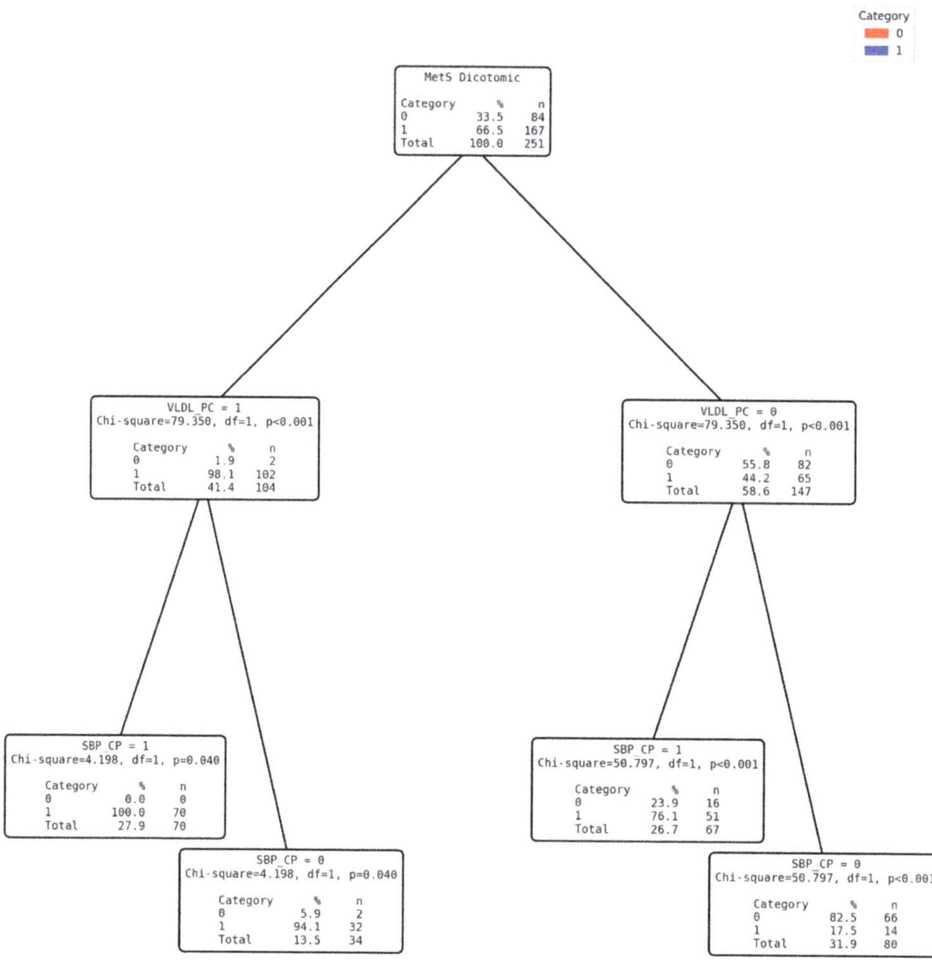


**Figure 4.** Clinical Decision Tree for MetS based on VLDL and SBP CP..

*3.4. Comparison of the Diagnostic Efficacy of Clinical Decision Trees*

As a final step, a comparative analysis of the three diagnostic trees (Table 5) was performed based on their diagnostic accuracy. Model 2 showed the highest sensitivity, with 92.22%, followed by Model 3, while Model 1 registered a slightly lower diagnostic accuracy.

On the other hand, specificity was highest for Model 3, with a value of 78.57%, followed by Model 1 and Model 2. AsimiMetSo, Model 3 also stood out for its Validity Index, with a value of 87.25%, nine points higher than Model 1, which had the lowest values.

In terms of Predictive Values, the PPV of Model 3 stood out with 89.47%. Model 2 showed a PPV of 82.80%, while Model 1 scored the lowest. However, the best Negative Predictive Value was evidenced by Model 2, with a value of 80%, followed, in that order, by Models 3 and 1,

Overall, and given that it was comparatively better than the rest on the basis of diagnostic accuracy metrics and, in particular, the Youden index, Model 3 was assessed as the most suitable for screening for STEMI in this type of population.

## 4. Discussion

The results obtained in this study reveal a high prevalence of MetS in the urban population of San Juan Bautista, reaching 47.9%, a figure considerably higher than that reported in other regions of Peru, where the average prevalence is around 31% (Ramírez et al., 2022), and well above the 19.7% found in rural Peruvian populations located below 1,000 m above sea level [37]. This finding highlights the severity of the problem and underscores the influence of changes in dietary habits and decreased physical activity in urban settings. The high proportion of abdominal obesity (66.5%) and dyslipidaemia (41.4%) observed in our sample aligns with the literature linking these factors to the development of MetS. Recent studies have confirmed that accelerated urbanisation in developing countries has intensified the risk factors associated with MetS, increasing its prevalence to 52% in certain urban areas [38,39].

The prevalence of MetS in this urban population is higher than that found in studies conducted in rural or mixed communities, which is consistent with research highlighting the impact of urbanisation and nutritional transition on the rise of metabolic diseases [40]. Furthermore, the proposed diagnostic model, based on simple variables such as SBP and VLDL levels, has proven to be effective and accessible, achieving a sensitivity of 91.6% and a specificity of 78.5%. These results are comparable to those reported by Fornari Laurindo et al. [41], who achieved a sensitivity of 89.4% and specificity of 75.2% using similar methods. Another study [42] also emphasized the need to adjust metabolic indicator cut-off points for different populations, supporting the relevance of adapted models like the one developed in this study.

The development of simple, cost-effective, and locally adapted diagnostic tools represents a significant advancement for the early detection of MetS in vulnerable urban populations. Implementing these models in primary healthcare centres could enhance the identification of at-risk individuals and facilitate the application of preventive interventions. For instance, the Triglyceride and Glucose (TyG) Index has emerged as a cost-effective diagnostic tool for various medical conditions, reflecting underlying insulin resistance, a key factor in many metabolic disorders [43]. Additionally, non-invasive methods utilizing machine learning models have been proposed for early and low-cost identification of MetS, demonstrating high sensitivity and convenience for large-scale screening [44]). Guzmán et al. [45] demonstrated that community interventions based on early detection of MetS can reduce the incidence of cardiovascular diseases by 25% and type 2 diabetes by 30%.

One of the main strengths of this study lies in the adaptation of the diagnostic model to the specific characteristics of the studied urban population. The use of easily obtainable and low-cost clinical variables increases the feasibility of its application in resource-limited settings. Additionally, the model shows an adequate balance between sensitivity and specificity. Recent studies have validated similar approaches, highlighting the importance of practical and adaptable models for MetS prevention [46].

Among the limitations, the relatively small sample size (n = 251) stands out, which could affect the generalizability of the results. Furthermore, the use of a non-probabilistic convenience sample and the focus on a specific urban Amazonian district may limit the applicability of these findings to broader populations. Additionally, this study focused primarily on the pathological and metabolic profile of the urban Amazonian population, without including variables such as dietary intake, physical activity levels, and stress management or alcohol consumption. These variables are critical in understanding the multifactorial nature of metabolic syndrome and its risk factors. Future studies should address these limitations by recruiting larger, more representative samples and incorporating lifestyle and behavioural data to provide a more comprehensive assessment of metabolic health. Furthermore, external validation of the diagnostic model in diverse demographic and geographic contexts is essential to confirm its generalizability and clinical applicability. Additionally, the model was validated in the same population in which it was developed, making it necessary to test its effectiveness in other urban populations. Likewise, the use of standard formulas to estimate certain biochemical markers may not accurately reflect the reality of this community. Recent research suggests the incorporation of emerging biomarkers to improve diagnostic accuracy [47]. Furthermore, the reliance on traditional anthropometric and biochemical variables in this study, while practical for resource-limited settings, may not capture the full spectrum of factors contributing to MetS. Advanced biomarkers, such as inflammatory markers or metabolomics, could provide deeper insights into the pathophysiology of MetS and enhance diagnostic precision. Additionally, the integration of digital health solutions, including wearable devices and mobile applications, offers opportunities for real-time monitoring, early detection, and personalised management of MetS. Future studies should explore these innovations to complement traditional diagnostic models and improve health outcomes in vulnerable populations [48].

Future research should focus on validating the proposed model in other urban populations with different sociodemographic characteristics. Moreover, it would be advisable to expand the sample size and consider the use of additional biomarkers to enhance diagnostic precision. The implementation of longitudinal studies would allow for the evaluation of the model's predictive capacity over the long term and its impact on the prevention of chronic diseases. These would also provide a deeper understanding of how risk factors evolve over time and how early detection through the proposed model could influence the natural history of MetS. In addition, tracking individual trajectories could help assess the model's capacity to predict long-term health outcomes, such as the onset of type 2 diabetes and cardiovascular diseases.Therefore, these research efforts are crucial for validating the model's utility beyond its current context and ensuring its effective applicability across diverse populations. Additionally, validating the model in urban populations with varying sociodemographic and cultural characteristics would allow for the identification of potential modifications needed to optimise its applicability and effectiveness in different settings. Integrating digital health technologies, such as wearable devices and mobile applications, could facilitate continuous monitoring and personalised management of individuals at risk of developing MetS [49]. Additionally, exploring the role of gut microbiota and its modulation may offer new therapeutic avenues for MetS management [50].

## 5. Conclusions

This study highlights the alarming prevalence of MetS in the urban population of San Juan Bautista, emphasizing the urgent need for targeted public health interventions. The diagnostic model developed, based on simple and cost-effective clinical variables such as systolic blood pressure and VLDL levels, demonstrated high diagnostic accuracy with a sensitivity of 91.6% and specificity of 78.5%. While the model shows promise as a practical and adaptable tool for early detection and prevention strategies in resource-limited urban settings, its findings should be interpreted within the context of the study's limitations. These include the cross-sectional design, which prevents causal inferences, the non-probabilistic sampling method, which limits generalizability, and the need for validation in other populations and geographic contexts. Future research should address these limitations to further refine and validate the model, ensuring its broader applicability and effectiveness in diverse settings.

Implementing such cost-effective diagnostic tools in primary healthcare services can significantly improve the early identification of individuals at risk, enabling timely interventions that could reduce the incidence of cardiovascular diseases and type 2 diabetes. However, to enhance its applicability and reliability, future studies should validate this model in diverse urban populations and incorporate emerging biomarkers for better diagnostic precision.

In conclusion, our findings underscore the necessity for proactive health policies that incorporate accessible diagnostic methods and preventive measures tailored to vulnerable urban populations. The integration of digital health technologies could further strengthen the monitoring and management of MetS, fostering more effective and sustainable public health outcomes.

**Author Contributions:** Conceptualization, J.M.A.-L. and M.R.-S.; methodology, J.M.A.-L.; software, M.G.-R.; validation, J.M.A.-L., M.d.R.J.-M. and R.M.-L.; formal analysis, J.M.A.-L.; investigation, M.d.R.J.-M.; resources, R.M.-L.; data curation, M.G.-R.; writing—original draft preparation, J.M.A.-L.; writing—review and editing, G.M.-R.; visualization, M.d.R.J.-M.; supervision, M.R.-S.; project administration, J.M.A.-L.; funding acquisition, M.R.-S. All authors have read and agreed to the published version of the manuscript.

**Funding:** This research received no external funding.

**Institutional Review Board Statement:** The study was conducted in accordance with the Declaration of Helsinki and was approved by the Cordoba Research Ethics Committee (Act 348, Reference 5610, approved on 15 March 2023).

**Informed Consent Statement:** Informed consent was obtained from all subjects involved in the study. Written informed consent has been obtained from the patient(s) to publish this paper.

**Data Availability Statement:** The data are not publicly available due to privacy or ethical restrictions.

**Conflicts of Interest:** The authors declare no conflicts of interest.

## References

1. Alberti, K.; Zimmet, P.; Shaw, J.E. Metabolic Syndrome—A New World-wide Definition. A Consensus Statement from the International Diabetes Federation. *Diabet. Med.* **2006**, *23*, 469–480. [CrossRef] [PubMed]
2. Mottillo, S.; Filion, K.B.; Genest, J.; Joseph, L.; Pilote, L.; Poirier, P.; Rinfret, S.; Schiffrin, E.L.; Eisenberg, M.J. The Metabolic Syndrome and Cardiovascular Risk: A Systematic Review and Meta-Analysis. *J. Am. Coll. Cardiol.* **2010**, *56*, 1113–1132. [CrossRef] [PubMed]
3. Reaven, G.M. Role of Insulin Resistance in Human Disease. *Diabetes* **1988**, *37*, 1595–1607. [CrossRef] [PubMed]
4. Mozaffarian, D.; Benjamin, E.J.; Go, A.S.; Arnett, D.K.; Blaha, M.J.; Cushman, M.; de Ferranti, S.; Després, J.P.; Fullerton, H.J.; Howard, V.J. Heart Disease and Stroke Statistics—2016 Update: A Report from the American Heart Association. *Circulation* **2016**, *133*, e38–e360. [CrossRef] [PubMed]
5. Popkin, B.M. The Nutrition Transition: An Overview of World Patterns of Change. *Nutr. Rev.* **2004**, *62*, S140–S143. [CrossRef]
6. Organización Panamericana de la Salud (OPS). *Obesity and Overweight in the Americas*; Pan American Health Organization: Washington, DC, USA, 2021.
7. Ministerio de Salud del Perú (MINSA). *Encuesta Demográfica y de Salud Familiar 2021*; Ministerio de Salud del Perú: Lima, Peru, 2021.
8. International Diabetes Federation (IDF). *IDF Diabetes Atlas*, 10th ed.; International Diabetes Federation: Brussels, Belgium, 2021.
9. Chan, J.C.; Malik, V.; Jia, W.; Kadowaki, T.; Yajnik, C.S.; Yoon, K.H.; Hu, F.B. Diabetes in Asia: Epidemiology, Risk Factors, and Pathophysiology. *JAMA* **2009**, *301*, 2129–2140. [CrossRef]
10. Popkin, B.M. The Nutrition Transition and Obesity in the Developing World. *J. Nutr.* **2001**, *131*, 871S–873S. [CrossRef]
11. Lee, C.M.; Huxley, R.; Wildman, R.; Woodward, M. Indices of Abdominal Obesity Are Better Discriminators of Cardiovascular Risk Factors than BMI: A Meta-Analysis. *J. Clin. Epidemiol.* **2008**, *61*, 646–653. [CrossRef]
12. Nyamdorj, R.; Qiao, Q.; Söderberg, S.; Pitkäniemi, J.; Zimmet, P.; Shaw, J.; Alberti, K.G. BMI Compared with Central Obesity Indicators in an Urban Amazonian Context. *Int. J. Obes.* **2021**, *32*, 801–808. [CrossRef]
13. Alberti, K.g.m.m.; Eckel, R.H.; Grundy, S.M.; Zimmet, P.Z.; Cleeman, J.I.; Donato, K.A.; Fruchart, J.-C.; James, W.P.T.; Loria, C.M.; Smith, S.C. Harmonizing the Metabolic Syndrome. *Circulation* **2009**, *120*, 1640–1645. [CrossRef]
14. Misra, A.; Khurana, L. Obesity-Related Non-Communicable Diseases: South Asians vs White Caucasians. *Int. J. Obes.* **2011**, *35*, 167–187. [CrossRef] [PubMed]
15. Chirif, A.C. Biodiversidad Amazónica y Gastronomía Regional. *Folia Amaz.* **2005**, *14*, 91–98. [CrossRef]

16. Browning, L.M.; Hsieh, S.D.; Ashwell, M. A Systematic Review of Waist-to-Height Ratio as a Screening Tool for the Prediction of Cardiovascular Disease and Diabetes: 0·5 Could Be a Suitable Global Boundary Value. *Nutr. Res. Rev.* **2010**, *23*, 247–269. [CrossRef] [PubMed]
17. Huxley, R.; Mendis, S.; Zheleznyakov, E.; Reddy, S.; Chan, J. Body Mass Index, Waist Circumference and Waist–Hip Ratio as Predictors of Cardiovascular Risk—A Review of the Literature. *Eur. J. Clin. Nutr.* **2010**, *64*, 16–22. [CrossRef] [PubMed]
18. Lear, S.A.; Humphries, K.H.; Kohli, S.; Birmingham, C.L. The Use of BMI and Waist Circumference as Surrogates of Body Fat Differs by Ethnicity. *Obesity* **2007**, *15*, 2817–2824. [CrossRef]
19. Misra, A.; Khurana, L. The Metabolic Syndrome in South Asians: Epidemiology, Determinants, and Prevention. *Metab. Syndr. Relat. Disord.* **2009**, *7*, 497–514. [CrossRef]
20. Lear, S.A.; James, P.T.; Ko, G.T.; Kumanyika, S. Appropriateness of Waist Circumference and Waist-to-Hip Ratio Cutoffs for Different Ethnic Groups. *Eur. J. Clin. Nutr.* **2010**, *64*, 42–61. [CrossRef]
21. Popkin, B.M. Global Nutrition Dynamics: The World Is Shifting Rapidly toward a Diet Linked with Noncommunicable Diseases. *Am. J. Clin. Nutr.* **2006**, *84*, 289–298. [CrossRef]
22. Marquez-Sandoval, F.; Macedo-Ojeda, G.; Viramontes-Hörner, D.; Fernández Ballart, J.D.; Salas-Salvadó, J.; Vizmanos, B. The Prevalence of Metabolic Syndrome in Latin America: A Systematic Review. *Public Health Nutr.* **2011**, *14*, 1702–1713. [CrossRef]
23. Popkin, B.M.; Adair, L.S.; Ng, S.W. Global Nutrition Transition and the Pandemic of Obesity in Developing Countries. *Nutr. Rev.* **2012**, *70*, 3–21. [CrossRef]
24. Rodríguez, M.G.; Saldaña, M.R.; Leyva, J.M.A.; Rojas, R.M.; Molina-Recio, G. The FINDRISC Questionnaire Capacity to Predict Diabetes Mellitus II, Arterial Hypertension and Comorbidity in Women from Low-and-Middle-Income Countries. *Health Care Women Int.* **2020**, *41*, 205–226. [CrossRef] [PubMed]
25. Alcaide-Leyva, J.M.; Romero-Saldaña, M.; García-Rodríguez, M.; Molina-Luque, R.; Jiménez-Mérida, R.; Molina-Recio, G. Development of a Predictive Model of Cardiovascular Risk in a Male Population from the Peruvian Amazon. *J. Clin. Med.* **2023**, *12*, 3199. [CrossRef] [PubMed]
26. Simental-Mendía, L.E.; Rodríguez-Morán, M.; Guerrero-Romero, F. A New Lipid Index for Identifying Metabolic Syndrome in the Mexican Population. *Eur. J. Intern. Med.* **2008**, *19*, 442–447. [CrossRef]
27. Guerrero-Romero, F.; Villalobos-Molina, R.; Jiménez-Flores, J.R.; Simental-Mendía, L.E. The TyG Index as a Cardiometabolic Risk Marker in Healthy Young Adults. *Acta Diabetol.* **2016**, *53*, 461–467. [CrossRef]
28. Rubio, M.; Moreno, C.; Cabrerizo, L. Guías Para El Tratamiento de Las Dislipemias En El Adulto: Adult Treatment Panel III (ATP-III). *Endocrinol. Nutr.* **2004**, *51*, 254–265. [CrossRef]
29. Schneider, H.J.; Klotsche, J.; Silber, S.; Stalla, G.; Wittchen, H. Measuring Abdominal Obesity: Effects of Height on Distribution of Cardiometabolic Risk Factors Risk Using Waist Circumference and Waist-to-Height Ratio. *Diabetes Care* **2011**, *34*, e7. [CrossRef]
30. Ashwell, M.; Gunn, P.; Gibson, S. Waist-to-height Ratio Is a Better Screening Tool than Waist Circumference and BMI for Adult Cardiometabolic Risk Factors: Systematic Review and Meta-analysis. *Obes. Rev.* **2012**, *13*, 275–286. [CrossRef]
31. Friedewald, W.T.; Levy, R.I.; Fredrickson, D.S. Estimation of the Concentration of Low-Density Lipoprotein Cholesterol in Plasma, without Use of the Preparative Ultracentrifuge. *Clin. Chem.* **1972**, *18*, 499–502. [CrossRef]
32. Norton, K.I. Standards for Anthropometry Assessment. In *Kinanthropometry and Exercise Physiology*; Routledge: Boca Raton, FL, USA, 2018; pp. 68–137. ISBN 1-315-38566-X.
33. Ladwig, G.B.; Ackley, B.J.; Makic, M.B.F. *Mosby's Guide to Nursing Diagnosis, Revised Reprint with 2021–2023 NANDA-I® Updates-E-Book*; Elsevier Health Sciences: Amsterdam, The Netherlands, 2021; ISBN 0-323-87547-5.
34. Manzini, J.L. Declaración de Helsinki: Principios Éticos Para La Investigación Médica Sobre Sujetos Humanos. *Acta Bioethica* **2000**, *6*, 321–334. [CrossRef]
35. Perú: Ley Nº 26.842 de 1997—Ley General de Salud. Available online: https://www.refworld.org/es/leg/legis/pleg/1997/es/130591 (accessed on 15 January 2025).
36. European Union. *Reglamento (UE) 2016/679 del Parlamento Europeo y del Consejo—De 27 de Abril de 2016—Relativo a la Protección de las Personas Físicas en lo Que Respecta al Tratamiento de Datos Personales y a la Libre Circulación de Estos Datos y Por el Que se Deroga la Directiva 95/46/CE (Reglamento General de Protección de Datos)*; European Union: Brussels, Belgium, 2016.
37. Pajuelo, J.; Sánchez-Abanto, J.; Torres, H.L.; Miranda, M. Prevalencia Del Síndrome Metabólico En Pobladores Peruanos Por Debajo de 1 000 y Por Encima de Los 3 000 Msnm. *An. Fac. Med.* **2012**, *73*, 101–106. [CrossRef]
38. Saklayen, M.G. The Global Epidemic of the Metabolic Syndrome. *Curr. Hypertens. Rep.* **2018**, *20*, 1–8. [CrossRef] [PubMed]
39. França, S.L.; Lima, S.S.; Vieira, J.R.D.S. Metabolic Syndrome and Associated Factors in Adults of the Amazon Region. *PLOS ONE* **2016**, *11*, e0167320. [CrossRef]
40. Bernabé-Ortiz, A.; Carrillo-Larco, R.M.; Gilman, R.H.; Checkley, W.; Smeeth, L.; Miranda, J.J.; CRONICAS Cohort Study Group. Impact of Urbanisation and Altitude on the Incidence of, and Risk Factors for, Hypertension. *Heart* **2017**, *103*, 827–833. [CrossRef] [PubMed]

41. Fornari Laurindo, L.; Minniti, G.; José Tofano, R.; Quesada, K.; Federighi Baisi Chagas, E.; Maria Barbalho, S. Detection of Metabolic Syndrome Using Insulin Resistance Indexes: A Cross-Sectional Observational Cohort Study. *Endocrines* **2023**, *4*, 257–268. [CrossRef]
42. Farinola, M.G.; Sganga, M. Puntos de Corte de Indicadores Antropométricos Para Hipertensión e Hiperglucemia En Adultos Argentinos. *Rev. Fac. Cienc. Médicas Univ. Nac. Córdoba* **2022**, *79*, 260–266. [CrossRef] [PubMed]
43. Xie, E.; Ye, Z.; Wu, Y.; Zhao, X.; Li, Y.; Shen, N.; Gao, Y.; Zheng, J. The Triglyceride-Glucose Index Predicts 1-Year Major Adverse Cardiovascular Events in End-Stage Renal Disease Patients with Coronary Artery Disease. *Cardiovasc. Diabetol.* **2023**, *22*, 292. [CrossRef]
44. Sghaireen, M.G.; Al-Smadi, Y.; Al-Qerem, A.; Srivastava, K.C.; Ganji, K.K.; Alam, M.K.; Khader, Y. Machine Learning Approach for Metabolic Syndrome Diagnosis Using Explainable Data-Augmentation-Based Classification. *Diagnostics* **2022**, *12*, 3117. [CrossRef]
45. Guzmán, A.; Navarro, E.; Obando, L.; Pacheco, J.; Quirós, K.; Vásquez, L.; Ramírez, F. Efectividad de Las Intervenciones Para Revertir El Diagnóstico Del Síndrome Metabólico: Actualización de Un Metaanálisis de Comparación Mixta de Tratamientos. *Biomédica* **2019**, *39*, 647–662. [CrossRef]
46. Houser, D.S.; Champagne, C.D.; Crocker, D.E. A Non-Traditional Model of the Metabolic Syndrome: The Adaptive Significance of Insulin Resistance in Fasting-Adapted Seals. *Front. Endocrinol.* **2013**, *4*, 164. [CrossRef]
47. Cho, Y.; Lee, S.Y. Useful Biomarkers of Metabolic Syndrome. *Int. J. Environ. Res. Public. Health* **2022**, *19*, 15003. [CrossRef]
48. Falahi, E.; Khalkhali, H.R.; Bagherniya, M.; Hashemi, R. Systematic Review of Metabolic Syndrome Biomarkers: A Panel for Early Detection, Management, and Risk Stratification. *Int. J. Endocrinol. Metab.* **2015**, *13*, e22848.
49. Lee, J.H.; Lee, K.H.; Kim, H.J.; Youk, H.; Lee, H.Y. Effective Prevention and Management Tools for Metabolic Syndrome Based on Digital Health-Based Lifestyle Interventions Using Healthcare Devices. *Diagnostics* **2022**, *12*, 1730. [CrossRef] [PubMed]
50. Croci, S.; D'Apolito, L.I.; Gasperi, V.; Catani, M.V.; Savini, I. Dietary Strategies for Management of Metabolic Syndrome: Role of Gut Microbiota Metabolites. *Nutrients* 2021. [CrossRef] [PubMed]

*nutrients*

MDPI

*Article*

# Anti-Fatigue Activity of Corn Protein Hydrolysate Fermented by Lactic Acid Bacteria

**Nan Hu, Jingyi Sun, Yujia Cao, Hongji Zhao, Meng Sun, Guanlong Li, Xiaolan Liu and Shanzi Cong ***

Heilongjiang Provincial Key Laboratory of Corn Deep Processing Theory and Technology, College of Food and Bioengineering, Qiqihar University, Qiqihar 161006, China
* Correspondence: congshanzi0612@126.com

**Abstract:** Objectives: This study aimed to clarify the effect of lactic acid bacteria-fermented corn protein hydrolysate (FCH) on fatigue in mice and explore the connection between fatigue-related indicators and intestinal microbial flora. Methods: The fatigue model of mice was constructed by exercise endurance experiment. The anti-fatigue level of FCH was evaluated by measuring physiological and biochemical indexes in mouse serum, liver and skeletal muscle. The relationship between FCH, intestinal flora and fatigue was explored through the analysis of intestinal microbial diversity in mice, and the anti-fatigue mechanism of FCH was further analyzed. Results: The results showed that the weight-bearing swimming time of mice was prolonged by 1.96 times, and the running time of mice was prolonged by 2.63 times in the high-dose FCH (FCH-H) group. Moreover, the lactic acid contents in the blood were reduced by 16.00%, and lactate dehydrogenase activity and urea nitrogen contents basically returned to the normal level. Meanwhile, the malondialdehyde contents were reduced by 31.24%, and superoxide dismutase activity and glutathione contents were increased by 1.84 times and 1.72 times, respectively. In addition, the glycogen contents of the body were restored, and the muscle glycogen and liver glycogen were increased by 1.81 and 5.81 times, respectively. Analysis of intestinal microbial flora diversity in mice showed that the highest relative abundance was *Lactobacillus*, and the FCH group could recover and even increase its relative abundance. *Lactobacillus* was significantly positively correlated with muscle glycogen and SOD. Conclusions: FCH can alleviate fatigue by regulating fatigue-related indicators and improving the intestinal microbial flora of the organism.

**Keywords:** corn protein hydrolysate; anti-fatigue; fermentation; gut microbiota; lactic acid bacteria

## 1. Introduction

The accelerating pace of modern life results in increased pressure and fatigue has become a common problem. Fatigue is a sub-health state, mainly due to physical or mental labor caused by increased energy consumption of various organs, resulting in a temporary decline in working ability and physical function [1,2]. Individuals who feel tired often manifest reduced exercise ability and work efficiency, and long-term fatigue often increases the incidence of various diseases, such as multiple sclerosis, Parkinson's disease, depression, etc., which seriously affects normal work and life [3,4].

At present, the methods for relieving fatigue mainly include sleep, tobacco, dietary supplements, etc. [5–7]. Dietary supplements can restore normal physical functions by ingesting nutrients needed by the body. According to reports, consuming foods rich in


https://doi.org/10.3390/nu17020199

polysaccharides, proteins, and peptides can effectively alleviate fatigue [8]. Wang et al. reported that the polypeptides extracted from sea cucumbers have good anti-fatigue function [9]. The high doses of sea cucumber peptides can prolong the exhaustive swimming time and forelimb grip strength of mice. Qiao et al. showed that the polysaccharides extracted from *Ribes stenocarpum* Maxim have strong anti-fatigue activity and can significantly increase the liver glycogen and muscle glycogen contents of mice [10]. Lu et al. found that fish protein hydrolysates can prolong the swimming time of mice, reduce the accumulation of lactic acid in the blood, and have a certain anti-fatigue function [11]. The above results clearly show that food supplementation is an effective means to relieve fatigue. Searching for foods that are inexpensive, abundant, contain anti-fatigue functional ingredients, and capable of being processed for enhancing contents of functional ingredients will become the main development direction of functional foods in the future.

Corn gluten meal is a byproduct of corn starch processing, with a protein content of over 60% and high hydrophobicity. It is commonly used as a raw material for animal feed. Corn gluten meal is limited in its application in food due to its lack of essential lysine and tryptophan for the human body [12]. By modifying corn gluten meal, not only can the amino acid composition of corn gluten meal be reshaped, but its physiological functions can also be improved, such as antioxidant activity, blood pressure-lowering effects, liver protection, and promotion of alcohol metabolism [13,14]. However, the modified corn gluten meal (corn protein hydrolysate, CPH) has a higher content of bitter peptides, resulting in a poorer flavor of the CPH [15]. Reprocessing CPH through fermentation can effectively improve its unpleasant flavor and further reduce its molecular weight, endowing it with stronger functionality and antioxidant properties [16]. Cui et al. used *Bacillus*, *Lactobacillus*, and *Hansenula* strains to co-ferment soybeans and studied the nutritional properties and anti-fatigue ability of the products and found that the contents of polypeptides, total phenols, and total flavonoids were significantly increased after fermentation, and its antioxidant activity was enhanced [17]. Moreover, fermented soybean products could increase the contents of liver glycogen in mice, alleviate the liver damage caused by exercise, and show a good anti-fatigue function [18]. Fang et al. studied the effects of soy protein hydrolysate fermented by *Lactobacillus acidophilus* on the anti-fatigue of mice and showed that the weight-bearing swimming time of the experimental group was significantly increased, indicating that the fermented soy protein hydrolysate had an anti-fatigue function [19]. Zhang et al. used lactic acid bacteria to ferment wheat protein hydrolysate and showed that it could increase the contents of liver glycogen and muscle glycogen in mice, prolong the exhaustive swimming time, and had an anti-fatigue ability [20]. These results show that plant-derived polypeptides have a good effect on relieving fatigue. In addition, lactic acid bacteria fermentation is also a good modification method for plant-derived polypeptides. At present, there are few reports on the potential anti-fatigue properties of FCH.

Numerous studies have shown that peptides have a certain positive impact on the body's anti-fatigue function. This study evaluated the anti-fatigue effect of FCH in mice. The anti-fatigue level of FCH was evaluated by measuring physiological and biochemical indexes in mouse serum, liver, and skeletal muscle. Finally, the relationship between FCH, intestinal flora, and fatigue was explored through the analysis of intestinal microbial diversity in mice, and the anti-fatigue mechanism of FCH was further analyzed. The objective of the current work is to provide a theoretical basis for the functional study of FCH.

## 2. Materials and Methods

### 2.1. Subsection

The preparation method of FCH was according to Cong et al. [21].

CPHs were prepared by enzymatic hydrolysis of corn protein meal by a two-enzyme method. The CPH was dissolved in deionized water (substrate concentration 20%, *w*/*v*) and sterilized (121 °C, 30 min). The fermentation conditions of FCH were as follows: the 3:1 ratio of Lactobacillus rhamnosus and Lactobacillus fermentosa for inoculation (4% with the viable count of lactic acid bacteria of about $10^6$ CFU/mL, *v*/*v*), CPH concentration of 20.50%, the addition of 5% fructose syrup (*v*/*v*), and the fermentation at 39 °C for 24 h.

### 2.2. Experimental Animal Design

Ninety-six healthy male ICRs (18–22 g, 4-week-old, Institute of Cancer Research) were purchased from Changchun Yisi Experimental Animal Research Center (Changchun, China) (permit number: SCXK (yue) 2023-0017). The animal experiment was approved on 21 March 2023 by the Animal Ethics Committee of the College of Food and Bioengineering, Qiqihar University (Approval No. 2023-005). The conditions of temperature and humidity were 25 ± 1 °C and 55 ± 5%, respectively. The mice were fed with free access to water and food.

The mice were randomly divided into 6 groups according to their body weight, with 16 mice per group. After adapting to the environment for one week, the mice swimming screening experiment was carried out, and the mice that could not swim or had uncoordinated swimming postures were excluded. Ten mice were selected in each group for the follow-up experiment. The 6 groups were the blank control group (BCG, normal saline), fatigue model group (FMG, normal saline), positive control group (CPH-M, 250 mg/kg·bw of CPH), low-dose group (FCH-L, 125 mg/kg·bw of FCH), medium-dose group (FCH-M, 250 mg/kg·bw of FCH), and high-dose group (FCH-H, 500 mg/kg·bw of FCH), of which the FMG group did not participate in the determination of exercise endurance. The experiment lasted 28 days, and the initial weight of the mice was recorded. Weight was weighed once a day before feeding. After intragastric administration and resting for 30 min, swimming training was performed. The first week of swimming training was 20 min, and after that, it was increased by 5 min per week.

### 2.3. Determination of Weight-Bearing Swimming Time and Running Time

After 30 min of intragastric administration on the 26th day, the tails of the mice were wound with a lead block (10% of body weight). Then, the mice were forced to swim in a water pool (25 ± 1 cm, 25 ± 1 °C). Weight-bearing swimming time was recorded when the head of the mice under the water was more than 8 s.

After 30 min of intragastric administration on the 27th day, the mice in each experimental group were placed on the rotating rod in turn, and the rotating speed was slowly adjusted to 15 r/min. The first three times were pre-experiments, and the timing starts from the fourth time. Running time was recorded when the mice fell from the rod due to muscle fatigue. If the mice did not fall from the rotating rod within 30 min, the running time was recorded as 30 min.

### 2.4. Determination of Anti-Fatigue Relevant Physiological and Biochemical Indexes in Mice

After 30 min of the last intragastric administration, the mice (excluding the BCG group) without load were forced to swim in a water pool (30 ± 1 °C) for 30 min. Then, the mice were removed and wiped dry. After resting for 20 min, blood samples were collected from the orbital sinuses of mice, and skeletal muscles and internal organs such as liver were obtained by autopsy. The organ index was calculated according to the following formula.

$$\text{Organ index (\%)} = \text{organ mass (g)}/\text{mouse body weight (g)} \times 100\%$$

The blood samples were placed at 4 °C overnight, centrifuged at 3000× g for 10 min, and the supernatant was serum. The liver and skeletal muscle were prepared into 10% liver homogenate and skeletal muscle homogenate with pre-cooled normal saline, centrifuged at 3000× g for 10 min. The concentrations of serum urea nitrogen (BUN), serum lactate (LA), serum lactate dehydrogenase (LDH), liver superoxide dismutase (SOD), liver glutathione (GSH), liver malondialdehyde (MDA), liver glycogen (LG), and muscle glycogen (MG) were determined using an assay kit (Jianglai Biotechnology Co., Ltd., Shanghai, China).

*2.5. Detection of Intestinal Microbial Flora in Mice*

The cecum samples were collected, 2 g per mice. The cecum samples were frozen in liquid nitrogen and then sent to Meiji Biomedical Technology Co., Ltd. (Shanghai, China). To determine the microbial diversity of mice cecum bacteria contents, the sample DNA was extracted using the TruSeqTM DNA Sample Prep Kit. After confirming purity, the V3–V4 region of the 16 S rDNA gene was amplified from DNA samples using the primer pair 338 F/806 R (338 F: 5′-ACTCCTACGGGAGGCAGCAG-3′, 806 R: 5′-GGACTACHVGGGTWTCTAAT-3′). The Illumina MiSeq platform was selected for sequencing, and the analysis method was the same as Hu et al. [22].

*2.6. Data Analysis*

The above tests were repeated at least three times, and the test results were expressed as mean ± standard deviation. Origin 2022 software was used to analyze the data and draw charts. SPSS Statistics 20.0 (IBM, Armonk, NY, USA) was used for significance analysis. The heatmap was visualized by TBtools V 2.01 (2023). Principal coordinates analysis (PCoA), statistical analysis, and mapping were performed with R language (version 3.3.1). Statistical analysis of different groups was performed using one-way analysis of variance (ANOVA) and Dunnett's multiple comparison tests. Statistical significance was set at * $p < 0.05$ or ** $p < 0.01$.

## 3. Results

*3.1. Effects of FCH on the Body Weight Change and Organ Index*

Body weight change and organ index can reflect whether the administration of CPH and FCH has an impact on the health of mice. The weight of the six experimental groups of mice showed a steady upward trend during the test schedule (Figure 1A). During the 4 weeks of the experiment, the weight of the mice in each group increased by an average of 11.58 g. At the end of the experiment, the weight of the mice in each group reached 40.42–42.81 g. There were no significant differences between the experimental groups and the BCG group ($p > 0.05$), and the trend of weight gain was consistent. There were no significant differences between the spleen, kidney, and liver indexes of the mice in each group ($p > 0.05$) (Figure 1B). In the thymus index, the FCH-H group was significantly higher than the CPH-M group and the FCH-M group ($p < 0.05$), and no significant differences with other groups ($p > 0.05$) were observed. In the heart index, the FCH-M group was significantly higher than the FMG group ($p < 0.05$), and no significant differences with other groups ($p > 0.05$) were observed. In addition, no significant abnormalities and death were observed in the mice during the experiment. The above results show that each dose group of the FCH and the CPH had no apparent effect on the health of the mice.

*3.2. Effect of FCH on Exercise Endurance*

The test of weight-bearing swimming and running time in mice is one of the main indicators to study the anti-fatigue effect (Figure 2A). With increased FCH dose, the weight-bearing swimming time and running time of mice showed a steady upward trend. In the mouse weight-bearing swimming test, the final weight-bearing swimming time of the BCG group could reach 46.36 s after swimming training within the test schedule. The CPH-M group, the FCH-L group, and the FCH-M group showed no significant differences from the BCG group ($p > 0.05$). With further increase in the concentration of FCH, the weight-bearing swimming time of mice in the FCH-H group was significantly improved ($p < 0.05$), reaching 1.96 times that of the BCG group. The same results were obtained in the mouse rotarod test. The running time for the BCG group was 4.78 min. Compared with the BCG group, the running times for the CPH-M group, the FCH-L group, and the FCH-M group were slightly improved, but there were no significant differences ($p > 0.05$). The FCH-H group showed improved running time, reaching 3.63 times that of the BCG group ($p < 0.05$). It is concluded that FCH can effectively improve the weight-bearing swimming and running time of mice within a certain concentration range.

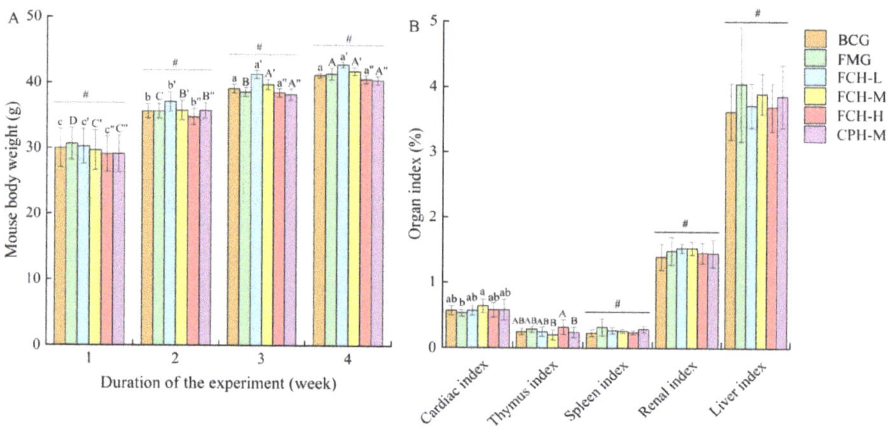


**Figure 1.** The effect of FCH on mice body weight and organ index. (**A**) The effect of FCH intervention on the body weight of mice. (**B**) The effect of FCH intervention on the organ index of mice. Data are shown as the mean ± SD ($n = 6$). Different large and lowercase letters in the figure indicate the significant difference between the groups ($p < 0.05$), and # indicates that there is no significant difference within the group ($p > 0.05$). BCG: blank control group; FMG: fatigue model group; CPH-M: medium dose group of CPH; FCH-L: low-dose group of FCH; FCH-M: medium-dose group of FCH; FCH-H: high-dose group of FCH.

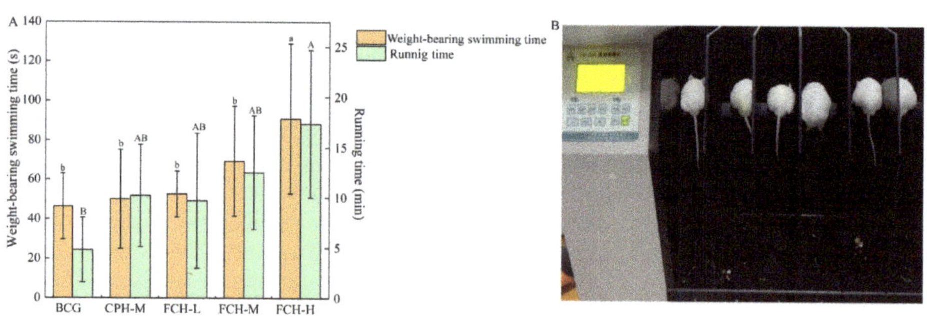


**Figure 2.** The effect of FCH on weight-bearing swimming and running time. (**A**) Mouse weight-bearing swimming and running time. (**B**) Mouse rotarod test process. Data are shown as the mean ± SD ($n = 6$). Different large and lowercase letters in the figure indicate significant differences between groups ($p < 0.05$). BCG: blank control group; CPH-M: medium-dose group of CPH; FCH-L: low-dose group of FCH; FCH-M: medium-dose group of FCH; FCH-H: high-dose group of FCH.

### 3.3. Effects of FCH on Anti-Fatigue Relevant Physiological and Biochemical Indexes in Mice

#### 3.3.1. Effect of FCH on Serum BUN, LA, and LDH Levels

The contents of BUN, LA, and LDH in mice are shown in Figure 3. The BUN contents of the BCG group were 4.46 ± 1.09 mmol/L, and the FMG group was 1.98 times that of the BCG group ($p < 0.05$). The BUN contents of the CPH-M group and the FCH groups were between the BCG group and the FMG group, at the level of 5.39–6.09 mmol/L. There was no significant difference between the other groups and the BCG group except for the FCH-L group ($p < 0.05$). The LA contents showed a similar trend to the BUN contents. The LA content of the FMG group was 8.06 ± 0.35 mmol/L, and the BCG group was 72.21% of the FMG group ($p < 0.05$). Compared with the FMG group, with increased FCH concentration, the LA content decreased significantly ($p < 0.05$). The LA content of the FCH-H group was 6.77 ± 0.13 mmol/L, which was 84.00% of the FMG group. The LA content of the CPH-M group was similar to the FCH-M group ($p > 0.05$). The LDH activity of the FMG group was 22.83 ± 3.34 ng/mL, and the BCG group was 61.54% of the FMG group ($p < 0.05$). With increased FCH concentrations, the LDH activities of FCH groups decreased significantly ($p < 0.05$), which were 81.52%, 71.66%, and 63.60%, respectively. The LDH activity of the FCH-H group was close to the BCG group ($p > 0.05$), and the CPH-M and FCH-M groups was similar ($p > 0.05$). Thus, FCH and CPH can effectively reduce the levels of BUN, LA, and LDH in the mice within a certain concentration range.

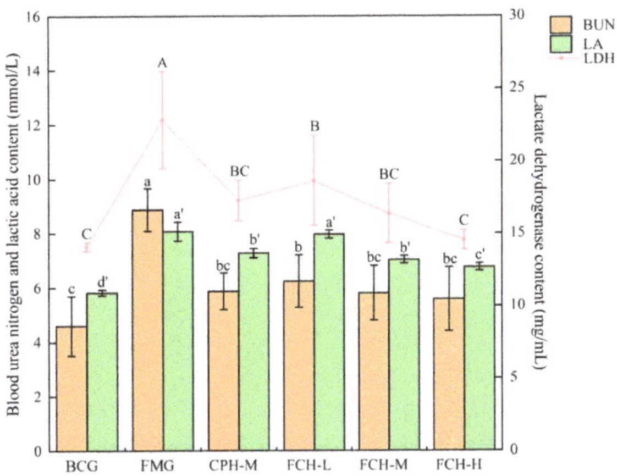


**Figure 3.** The effect of FCH on BUN, LA, and LDH. Data are shown as the mean ± SD ($n = 6$). Different large and lowercase letters in the figure indicate significant differences between groups ($p < 0.05$). BUN: urea nitrogen; LA: lactate; LDH: lactic dehydrogenase; BCG: blank control group; FMG: fatigue model group; CPH-M: medium dose group of CPH; FCH-L: low-dose group of FCH; FCH-M: medium-dose group of FCH; FCH-H: high-dose group of FCH.

#### 3.3.2. Effects of FCH on MG and LG

The contents of MG and LG in mice were shown in Figure 4. The MG content of the FMG group was 0.117 ± 0.002 mg/g, the BCG group was 1.29 times that of the FMG group ($p < 0.05$), and the MG content for the CPH-M group was between the FMG group and the BCG group ($p < 0.05$). With increased FCH concentrations, the MG contents of the FCH groups increased significantly, which were 1.36 times, 1.68 times, and 1.81 times that of the FMG group, respectively ($p < 0.05$). The LG content of the FMG group was 0.32 ± 0.005 mg/g, and the BCG group was 2.88 times that of the FMG group ($p < 0.05$). With increased FCH concentrations, the LG content of the FCH groups increased significantly, which was 2.03 times, 3.72 times, and 6.81 times that of the FMG group, respectively

($p < 0.05$). The LG contents of the CPH-M group was between the FMG group and the FMG-M group ($p < 0.05$). It is concluded that FCH and CPH can effectively increase the contents of MG and LG in mice within a certain concentration range, and the effect of FCH was significantly better than that of CPH.

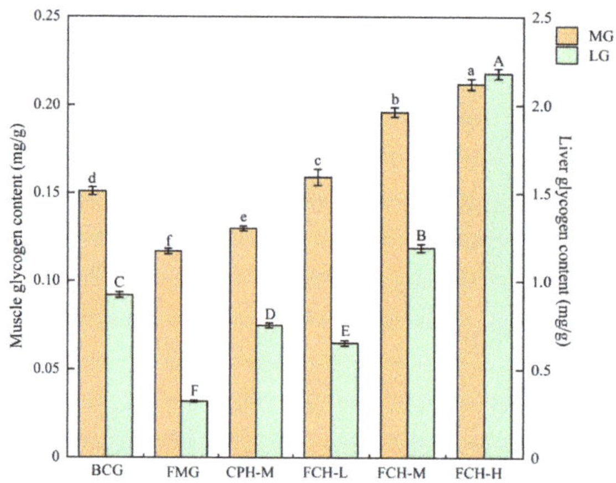


**Figure 4.** The effect of FCH on MG and LG. Data are shown as the mean ± SD ($n$ = 6). Different large and lowercase letters in the figure indicate significant differences between groups ($p < 0.05$). MG: muscle glycogen; LG: liver glycogen; BCG: blank control group; FMG: fatigue model group; CPH-M: medium dose group of CPH; FCH-L: low-dose group of FCH; FCH-M: medium-dose group of FCH; FCH-H: high-dose group of FCH.

### 3.3.3. Effects of FCH on Liver SOD, MDA, and GSH

The SOD activity and GSH contents of mice were shown in Figure 5A. The SOD activity test revealed that the SOD activity of the FMG group was 192.02 ± 15.6 U/mL, and the BCG group was 1.38 times that of the FMG group ($p < 0.05$). With increased FCH concentrations, the SOD activities of FCH groups were significantly increased, which were 1.55 times, 1.60 times, and 1.84 times that of the FMG group, respectively ($p < 0.05$). The GSH content of the FMG group was 3.05 ± 0.16 mg/mL, and the BCG group was 1.82 times that of the FMG group ($p < 0.05$). Compared with the FMG group, the GSH content of the FCH-M group and the FCH-H group was increased by 1.63 times and 1.72 times, respectively ($p < 0.05$), and the FCH-H group was close to the BCG group ($p > 0.05$). The GSH content of the CPH-M group was at the intermediate level of the FCH-L group and the FCH-M group ($p < 0.05$).

The MDA content of mice was shown in Figure 5B. The MDA content of FMG group was 27.18 ± 0.9 mmol/mL, and the BCG group was 64.61% of the FMG group ($p < 0.05$). Compared with the FMG group, MDA contents of the FCH-M group and FCH-H group were significantly reduced, being 78.66% and 68.76% of the FMG group, respectively ($p < 0.05$), and the FCH-H group was similar to the BCG group ($p > 0.05$). These results indicate that FCH and CPH could effectively increase SOD activity, as well as the MDA and GSH contents of mice within a certain concentration range, and the effect of FCH on GSH contents was better than CPH.

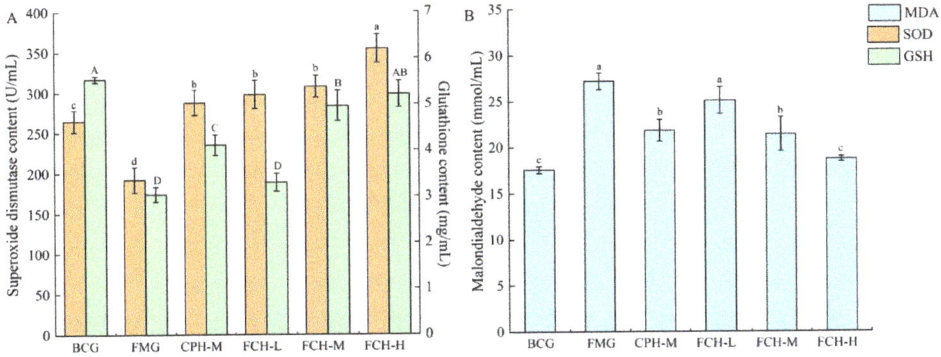


**Figure 5.** The effects of FCH on SOD, GSH, and MDA. (**A**) SOD and GSH contents in mouse liver. (**B**) MDA content in mouse liver. Data are shown as the mean ± SD ($n$ = 6). Different large and lowercase letters in the figure indicate significant differences between groups ($p < 0.05$). MDA: Malondialdehyde; SOD: Superoxide dismutase; GSH: Glutathione; BCG: blank control group; FMG: fatigue model group; CPH-M: medium dose group of CPH; FCH-L: low-dose group of FCH; FCH-M: medium-dose group of FCH; FCH-H: high-dose group of FCH.

### 3.4. *Effects of FCH on Intestinal Microbial Flora*

#### 3.4.1. Bacterial Alpha Diversity Analysis of Intestinal Microbial Flora in Mice

The Shannon index and Simpson index were used to compare the species diversity of mice intestinal bacteria (Figure 6A). The Shannon index and Simpson index of the 6 groups ranged from 4.18 to 4.72 and 0.025 to 0.054, respectively, and there was no significant difference ($p > 0.05$). The ACE index and Chao 1 index were used to evaluate the species richness (Figure 6B). The ACE index of the 6 groups ranged from 653.26 to 740 and for the Chao 1 index ranged from 654.62 to 732, with no significant difference ($p > 0.05$). It can be concluded that FCH and CPH had no significant effect on changes in the bacterial diversity and abundance of mice intestinal microbial flora.

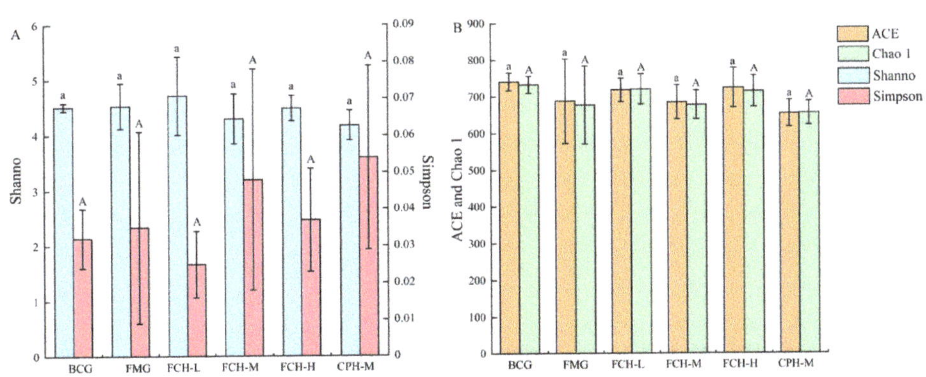


**Figure 6.** Alpha diversity index of mice intestinal microbial flora. (**A**) Shannon and Simpson index; (**B**) ACE and Chao 1 index. Data are shown as the mean ± SD ($n$ = 6). Different large and lowercase letters in the figure indicate significant differences between groups ($p < 0.05$). BCG: blank control group; FMG: fatigue model group; CPH-M: medium dose group of CPH; FCH-L: low-dose group of FCH; FCH-M: medium-dose group of FCH; FCH-H: high-dose group of FCH.

#### 3.4.2. Bacterial Beta Diversity Analysis of Intestinal Microbial Flora

The β-diversity (intergroup diversity) of intestinal microbial flora in mice was analyzed by the PCoA method. The distance between the sample points represented the similarity of the microbial communities in the samples, and the closer the distance, the higher the similarity (Figure 7). Under the influence of PC1 and PC2, the six groups formed completely different taxonomic clusters. It is evident that exercise fatigue, FCH, and CPH had a greater impact on the structure of the intestinal microbial flora in mice. There was a certain intersection between the BCG group and the FMG group in Figure 7, indicating that there were certain individual differences in the microbial diversity of the intestinal microbial flora in mice. However, FCH groups had basically no intersection with the FMG group, and the FCH-L and FCH-M groups are more tended to than the BCG group. The FCH-H group had no intersection with the BCG group and the FMG group, but it was more tended to than the BCG group. The results showed that a certain concentration of FCH could effectively regulate the intestinal microbiota of mice to achieve a normal state. The intersection between the CPH group and the FMG group was very small, indicating that a certain concentration of CPH can also improve the poor state of intestinal microbiota caused by fatigue.

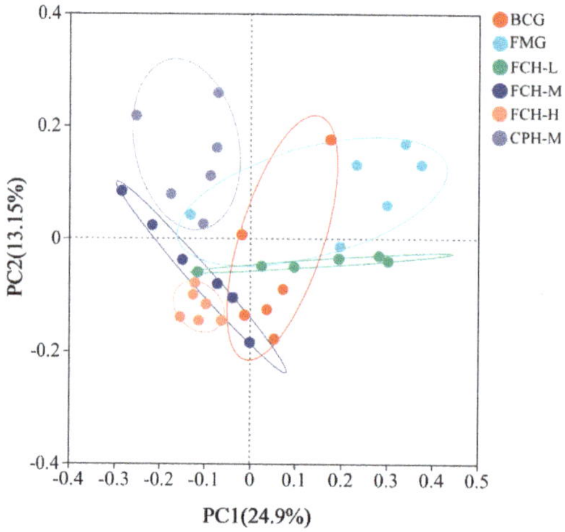


**Figure 7.** Beta diversity index of intestinal microbial flora. BCG: blank control group; FMG: fatigue model group; CPH-M: medium dose group of CPH; FCH-L: low-dose group of FCH; FCH-M: medium-dose group of FCH; FCH-H: high-dose group of FCH.

### 3.4.3. Classification and Analysis of Intestinal Microbial Flora

Figure 8 shows the phylum- and genus-level bacterial community structure of the intestinal microbial flora in mice.

The relative abundance of Firmicutes was 62.49%, ranking first in phylum-level relative abundance (Figure 8A). The relative abundance of Firmicutes in the BCG group and the FMG group was 62.49% and 45.70%, respectively. The relative abundances of Firmicutes in the CPH-M group and the FCH groups were 64.82%, 63.58%, 66.31%, and 69.63%, respectively, which were higher than the BCG group and the FMG group. The relative abundance of Bacteroides was 40.11%, ranking second. The relative abundance of Bacteroides in the BCG group was 27.62% and in the FMG group was 40.11%. The relative abundance of Bacteroidetes in the CPH-M group and the FCH groups were 21.60%, 31.18%, 21.47%, and 17.75%, respectively, which were lower than the FMG group and closer to the BCG group. The third-highest relative abundance belonged to Actinomycetes, with a relative abundance of 9.06%. The relative abundance of Actinomycetes in the BCG group was 2.16%, while for the FMG group it was 9.06%. The relative abundances of Actinomycetes in the CPH-M group and the FCH groups were 8.90%, 2.60%, 5.55% and 5.57%, respectively, in between the FMG group and the BCG group. The relative abundance of the rest of the bacterial population was less than 5%, and the relative effect was small.

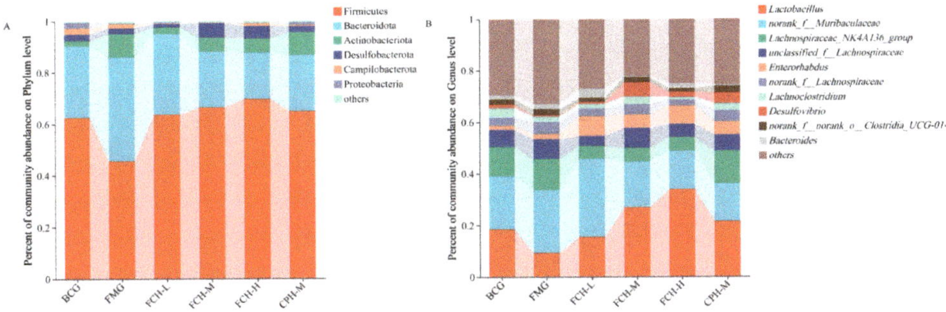


**Figure 8.** The phylum- (**A**) and genus- (**B**) level bacterial community structure of the intestinal microbial flora. BCG: blank control group; FMG: fatigue model group; CPH-M: medium dose group of CPH; FCH-L: low-dose group of FCH; FCH-M: medium-dose group of FCH; FCH-H: high-dose group of FCH.

The relative abundance of *Lactobacillus* was the highest in genus-level relative abundance (Figure 8B). The BCG group was 18.41% and the FMG group was only 9.19%. The CPH-M group and the FCH groups were 21.42%, 15.42%, 26.77%, and 33.78%, respectively, which were higher than the BCG group and the FMG group. The second highest relative abundance was *Muribaculaceae*, and the relative abundance of the BCG group and the FMG group was similar, with 20.32% and 24.18%, respectively. The CPH-M group and the FCH groups were 14.43%, 30.12%, 17.57%, and 14.88%, respectively. The third-highest relative abundance belonged to the *Lachnospiraceae_NK4A136_group*, and the BCG and FMG groups was still similar, with 11.60% and 12.31%, respectively. The CPH-M group was 12.94%, which was close to the BCG group and the FMG group. The FCH groups were lower than the BCG group and the FMG group, with 5.13%, 5.60%, and 5.38%, respectively. The relative abundance of *unclassified_f_Lachnospiraceae* in the BCG group and the FMG group was similar, being 6.66% and 7.58%, respectively. The CPH-M group, the FCH-M group, and the FCH-H group were closer to the BCG group and the FMG group, with 6.20%, 7.65%, and 5.10%, respectively. The FCH-L group was 3.83%, which was slightly lower than other groups. The relative abundance of the remaining bacteria was less than 5%.

#### 3.4.4. Correlation Analysis Between Intestinal Microbial Flora and Fatigue-Related Biochemical Indexes

The change in intestinal microbial flora in mice may be related to fatigue status. By analyzing the relationship between intestinal microbial flora and fatigue indexes in mice, the correlation between intestinal microbial flora and fatigue in mice was revealed (Figure 9). *Lactobacillus* was significantly positively correlated with MG and SOD, *Desulfovibrio* was significantly positively correlated with SOD ($p < 0.05$), and *Desulfovibrio* was highly significant positive correlated with MG ($p < 0.01$). However, *Muribaculaceae* was significantly negatively correlated with SOD ($p < 0.05$) and highly significantly negatively correlated with MG content ($p < 0.01$).

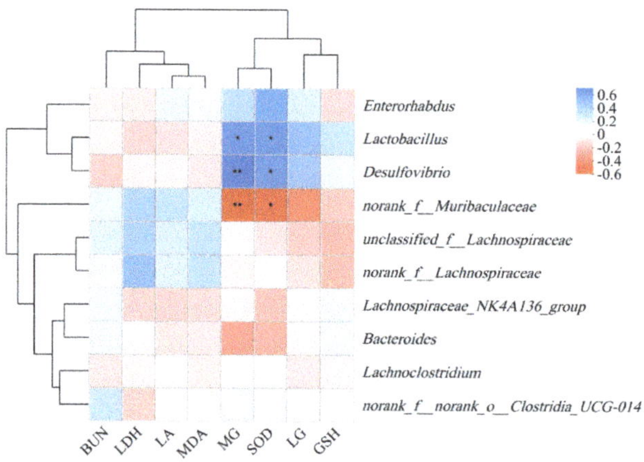


**Figure 9.** Correlation clustering heat map between intestinal microbial flora and fatigue indexes. * Indicates significant difference ($p < 0.05$), ** Indicates extremely significant difference ($p < 0.01$). BUN: urea nitrogen; LDH: lactate dehydrogenase; LA: lactate; MDA: malondialdehyde; MG: muscle glycogen; SOD: superoxide dismutase; LG: liver glycogen; GSH: glutathione.

## 4. Discussion

The purpose of this study was to explore the anti-fatigue effect of FCH. The reduction in exercise endurance is the most intuitive manifestation of organism fatigue [23]. This study first tested the ability of mice to weight-bearing swimming and running. From the perspective of exercise performance, feeding FCH and CPH could significantly prolong the time of weight-bearing swimming and running of mice. Among them, the FCH-H group was extended by 44.58 s and 12.57 min, respectively. FCH and CPH were shown to have apparent anti-fatigue effects at a certain concentration. Fang et al. reported that mice fed with fermented soybean protein peptides showed an increase of 35.78% for the weight-bearing swimming time [19]. Zhang et al. reported the doubling of the running time of mice after 4 weeks of administration of the peptide isolated from *Hippocampus abdominalis* [24]. The above results are consistent with the findings of this study, showing that the peptides can relieve exercise fatigue within a certain concentration, and the effect of lower molecular weight peptides is more obvious. Compared with CPH, FCH contains large number of functional short peptides with lower molecular weight, which can participate in regulating sugar metabolism, reducing protein consumption in muscles, thereby reducing urea production and achieving an anti-fatigue effect [25,26].

When the organism does not acquire energy replenishment in time after intense exercise, proteins will decompose to form blood urea nitrogen, while it will also accelerate the glycolysis process to produce a large amount of LA, which increases the concentration of LA or H+ in the muscles and causes muscle fatigue [27,28]. This study found that feeding a certain concentration of FCH by gavage can reduce the levels of BUN and LA in mice, indicating that long-term intake of a certain concentration of FCH can effectively relieve organism fatigue. Wang et al. reported that gavage mice with mackerel peptides for 4 weeks reduced the levels of BUN and LA by 0.88 mmol/L and 180.86 ug/L, respectively [29]. Yin et al. showed that gavage mice with the Young Yum Pill for 3 weeks, the BUN and LA contents were reduced by 29% and 50%, respectively [30]. Compared with mackerel peptides and the Young Yum Pill, FCH can increase the glycogen reserve of mice and reduce the catabolism of proteins in mice, thereby achieving a better anti-fatigue effect [31]. The two forms of glycogen reserve in the organism are LG and MG, and the storage of energy determines the tolerance of exercise. When the organism has insufficient blood sugar during intense exercise, it needs to consume reserve glycogen to maintain blood sugar levels to meet the needs of the organism [32]. FCH can significantly increase the organism's glycogen reserves. The contents of MG and LG in the FCH groups were significantly higher than the FMG group, and significantly higher than the BCG group at a certain concentration. Meanwhile, the increase in LG contents in mice was higher than that in the MG contents. This may be due to the fact that the organism preferentially consumes MG under the condition of stable blood sugar [33]. Therefore, the accumulation of LG in mice was higher than that of MG, similar to the results of Feng et al. and Lu et al. [33,34].

Strenuous exercise or muscle injury can cause LDH in skeletal muscle to penetrate into the blood, and LDH can catalyze the conversion of pyruvate to LA, reducing exercise tolerance [10]. This study showed that the FCH groups and the CPH group can significantly reduce the LDH activity in the blood, of which the FCH-H group has approached the level of the BCG group. Chen et al. showed that mice fed with spirulina peptides for 4 weeks had a 53.5% decrease in LDH activities [35]. Liu et al. reported that mice fed with peanut oligopeptides for 30 days had a 50% decrease in LDH activities [36]. By contrast, FCH can reduce the level of LDH in the blood more effectively. This may be related to the higher contents of branched-chain amino acids and phenylalanine in FCH [37]. It has been reported that branched-chain amino acids in CPH can promote the synthesis of skeletal muscle protein, repair skeletal muscle damage, and reduce LDH exudation, while hydrophobic amino acid residues such as Ala and Leu contained in CPH have the effect of scavenging free radicals and preventing lipid oxidation [38]. After strenuous exercise, the organism produces large number of free radicals, triggers lipid peroxidation, increases MDA contents, changes the permeability of cell membranes and, thus, leading to fatigue. In this study, FCH can effectively reduce MDA contents, and there is no significant difference between the FCH-H group and the BCG group. Zhong et al. showed that mice fed with soft-shelled turtle peptides for 30 days resulted in a 40.4% decrease in MDA contents [39]. Ye et al. reported that mice fed with sea cucumber peptides for 4 weeks had a 50% reduction in MDA [40]. The effect of FCH on MDA content reduction is better than that of soft-shelled turtle peptides and sea cucumber peptides. This may be due to the stronger antioxidant activity of CPH contributed by lactic acid bacteria fermentation, which accelerates the scavenging of superoxide free radicals in the organism, antagonizes the reactive oxygen clusters continuously generated by skeletal muscles during strong contraction, and reduces the loss of superoxide dismutase or due to the increase in SOD enzyme activity and GSH contents, resulting in the increase in the organism's antioxidant activity and reducing the free radicals produced by strenuous exercise [41–45]. The results reported in this study are consistent with the previous findings cited above.

The intestinal microbial flora of mice was further measured to explore the relationship between FCH and fatigue in mice. Although there was no significant difference in the alpha diversity of the six groups ($p > 0.05$). However, the beta diversity showed that FCH and CPH could effectively regulate the intestinal microbiota of mice to keep in a normal state (Figure 7). Among the intestinal microbial flora of mice, the relative abundances of Firmicutes (45.70–69.63%) and Bacteroides (17.75–40.11%) were the highest. The abundance of Firmicutes in the FMG group was lower than the BCG group, and the abundance of Bacteroides was higher than the BCG group. By feeding a certain concentration of FCH, the relative abundance of Firmicutes in the intestinal tract of mice increased significantly, and the relative abundance of Bacteroidetes gradually decreased. Firmicutes mainly include a variety of beneficial bacteria, while Bacteroidetes are closely related to metabolic diseases in the organism [46]. In this study, the ratio of Firmicutes to Bacteroidetes in the FCH-H group was closer to the BCG group. It is concluded that FCH can achieve the purpose of anti-fatigue by regulating the homeostasis of the level of intestinal flora in mice. At the genus level, the relative abundance of *Lactobacillus* (9.19–33.78%) was the highest. The abundance of *Lactobacillus* in the BCG group was significantly higher than the FMG group. By feeding FCH, the relative abundance of *Lactobacillus* in the intestines of mice was significantly increased, the FCH groups were higher than the FMG group. Fang et al. also obtained similar results in the fatigue intervention experiment of fermented soy protein peptide in mice. Fermented products of *Lactobacillus* can improve the intestinal flora, increase the abundance of probiotics in the intestines of tired mice, and, thus, affect system metabolism by changing the host metabolome, so as to improve the organism's metabolic capacity and anti-fatigue ability [17,19,47,48]. The increase in *Lactobacillus* contents in the intestines can significantly increase the contents of short fatty acids, activate peroxisome proliferators and receptor gamma coactivator 1$\alpha$ (PGC-1$\alpha$), increase the production of ATP, provide energy for exercise, and improve exercise endurance performance [48]. In the correlation analysis, it was also found that *Lactobacillus* was significantly positively correlated with MG. It has been reported that *Lactobacillus* can affect the composition of intestinal microorganisms, regulate the genes related to glycogen synthesis in tissues (GSK-3$\beta$ and Akt), and, thereby, affect the glycogen contents of the organism [49].

In conclusion, long-term intake of a certain concentration of FCH can effectively relieve organism fatigue. FCH can play an anti-fatigue effect by regulating the intestinal microbial flora of mice, and the anti-fatigue effect of FCH is better than that of CPH.

## 5. Conclusions

Long-term ingestion of a certain amount of peptide can effectively relieve fatigue caused by exercise. However, due to the different molecular weights of various peptides, there are also obvious differences in the effects on fatigue. This study aimed to reveal the effect of FCH on organism fatigue and explore the relationship between intestinal microorganisms and fatigue-related indicators. From the perspective of the exercise state of mice, ingesting FCH for 4 weeks could effectively improve the exercise endurance of mice as confirmed in the weight-bearing swimming and rotarod test of mice. In the determination of biochemical indicators, it was found that FCH could effectively reduce the contents of LA and LDH in the blood and restore the content of BUN to normal levels. Moreover, the activities of SOD and GSH were increased to varying degrees, and the contents of MDA were reduced significantly, while the glycogen reserve of the organism was restored. MG and LG were increased to varying degrees, and most experimental groups had exceeded the level of the BCG group. The results showed that both FCH and CPH had certain anti-fatigue effects. For the same dose, the effect of FCH was better than CPH. In the analysis of intestinal microorganisms in mice, *Lactobacillus* was the most abundant relative bacteria, followed by *norank_f_Muribaculaceae*. Different concentrations of FCH could restore or even increase the relative abundance of *Lactobacillus* and reduce the abundance of *norank_f_Muribaculaceae*. In the association analysis, *Lactobacillus* was significantly positively correlated with MG and SOD, while *norank_f_Muribaculaceae* was significantly negatively correlated with SOD and was significantly negatively correlated with MG. Fatigue of the organism may be related to the ratio of *Lactobacillus* and *norank_f_Muribaculaceae*, but the specific mechanism involved needs to be revealed by further experiments.

**Author Contributions:** N.H. performed the experiments and wrote the main manuscript text; S.C. and X.L. provided the idea and wrote the main manuscript text; J.S., Y.C. H.Z., M.S. and G.L. performed the experiments and processed the data. All authors have read and agreed to the published version of the manuscript.

**Funding:** This work was supported by grants from the Heilongjiang Provincial Foundation for the Characteristic Discipline of Processing Technology of Plant Foods (No. YSTSXK202406).

**Institutional Review Board Statement:** The animal experiment was approved on 21 March 2023 by the Animal Ethics Committee of the College of Food and Bioengineering, Qiqihar University (Approval No. 2023-005).

**Informed Consent Statement:** Not applicable.

**Data Availability Statement:** Data is contained within the article.

**Conflicts of Interest:** The authors declare that they have no known competing financial interests or personal relationships that could have appeared to influence the work reported in this paper.

## Abbreviations

The following abbreviations are used in this manuscript:

| | |
|---|---|
| FCH | Lactic acid bacteria-fermented corn protein hydrolysate |
| CPH | Corn protein hydrolysates |
| BCG | Blank control group |
| FMG | Fatigue model group |
| CPH-M | Medium dose group of CPH |
| FCH-L | Low-dose group of FCH |
| FCH-M | Medium dose group of FCH |
| FCH-H | High dose group of FCH |
| BUN | Urea nitrogen |
| LA | Lactate |
| LDH | Lactic dehydrogenase |
| MG | Muscle glycogen |
| LG | Liver glycogen |
| MDA | Malondialdehyde |
| SOD | Superoxide dismutase |
| GSH | Glutathione |
| PCoA | Principal coordinates analysis |
| ACE | Abundance-based coverage estimator |
| ICR | Institute of cancer research |

## References

1. Luo, C.H.; Xu, X.R.; Wei, X.C.; Feng, W.W.; Huang, H.Z.; Liu, H.Y.; Xu, R.C.; Lin, J.Z.; Han, L.; Zhang, D.K. Natural medicines for the treatment of fatigue: Bioactive components, pharmacology, and mechanisms. *Pharmacol. Res.* **2019**, *148*, 104409. [CrossRef] [PubMed]
2. Lock, A.M.; Bonetti, D.L.; Campbell AD, K. The psychological and physiological health effects of fatigue. *Occup. Med.* **2018**, *68*, 502–511. [CrossRef] [PubMed]
3. Matura, L.A.; Malone, S.; Jaime-Lara, R.; Riegel, B. A systematic review of biological mechanisms of fatigue in chronic illness. *Biol. Res. Nurs.* **2018**, *20*, 410–421. [CrossRef]
4. Guest, A.J.; Clemes, S.A.; King, J.A.; Chen, Y.L.; Ruettger, K.; Sayyah, M.; Sherry, A.; Varela-Mato, V.; Paine, N.J. Attenuated cardiovascular reactivity is related to higher anxiety and fatigue symptoms in truck drivers. *Psychophysiology* **2021**, *58*, e13872. [CrossRef]
5. Francoeur, R.B. Using an innovative multiple regression procedure in a cancer population (Part II): Fever, depressive affect, and mobility problems clarify an influential symptom pair (pain–fatigue/weakness) and cluster (pain–fatigue/weakness–sleep problems). *OncoTargets Ther.* **2014**, *8*, 57–72. [CrossRef]
6. Sreenivasan, S.T.; Nattala, P.; Rao, G.N.; Sridaramurthy, M.K. "So what if I use tobacco or alcohol? It won't hurt me!" How women perceive substance use: Insights from a community study in India. *Arch. Women's Ment. Health* **2022**, *25*, 129–136. [CrossRef]
7. Cui, P.B.; Li, M.Y.; Yu, M.X.; Liu, Y.F.; Ding, Y.T.; Liu, W.L.; Liu, J.H. Advances in sports food: Sports nutrition, food manufacture, opportunities and challenges. *Food Res. Int.* **2022**, *157*, 111258. [CrossRef]
8. Xiao, M.F.; Lin, L.; Chen, H.P.; Ge, X.D.; Huang, Y.; Zheng, Z.P.; Li, S.M.; Pan, Y.Y.; Liu, B.; Zeng, F. Anti-fatigue property of the oyster polypeptide fraction and its effect on gut microbiota in mice. *Food Funct.* **2020**, *11*, 8659–8669. [CrossRef]

9. Wang, Q.Q.; Shi, J.Y.; Zhong, H.; Zhuang, J.C.; Zhang, J.H.; Wang, J.; Zhang, X.; Feng, F.Q. Abdullah High-degree hydrolysis sea cucumber peptides improve exercise performance and exert antifatigue effect via activating the NRF2 and AMPK signaling pathways in mice. *J. Funct. Foods* **2021**, *86*, 104677. [CrossRef]
10. Qiao, Y.B.; Ye, Y.; Cai, T.X.; Li, S.; Liu, X.Q. Anti-fatigue activity of the polysaccharides isolated from Ribes stenocarpum Maxim. *J. Funct. Foods* **2022**, *89*, 104947. [CrossRef]
11. Lu, B.X. Evaluating the efficacy of fish proteins for the amelioration of extreme exercise-induced fatigue leading to death in mice. *Curr. Top. Nutraceutical Res.* **2020**, *18*, 52–55. [CrossRef]
12. Jing, Y.; Liu, X.L.; Wang, J.Y.; Ma, Y.Q.; Zheng, X.Q. Production of corn protein hydrolysate with glutamine-rich peptides and its antagonistic function in ulcerative colitis in vivo. *Foods* **2022**, *11*, 3359. [CrossRef] [PubMed]
13. Shen, Y.T.; Hu, R.J.; Li, Y.H. Antioxidant and emulsifying activities of corn gluten meal hydrolysates in oil-in-water emulsions. *J. Am. Oil Chem. Soc.* **2020**, *97*, 175–185. [CrossRef]
14. Kopparapu, N.K.; Duan, Y.J.; Huang, L.H.; Katrolia, P. Review on utilisation of corn gluten meal, a by-product from corn starch industry for production of value-added products. *Int. J. Food Sci. Technol.* **2022**, *57*, 5592–5599. [CrossRef]
15. Liu, B.Y.; Li, N.N.; Chen, F.S.; Zhang, J.S.; Sun, X.R.; Xu, L.; Fang, F. Review on the release mechanism and debittering technology of bitter peptides from protein hydrolysates. *Compr. Rev. Food Sci. Food Saf.* **2022**, *21*, 5153–5170. [CrossRef]
16. Mirzapour-Kouhdasht, A.; McClements, D.J.; Taghizadeh, M.S.; Niazi, A.; Garcia-Vaquero, M. Strategies for oral delivery of bioactive peptides with focus on debittering and masking. *NPJ Sci. Food* **2023**, *7*, 22. [CrossRef]
17. Cui, J.W.; Shi, C.; Xia, P.B.; Ning, K.; Xiang, H.Y.; Xie, Q.H. Fermented deer blood ameliorates intense exercise-induced fatigue via modulating small intestine microbiota and metabolites in mice. *Nutrients* **2021**, *13*, 1543. [CrossRef]
18. Cui, J.W.; Xia, P.B.; Zhang, L.L.; Hu, Y.; Xie, Q.H.; Xiang, H.Y. A novel fermented soybean, inoculated with selected *Bacillus*, *Lactobacillus* and *Hansenula* strains, showed strong antioxidant and anti-fatigue potential activity. *Food Chem.* **2020**, *333*, 127527. [CrossRef]
19. Fang, L.; Zhang, R.X.; Wei, Y.; Ling, K.; Lu, L.; Wang, J.; Pan, X.C.; Cai, M.Y. Anti-fatigue effects of fermented soybean protein peptides in mice. *J. Sci. Food Agric.* **2022**, *102*, 2693–2703. [CrossRef]
20. Zhang, R.X.; Zhang, J.T.; Liu, Y.; Fang, L.; Wei, Y.; Gu, R.Z.; Lin, M.; Chen, L.; Zhou, Z.F. The effect of fermented wheat protein hydrolysate on the exercise performance in mice. *J. Funct. Foods* **2022**, *97*, 105217. [CrossRef]
21. Cong, S.Z.; Cao, Y.J.; Zhang, X.X.; Li, G.L.; Liu, X.L.; Hu, N. Optimization of technological conditions and antioxidant activity of corn protein hydrolysates fermented by lactic acid bacteria. *Food Res. Dev.* **2024**, *45*, 152–162. [CrossRef]
22. Hu, N.; Lei, M.; Zhao, X.L.; Wang YY, F.; Zhang, Y.; Wang, S. Analysis of microbiota in Hainan Yucha during fermentation by 16S rRNA gene high-throughput sequencing. *J. Food Process. Preserv.* **2020**, *44*, e14523. [CrossRef]
23. Burt, D.; Lamb, K.; Nicholas, C.; Twist, C. Effects of muscle-damaging exercise on physiological, metabolic, and perceptual responses during two modes of endurance exercise. *J. Exerc. Sci. Fit.* **2012**, *10*, 70–77. [CrossRef]
24. Zhang, Y.Y.; Ryu, B.M.; Cui, Y.H.; Li, C.Y.; Zhou, C.X.; Hong, P.Z.; Lee, B.; Qian, Z.J. A peptide isolated from *Hippocampus abdominalis* improves exercise performance and exerts anti-fatigue effects via AMPK/PGC-1$\alpha$ pathway in mice. *J. Funct. Foods* **2019**, *61*, 103489. [CrossRef]
25. Jiao, Y.; Chen, H.D.; Han, H.; Chang, Y. Development and utilization of corn processing by-products: A review. *Foods* **2022**, *11*, 3709. [CrossRef]
26. Ramanjaneya, M.; Bettahi, I.; Jerobin, J.; Chandra, P.; Khalil, C.A.; Skarulis, M.; Atkin, S.L.; Abou-Samra, A.B. Mitochondrial-derived peptides are down regulated in diabetes subjects. *Front. Endocrinol.* **2019**, *10*, 331. [CrossRef]
27. Wang, X.Q.; Xing, R.E.; Chen, Z.Y.; Yu, H.H.; Li, R.F.; Li, P.C. Effect and mechanism of mackerel (*Pneumatophorus japonicus*) peptides for anti-fatigue. *Food Funct.* **2014**, *5*, 2113–2119. [CrossRef]
28. Hargreaves, M.; Spriet, L.L. Skeletal muscle energy metabolism during exercise. *Nat. Metab.* **2020**, *2*, 817–828. [CrossRef]
29. Wang, J.; Sun, C.X.; Zheng, Y.; Pan, H.L.; Zhou, Y.F.; Fan, Y.Y. The effective mechanism of the polysaccharides from *Panax ginseng* on chronic fatigue syndrome. *Arch. Pharmacal Res.* **2014**, *37*, 530–538. [CrossRef]
30. Yin, C.L.; Fu, X.Q.; Chou, J.Y.; Li, J.K.; Chen, Y.J.; Bai, J.X.; Wu, J.Y.; Wu, Y.; Wang, X.Q.; Yu, Z.L. A proprietary herbal drug Young Yum Pill ameliorates chronic fatigue syndrome in mice. *Phytomedicine* **2021**, *88*, 153602. [CrossRef]
31. Feng, Z.Y.; Wei, Y.; Xu, Y.G.; Zhang, R.X.; Li, M.L.; Qin, H.M.; Gu, R.Z.; Cai, M.Y. The anti-fatigue activity of corn peptides and their effect on gut bacteria. *J. Sci. Food Agric.* **2022**, *102*, 3456–3466. [CrossRef] [PubMed]
32. Yu, J.H.; Cao, Y.; He, F.; Xiang, F.; Wang, S.Z.; Ke, W.B.; Wu, W. Polysaccharides from *Artemisia argyi* leaves: Environmentally friendly ultrasound-assisted extraction and antifatigue activities. *Ultrason. Sonochem.* **2024**, *107*, 106932. [CrossRef] [PubMed]
33. Lu, X.D.; Chen, J.Q.; Huang, L.Y.; Ou, Y.J.; Wu, J.R.; Guo, Z.B.; Zheng, B.D. The anti-fatigue effect of glycoprotein from hairtail fish (*Trichiurus lepturus*) on BALB/c mice. *Foods* **2023**, *12*, 1245. [CrossRef]
34. Feng, T.; Huang, Y.Y.; Tang, Z.H.; Wei, D.D.; Mo, J.M. Anti-fatigue effects of pea (*Pisum sativum* L.) peptides prepared by compound protease. *J. Food Sci. Technol.* **2021**, *58*, 2265–2272. [CrossRef]

35. Chen, Y.H.; Wang, F.; Zhou, J.W.; Niu, T.T.; Xuan, R.R.; Chen, H.M.; Wu, W. In vivo antifatigue activity of Spirulina peptides achieved by their antioxidant activity and by acting on fat metabolism pathway in mice. *Nat. Prod. Commun.* **2020**, *15*, 1934578X20946233. [CrossRef]
36. Liu, R.; Li, Z.; Yu, X.C.; Hu, J.N.; Zhu, N.; Liu, X.R.; Hao, Y.T.; Kang, J.W.; Li, Y. The effects of peanut oligopeptides on exercise-induced fatigue in mice and its underlying mechanism. *Nutrients* **2023**, *15*, 1743. [CrossRef]
37. Wang, Y.C.; Song, X.J.; Feng, Y.G.; Cui, Q. Changes in peptidomes and Fischer ratios of corn-derived oligopeptides depending on enzyme hydrolysis approaches. *Food Chem.* **2019**, *297*, 124931. [CrossRef]
38. White, J.P. Amino acid trafficking and skeletal muscle protein synthesis: A case of supply and demand. *Front. Cell Dev. Biol.* **2021**, *9*, 656604. [CrossRef]
39. Zhong, H.; Shi, J.Y.; Zhang, J.H.; Wang, Q.Q.; Zhang, Y.P.; Yu, P.; Guan, R.F.; Feng, F.Q. Soft-shelled turtle peptide supplementation modifies energy metabolism and oxidative stress, enhances exercise endurance, and decreases physical fatigue in mice. *Foods* **2022**, *11*, 600. [CrossRef]
40. Ye, J.; Shen, C.H.; Huang, Y.Y.; Zhang, X.Q.; Xiao, M.T. Anti-fatigue activity of sea cucumber peptides prepared from *Stichopus japonicus* in an endurance swimming rat model. *J. Sci. Food Agric.* **2017**, *97*, 4548–4556. [CrossRef]
41. Bian, X.Y.; Wang, Y.W.; Yang, R.R.; Ma, Y.Y.; Dong, W.Y.; Guo, C.J.; Gao, W.N. Anti-fatigue properties of the ethanol extract of Moringa oleifera leaves in mice. *J. Sci. Food Agric.* **2023**, *103*, 5500–5510. [CrossRef] [PubMed]
42. Peng, F.; Yin, H.Y.; Du, B.; Niu, K.; Ren, X.; Yang, Y.D. Anti-fatigue activity of purified flavonoids prepared from chestnut (*Castanea mollissima*) flower. *J. Funct. Foods* **2021**, *79*, 104365. [CrossRef]
43. Nasri, R.; Abdelhedi, O.; Nasri, M.; Jridi, M. Fermented protein hydrolysates: Biological activities and applications. *Curr. Opin. Food Sci.* **2022**, *43*, 120–127. [CrossRef]
44. Peng, Y.F.; Zhao, L.L.; Hu, K.; Yang, Y.J.; Ma, J.; Zhai, Y.Q.; Jiang, Y.; Zhang, D.J. Anti-fatigue effects of *Lycium barbarum* polysaccharide and effervescent tablets by regulating oxidative stress and energy metabolism in rats. *Int. J. Mol. Sci.* **2022**, *23*, 10920. [CrossRef]
45. Zhu, S.; Yang, W.; Lin, Y.; Du, C.D.; Huang, D.J.; Chen, S.W.; Yu, T.; Cong, X. Antioxidant and anti-fatigue activities of selenium-enriched peptides isolated from *Cardamine violifolia* protein hydrolysate. *J. Funct. Foods* **2021**, *79*, 104412. [CrossRef]
46. Johnson, E.L.; Heaver, S.L.; Walters, W.A.; Ley, R.E. Microbiome and metabolic disease: Revisiting the bacterial phylum Bacteroidetes. *J. Mol. Med.* **2017**, *95*, 1–8. [CrossRef]
47. Wieërs, G.; Belkhir, L.; Enaud, R.; Leclercq, S.; Philippart de Foy, J.M.; Dequenne, I.; de Timary, P.; Cani, P.D. How probiotics affect the microbiota. *Front. Cell. Infect. Microbiol.* **2020**, *9*, 454. [CrossRef]
48. Lee, M.C.; Hsu, Y.J.; Ho, H.H.; Kuo, Y.W.; Lin, W.Y.; Tsai, S.Y.; Chen, W.L.; Lin, C.L.; Huang, C.C. Effectiveness of human-origin *Lactobacillus plantarum* PL-02 in improving muscle mass, exercise performance and anti-fatigue. *Sci. Rep.* **2021**, *11*, 19469. [CrossRef]
49. Nay, K.; Jollet, M.; Goustard, B.; Baati, N.; Vernus, B.; Pontones, M.; Lefeuvre-Orfila, L.; Bendavid, C.; Rué, O.; Mariadassou, M.; et al. Gut bacteria are critical for optimal muscle function: A potential link with glucose homeostasis. *Am. J. Physiol. Endocrinol. Metab.* **2019**, *317*, E158–E171. [CrossRef]

*nutrients*

MDPI

*Article*

# Daily Orange Consumption Reduces Hepatic Steatosis Prevalence in Patients with Metabolic Dysfunction-Associated Steatotic Liver Disease: Exploratory Outcomes of a Randomized Clinical Trial

**Maria Notarnicola [1,*], Valeria Tutino [1], Valentina De Nunzio [1], Anna Maria Cisternino [2], Miriam Cofano [1], Rossella Donghia [3], Vito Giannuzzi [4], Marianna Zappimbulso [4], Rosa Anna Milella [5], Gianluigi Giannelli [6,†] and Luigi Fontana [7,8,†]**

1 Laboratory of Nutritional Biochemistry, National Institute of Gastroenterology—IRCCS "Saverio de Bellis", Castellana Grotte, 70013 Bari, Italy; valeria.tutino@irccsdebellis.it (V.T.); valentina.denunzio@irccsdebellis.it (V.D.N.); miriam.cofano@irccsdebellis.it (M.C.)

2 Ambulatory of Clinical Nutrition, National Institute of Gastroenterology—IRCCS "Saverio de Bellis", Castellana Grotte, 70013 Bari, Italy; annamaria.cisternino@irccsdebellis.it

3 Data Science Unit, National Institute of Gastroenterology—IRCCS "Saverio de Bellis", Castellana Grotte, 70013 Bari, Italy; rossella.donghia@irccsdebellis.it

4 Unit of Gastroenterology, National Institute of Gastroenterology—IRCCS "Saverio de Bellis", Castellana Grotte, 70013 Bari, Italy; vito.giannuzzi@irccsdebellis.it (V.G.); marianna.zappimbulso@irccsdebellis.it (M.Z.)

5 Research Centre for Viticulture and Enology, 70010 Turi, Italy; rosaanna.milella@crea.gov.it

6 Scientific Direction National Institute of Gastroenterology—IRCCS "Saverio de Bellis", Castellana Grotte, 70013 Bari, Italy; gianluigi.giannelli@irccsdebellis.it

7 Charles Perkins Centre, Faculty of Medicine and Health, The University of Sydney, Sydney, NSW 2006, Australia; luigi.fontana@sydney.edu.au

8 Department of Endocrinology, Royal Prince Alfred Hospital, Sydney, NSW 2050, Australia

* Correspondence: maria.notarnicola@irccsdebellis.it

† These authors contributed equally to this work.

**Abstract: Background**: Consumption of flavonoid-rich orange juice has been shown to reduce adiposity and liver steatosis in murine models of diet-induced obesity. However, little is known about the effects of whole orange intake, independent of body weight changes, on liver function and steatosis in individuals with metabolic dysfunction-associated steatotic liver disease (MASLD). The goal is to understand the direct impact of orange consumption on metabolic health. **Methods**: Sixty-two men and women aged 30–65 with MASLD (Controlled Attenuation Parameter, (CAP) > 275 dB/m) were randomly assigned to consume either 400 g of whole oranges or non-citrus fruits daily for 4 weeks. Baseline evaluations included medical assessments, blood tests, and body composition. Liver health was assessed using transient elastography (FibroScan®) for steatosis and fibrosis, conducted by blinded personnel. This clinical trial was registered at ClinicalTrials.gov (NCT05558592). **Results**: After 4 weeks of orange supplementation, liver steatosis decreased in the treatment group, with 70.9% showing steatosis compared to 100% in controls ($p < 0.004$), indicating a 30% reduction in liver disease prevalence. There were no significant changes in fibrosis or plasma liver enzymes, though plasma gamma glutaril transferase (GGT) levels decreased significantly. Body weight, waist circumference, body composition, lipid profile, fasting glucose, insulin, and C-reactive protein levels remained unchanged. Dietary analysis revealed no change in caloric intake, but vitamins C, A, thiamine, and riboflavin increased in the orange group. **Conclusions**: Our findings suggest that phytochemical-rich foods, especially whole fruits like oranges, may enhance liver function as an adjunct treatment for MASLD. The notable reduction in liver steatosis prevalence occurred independently of body weight changes. Further studies are needed to investigate the long-term effects of orange supplementation on steatosis and fibrosis progression and to identify the specific bioactive compounds and mechanisms involved.

**Keywords:** MASLD; phytochemical food; CAP; steatosis; oranges

## 1. Introduction

Diets enriched with flavonoids have been closely associated with the prevention and treatment of various metabolic diseases, including obesity, dyslipidemia, insulin resistance, hepatic steatosis, type 2 diabetes, cancer, and atherosclerosis.

Flavonoids exhibit potential health benefits due to their antioxidant, anti-inflammatory, and hypolipidemic properties, making them promising nutraceutical agents for handling various pathological conditions [1–3].

Flavonoids are phytochemicals found abundantly in vegetables and fruits, particularly in citrus fruits, especially in the albedo and membranes separating orange segments [1]. Key flavonoids include narirutin, naringenin, and tangerine, with hesperidin being the major component. Known for their antioxidant, anti-inflammatory, and hypolipidemic properties, flavonoids have been hypothesized to offer significant metabolic health benefits [2,4].

Moreover, in vitro, flavonoids extracted from oranges of the "Tacle" variety have demonstrated an inhibitory action on cholesterol synthesis and biomarkers levels involved in inflammation [5]. Under normal conditions, adipose tissue stores lipids in the form of triglycerides, whereas during obesity, hyperlipidemia causes excessive infiltration by macrophages in the adipose tissue and liver, resulting in the production of proinflammatory cytokines, such as tumor necrosis factor (TNF-α), interleukin 6 (IL-6), and inducible nitric oxide synthase (iNOS) [6,7], associated with systemic inflammation and atherogenesis [8,9].

For instance, protocatechuic acid administration for 10 weeks reduced lipogenic enzyme expression and hepatic lipid accumulation in high-fat-diet mice [10]. Preliminary clinical trial data suggest that 2 weeks of orange juice consumption positively affects lipid metabolism, particularly triglyceride-specific fatty acid chains and cholesterol esters in individuals with obesity and insulin resistance [11]. However, the interpretation of data from these preclinical and clinical studies is often confounded by lifestyle and weight changes among subjects randomized to consume orange juice.

Consumption of juice from anthocyanin-rich oranges for 12 weeks has demonstrated multiple beneficial effects in murine models of diet-induced obesity, including preventing weight gain, improving insulin sensitivity, reducing serum total cholesterol and triglycerides, lowering liver enzymes, and reversing liver steatosis [12,13]. These benefits are believed to be mediated through the induction of peroxisome proliferator-activated receptor-α (PPAR-α) and its target gene acyl-CoA oxidase, a key enzyme involved in lipid oxidation. However, the specific effects of orange fruit intake, independent of weight loss, on individuals with metabolic dysfunction-associated fatty liver disease (MASLD) remain largely unknown, particularly concerning liver function, steatosis, and fibrosis as assessed by vibration-controlled elastography (VCTE) using FibroScan®.

Recent evidence suggests that hesperidin may potentially improve non-alcoholic fatty liver disease (NAFLD) by exerting hypoglycemic effects, promoting fatty acid β-oxidation through activating silent information regulator 1 (SIRT1)/ peroxisome proliferator-activated receptor gamma coactivator 1α (PGC1α), and, finally, modifying lipid profiles [14].

NAFLD, now known as metabolic dysfunction-associated fatty liver disease (MAFLD), represents the most common cause of chronic liver disease worldwide, with a 20–30% prevalence in Western countries [15].

MAFLD, unlike the term NAFLD, emphasizes metabolic risk and focuses on alterations in glucose (insulin resistance) and lipid metabolism (lipotoxicity, oxidative stress, etc.) as well as the significant role of inflammatory processes in hepatocytes [16,17].

In this scenario, the main aim of this randomized clinical trial was to investigate the effects of 4-week consumption of "Navelina" whole oranges, independent of weight changes, on metabolic and liver function in 62 middle-aged overweight men and women diagnosed with MAFLD.

To isolate the independent effects of orange supplementation on metabolic and liver function, each subject was contacted by one of the investigators at least once every week by phone to review their medical condition and reinforce the importance of maintaining their usual food intake and physical activity, ensuring stable body weight. We hypothesized that ingesting the entire fruit, including its flavonoid-rich albedo, would offer favorable effects on liver function and steatosis, independent of weight modifications. This focus is crucial as it aims to understand the direct impact of orange fruit consumption on metabolic health, removing the confounding variable of weight change.

## 2. Materials and Methods

### *2.1. Orange*

The "Navelina" variety oranges used in this study were biological oranges purchased by a BioFarm from the Cosenza (Calabria Region, Italy).

The physicochemical properties, polyphenol content, and total antioxidant activity of oranges were analyzed by the Council for Agricultural Research and Economics (CREAVE), Turi, BA, Italy. Polyphenolic profiles were determined by high-performance liquid chromatography (HPLC) 1100 (Agilent Technologies, Palo Alto, CA, USA) equipped with a diode array detector (DAD) analysis (Table 1).

**Table 1.** Physicochemical properties, polyphenol content, and total antioxidant activity of "Naveline" oranges.

| **Physicochemical Properties of Navelina Orange** | |
|---|---|
| Fruit weight (g) | 192.85 ± 25.59 |
| Equatorial diameter (mm) | 74.83 ± 2.14 |
| Fruit height (mm) | 75.83 ± 3.43 |
| pH | 3.46 ± 0.17 |
| TA (g citric acid/L) | 8.92 ± 1.14 |
| TSS (° Brix) | 9.75 ± 0.57 |
| Maturity index (TSS/TAA) | 11.09 ± 1.70 |
| Polyphenols and total antioxidant activity of Navelina orange | |
| Total phenolic content (mg/kg flesh tissue) | 1061.1 ± 136.8 |
| Total phenolic content (mg/L juice) | 134.0 ± 12.00 |
| Hesperidin mg/L juice | 505.7 ± 51.60 |
| DPPH (mM TE/L juice) | 7.90 ± 0.20 |
| DPPH (mM TE/kg FW) | 63.20 ± 3.70 |
| ORAC (mM TE/kg FW) | 155.40 ± 12.10 |

As mean and standard deviation (M ± SD).

### *2.2. Participants*

Seventy men and women aged 30–65 years diagnosed with MAFLD were recruited from the outpatient nutrition clinic of the National Institute of Gastroenterology "S. de Bellis" between February 2023 and November 2023. Inclusion criteria required participants to exhibit liver steatosis (CAP score > 275 dB/m) along with either overweight status (Body Mass Index, BMI > 25), type 2 diabetes, and/or metabolic syndrome. All of the subjects had had a stable weight (with fluctuations of no more than 2 percent of the body weight) for at least two months and had been sedentary (exercising for less than one hour per week) for at least six months before entering the study. Approval for this study was obtained from the Human Studies Committee of the IRCCS Oncological Hospital—Giovanni Paolo II, Bari, Italy (Approval Number #184 del 13 May 2022).

All participants provided informed consent following the principles outlined in the Declaration of Helsinki. The CONSORT diagram illustrating participant enrollment is depicted in Figure 1. This clinical trial was registered at ClinicalTrials.gov (NCT05558592).

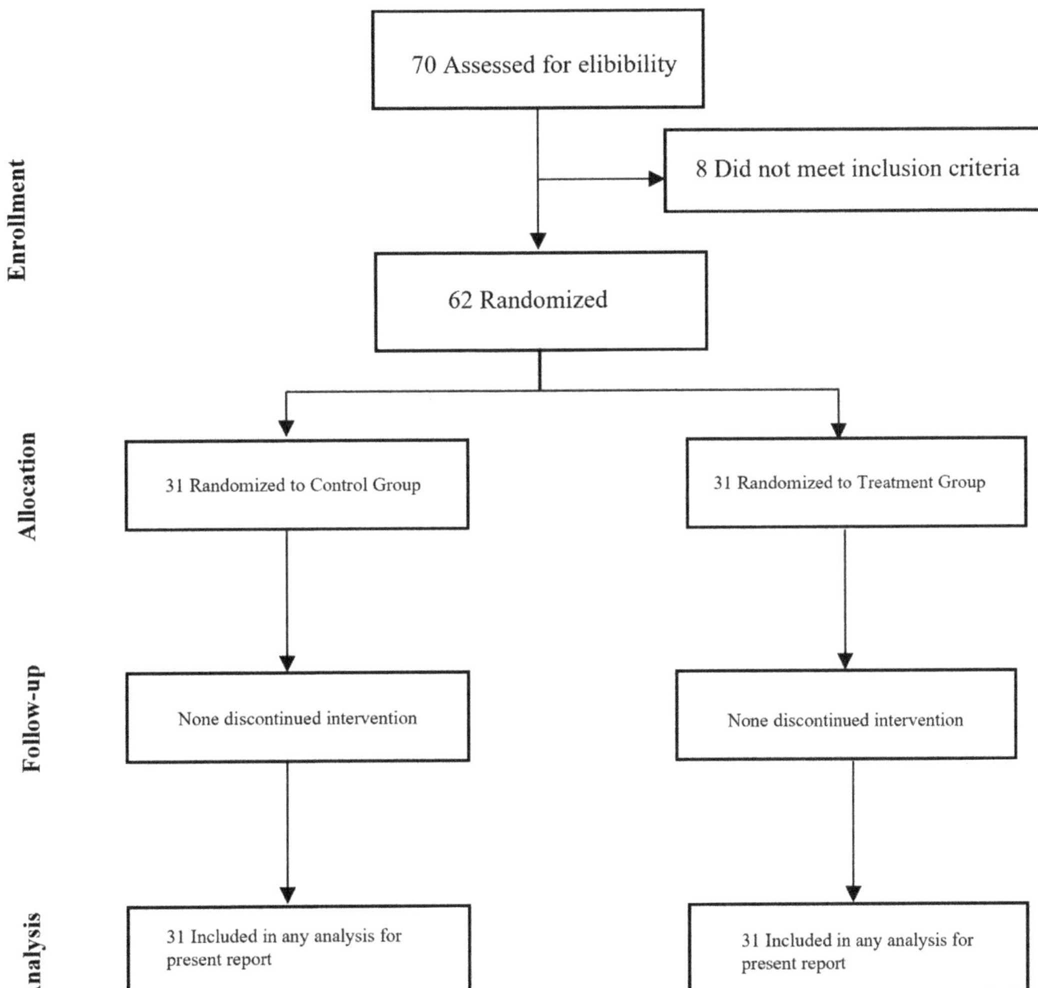


**Figure 1.** CONSORT flow diagram.

### 2.3. Study Design

At baseline, all participants underwent a comprehensive medical and nutritional assessment, including routine blood tests. Potential subjects were excluded if they had a history of gastroesophageal disease, chronic inflammatory disease, a recent history or evidence of malignancy, anticoagulant therapy use, or adherence to a special diet. Eligible participants were randomly assigned to one of two groups: consuming 400 g of oranges (net of waste) daily for 4 weeks or consuming 400 g of non-citrus fruits daily. The "Navelina" variety oranges used in this study were sourced organically from a BioFarm in the Calabria Region, Italy. The physicochemical properties, polyphenol content, and total antioxidant activity of the oranges were analyzed by the Research Center for Viticulture and Enology of Council for Agricultural Research and Economics (CREAVE) in Turi (BA), Italy. Analysis of polyphenolic profiles was conducted using high-performance liquid chromatography (HPLC) 1100 (Agilent Technologies, Palo Alto, CA, USA) equipped with a diode array detector (DAD) as shown in Table 1.

All study participants were provided with dietary guidelines, which included recommendations to restrict the intake of alcohol, caffeine, and foods rich in vitamin C (Supplementary Table S1). A total of 62 research volunteers (17 females and 45 males) began the intervention. Each subject was contacted by an investigator at least once a week via phone. During these calls, the investigator reviewed the participant's medical condition, reinforced the importance of adhering to their usual diet and physical activity levels, and emphasized the necessity of maintaining a stable body weight throughout the study. This regular communication was designed to ensure that any observed effects could be attributed specifically to orange consumption rather than changes in weight or other lifestyle factors. All study personnel performing assessments were masked to treatment assignment. Participants were advised to maintain their usual dietary and physical activity habits throughout the study.

### 2.4. Anthropometrics and Dietary Assessment

Body weight was measured in duplicate in the morning following a 12 h fast with the subject wearing a hospital gown and no shoes. Height and waist circumference were measured twice using a wall-mounted stadiometer and tape measure. BMI was calculated as weight divided by the square of height (kg/m$^2$). Changes in body weight and body fat mass were assessed by bioelectrical impedance analysis—BIA (BIA 101, Akern SRL, Pontassieve, Italy). The phase angle (PhA) was calculated using the arctangent of the extracellular water (ECW) ratio, directly derived from Rz and Xc values with Bodygram PLUS Software v. 1.0 (Akern SRL, Pontassieve, Italy) utilizing medically validated algorithms. Seven-day food diaries were used to estimate self-reported intake. Participants received detailed instructions on how to weigh, measure, and record all food and beverages consumed during the collection. Research dietitians reviewed the diaries with participants and then analyzed them using MetaDIETA Professional 4.0.1 (Meteda, Rome, Italy).

### 2.5. Blood Analyses

Venous blood was sampled for metabolic and hormone concentrations after an overnight fast. Samples were collected in serum and edetic acid plasma tubes, immediately centrifuged to separate the plasma, aliquoted, and stored in a −80 °C freezer until use. All serum and plasma samples were analyzed by the Core Laboratory at the National Institute of Gastroenterology "S. de Bellis"; technicians performing assessments were masked to treatment assignment.

### 2.6. Liver Fibroscan®

Non-invasive transient elastography (FibroScan®, Echo-Sens, Paris, France) was performed to evaluate hepatic steatosis and fibrosis after fasting for at least 4 h. All FibroScan® measurements were taken by highly trained technicians who were masked to treatment assignment. Steatosis was assessed by CAP (dB/m), and liver stiffness was measured in kPa.

### 2.7. Statistical Analysis

All participants who provided both baseline and 4-week data were included in the analyses. Data are presented as mean and standard deviation (M ± SD) for continuous variables at each time point and for the change between baseline and 4 weeks, while data are presented as frequency and percentages (%) for categories. Baseline characteristics were compared between groups with the Chi-square test employed for categorical variables as needed, while the Wilcoxon rank was used for continuous variables. The Wilcoxon matched-pairs signed-rank or McNemar's test was applied for continuous or categorical parameters to evaluate variations after and before 4 weeks of observation. To test the association between the independent groups, the Chi-square test was employed for categorical variables as needed, while the Mann–Whitney test was used for continuous variables. All statistical tests were two-tailed, and significance was accepted at $p < 0.05$. All analyses were performed using StataCorp. 2023 software, version 18 (College Station, TX, USA: StataCorp LLC), while RStudio ("Chocolate Cosmos" Release) was used for the plots.

## 3. Results

### 3.1. Study Participants

A total of 70 participants were screened for eligibility, with 62 being randomized and starting the intervention. All participants completed the 4-week intervention (Figure 1).

Subjects randomized to the orange supplementation group ($n = 31$; age 51.8 ± 10.3 years) and the control group ($n = 31$; age 50.1 ± 9.8 years) had similar baseline characteristics, except for higher plasma concentrations of total cholesterol and GGT levels and lower HDL cholesterol in the treatment group (Table 2).

**Table 2.** Baseline study subjects' characteristics ($n = 62$).

| Parameters [1] | Control ($n = 31$) | Treatment ($n = 31$) | $p$ [2] |
|---|---|---|---|
| Age (yrs) | 50.06 ± 9.77 | 51.77 ± 10.31 | 0.45 |
| Gender (M) (%) | 21 (67.74) | 24 (77.42) | 0.39 [3] |
| *Anthropometric parameters* | | | |
| Weight (kg) | 91.95 ± 11.42 | 91.98 ± 9.96 | 0.99 |
| BMI (kg/m$^2$) | 32.31 ± 4.14 | 32.07 ± 4.25 | 0.97 |
| Neck circumference (cm) | 42.36 ± 11.17 | 39.61 ± 8.05 | 0.91 |
| Waist circumference (cm) | 108.60 ± 12.83 | 108.32 ± 12.72 | 0.53 |
| Hip circumference (cm) | 112.88 ± 10.02 | 109.77 ± 23.88 | 0.76 |
| Whole body phA° | 6.43 ± 0.66 | 6.11 ± 1.76 | 0.99 |
| FFM (kg) | 62.45 ± 9.50 | 58.40 ± 17.89 | 0.81 |
| FM (kg) | 30.49 ± 10.34 | 29.59 ± 15.94 | 0.44 |
| *Biochemical parameters* | | | |
| Total cholesterol (mg/dL) | 183.26 ± 42.88 | 202.29 ± 40.25 | 0.05 |
| HDL cholesterol (mg%) | 51.44 ± 10.43 | 47.10 ± 13.15 | 0.05 |
| LDL cholesterol (mg/dL) | 119.18 ± 39.86 | 132.11 ± 37.64 | 0.16 |
| Triglycerides (mg/dL) | 121.45 ± 70.41 | 132.10 ± 53.32 | 0.14 |
| Fasting glucose (mg/GI) | 94.71 ± 9.45 | 101.00 ± 21.62 | 0.27 |
| Fasting insulin (µUI/mL) | 15.24 ± 7.03 | 16.08 ± 8.55 | 0.58 |
| HOMA-IR | 3.58 ± 2.13 | 4.10 ± 2.50 | 0.39 |
| AST (U/L) | 23.48 ± 7.83 | 23.42 ± 9.93 | 0.70 |
| ALT (U/L) | 30.35 ± 15.74 | 36.68 ± 23.74 | 0.20 |
| GGT (U/L) | 29.71 ± 10.78 | 40.48 ± 23.01 | 0.05 |
| Alkaline phosphatase (U/L) | 69.77 ± 21.00 | 67.64 ± 19.99 | 0.76 |
| CRP (mg/dL) | 0.29 ± 0.23 | 0.34 ± 0.43 | 0.52 |
| Ferritin (ng/mL) | 191.35 ± 95.77 | 241.05 ± 170.98 | 0.48 |

[1] As mean and standard deviation for continuous variables and as frequency and percentage (%) for categorical. [2] Wilcoxon rank-sum test (Mann–Whitney) or [3] Chi-square test where necessary. Abbreviations: BMI, body mass index; Rz, resistance; XC, reactance; phA, phase angle; BCM, body cell mass; FFM, free fat mass; FM, fat mass; TBW, total body water; ECW, extracellular water; CAP, controlled attenuation parameter; RBC, red blood cell; AST, Aspartate Aminotransferase; Alanine Transaminase; ALT, Alanine Transaminase; GGT, Gamma-Glutamyl Transferase; HDL, high-density lipoprotein; LDL, low-density lipoprotein; HOMA, homeostatic model assessment; CRP, C-reactive protein.

The analysis of an adherence questionnaire demonstrated compliance with the recommended diet. The macronutrients contained in the diet used and daily calorie consumption are shown in Supplementary Figure S1.

### 3.2. Orange Supplementation Does Not Affect Body Composition or Key Cardiometabolic Markers

After 4 weeks of orange supplementation, body weight, waist circumference, and body composition measured by BIA (fat mass and fat-free mass) did not change (Table 3).

**Table 3.** Anthropometric parameters before and after intervention.

| Parameters [1] | Group | | Between-Group [2] |
|---|---|---|---|
| | Control | Treatment | |
| Weight (kg) | | | |
| Baseline | 91.95 ± 11.42 | 91.98 ± 9.96 | |
| 28 Days | 91.03 ± 11.47 | 91.26 ± 9.53 | |
| Change | −0.010 ± 0.017 | −0.007 ± 0.021 | 0.43 |
| Within-Group [3] | 0.30 | 0.26 | |
| BMI (kg/m$^2$) | | | |
| Baseline | 32.31 ± 4.14 | 32.07 ± 4.25 | |
| 28 Days | 31.93 ± 4.35 | 31.95 ± 4.28 | |
| Change | −0.012 ± 0.019 | −0.003 ± 0.030 | 0.17 |
| Within-Group [3] | 0.42 | 0.57 | |
| Neck Circumference (cm) | | | |
| Baseline | 42.36 ± 11.17 | 39.61 ± 8.05 | |
| 28 Days | 39.78 ± 3.54 | 39.27 ± 8.04 | |
| Change | −0.035 ± 0.110 | −0.044 ± 0.182 | 0.19 |
| Within-Group [3] | 0.07 | 0.15 | |
| Waist circumference (cm) | | | |
| Baseline | 108.60 ± 12.83 | 108.32 ± 12.72 | |
| 28 Days | 107.57 ± 12.51 | 107.32 ± 12.13 | |
| Change | −0.009 ± 0.015 | −0.009 ± 0.018 | 0.91 |
| Within-Group [3] | 0.45 | 0.05 | |
| Hip circumference (cm) | | | |
| Baseline | 112.88 ± 10.02 | 109.77 ± 23.88 | |
| 28 Days | 112.19 ± 9.85 | 111.86 ± 11.30 | |
| Change | −0.006 ± 0.014 | −0.010 ± 0.023 | 0.68 |
| Within-Group [3] | 0.04 | 0.04 | |
| Whole Body phA° | | | |
| Baseline | 6.43 ± 0.66 | 6.11 ± 1.76 | |
| 28 Days | 6.48 ± 0.75 | 6.32 ± 1.39 | |
| Change | 0.009 ± 0.060 | 0.004 ± 0.069 | 0.56 |
| Within-Group [3] | 0.56 | 0.85 | |
| FFM (kg) | | | |
| Baseline | 62.45 ± 9.50 | 58.40 ± 17.89 | |
| 28 Days | 62.38 ± 10.08 | 61.19 ± 15.53 | |
| Change | −0.002 ± 0.042 | 0.013 ± 0.053 | 0.49 |
| Within-Group [3] | 0.14 | 0.58 | |
| FM (kg) | | | |
| Baseline | 30.49 ± 10.34 | 29.59 ± 15.94 | |
| 28 Days | 29.37 ± 10.80 | 28.99 ± 13.36 | |
| Change | −0.041 ± 0.116 | −0.032 ± 0.097 | 0.97 |
| Within-Group [3] | 0.14 | 0.14 | |

[1] As mean and standard deviation for continuous variables and as frequency and percentage (%) for categorical. [2] Wilcoxon rank-sum test (Mann–Whitney); [3] Wilcoxon matched-pairs signed-rank test. Abbreviations: BMI, body mass index; Rz, resistance; XC, reactance; phA, phase angle; BCM, body cell mass; FFM, free fat mass; FM, fat mass.

Analysis of multiple 7-day food diaries indicated no significant change in daily caloric intake before and after the 28-day period (2026.91 ± 230.67 vs. 2036.65 ± 242.16, respectively, $p = 0.15$). Analysis of 7-day food diaries showed a significant increase in several key vitamins, including vitamin C, vitamin A, thiamine, and riboflavin, in the treatment group (Figure 2).

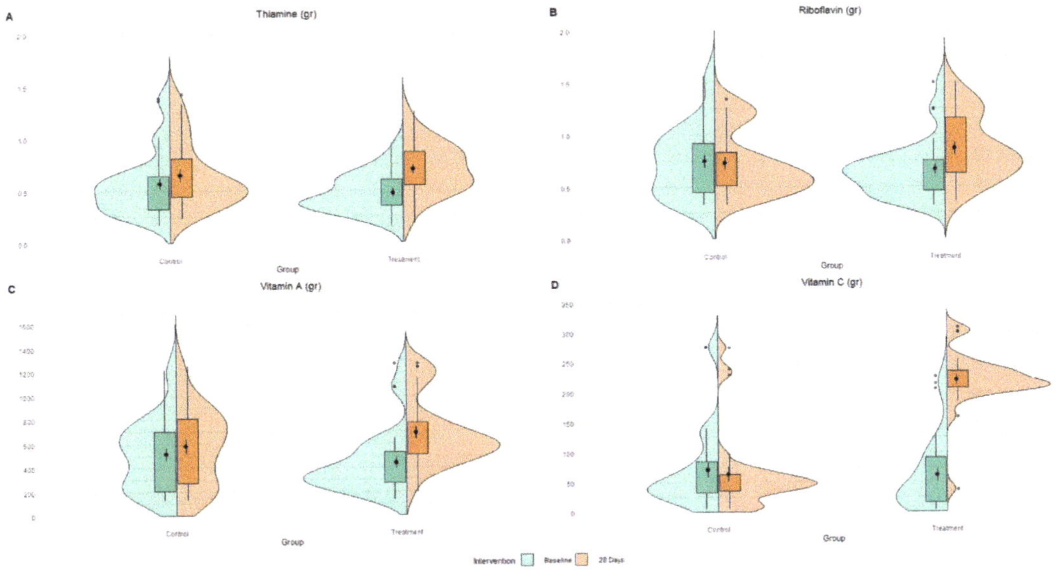


**Figure 2.** Changes in specific nutrient intake. Split-violin plots of vitamins, thiamine (**A**), riboflavin (**B**), vitamin A (**C**), and vitamin C (**D**) distribution between treatment time and groups.

Plasma substrates and hormones (glucose, insulin, and plasma lipids), markers of inflammation (C-reactive protein [CRP] and ferritin), and the homeostasis model assessment of insulin resistance (HOMA-IR) score did not change after orange supplementation (Table 4).

**Table 4.** Metabolic parameters before and after intervention.

| Parameters [1] | Group | | Between-Group [2] |
|---|---|---|---|
| | **Control** | **Treatment** | |
| Total Cholesterol (mg/dL) | | | |
| Baseline | 183.26 ± 42.88 | 202.29 ± 40.25 | |
| 28 Days | 186.03 ± 35.94 | 193.39 ± 40.83 | |
| Change | 0.033 ± 0.134 | −0.033 ± 0.145 | 0.07 |
| Within-Group [3] | 0.85 | 0.28 | |
| LDL Cholesterol (mg/dL) | | | |
| Baseline | 119.18 ± 39.86 | 132.11 ± 37.64 | |
| 28 Days | 121.22 ± 39.23 | 130.94 ± 35.58 | |
| Change | 0.046 ± 0.217 | 0.012 ± 0.160 | 0.69 |
| Within-Group [3] | 0.10 | 0.47 | |
| HDL Cholesterol (mg/dL) | | | |
| Baseline | 51.44 ± 10.43 | 47.10 ± 13.15 | |
| 28 Days | 51.80 ± 11.94 | 47.53 ± 10.74 | |
| Change | 0.007 ± 0.101 | 0.034 ± 0.173 | 0.92 |
| Within-Group [3] | 0.20 | 0.72 | |
| Triglycerides (mg/dL) | | | |
| Baseline | 121.45 ± 70.41 | 132.10 ± 53.32 | |
| 28 Days | 112.29 ± 70.34 | 123.06 ± 53.55 | |
| Change | −0.056 ± 0.257 | −0.032 ± 0.267 | 0.66 |
| Within-Group [3] | 0.14 | 0.72 | |

**Table 4.** *Cont.*

| Parameters [1] | Group | | Between-Group [2] |
|---|---|---|---|
| | Control | Treatment | |
| Fasting Glucose (mg/dL) | | | |
| Baseline | 94.71 ± 9.45 | 101.00 ± 21.62 | |
| 28 Days | 95.71 ± 9.22 | 99.59 ± 26.83 | |
| Change | 0.012 ± 0.057 | −0.018 ± 0.074 | 0.09 |
| Within-Group [3] | 0.18 | 0.72 | |
| Fasting Insulin (μUI/mL) | | | |
| Baseline | 15.24 ± 7.03 | 16.08 ± 8.55 | |
| 28 Days | 15.53 ± 8.21 | 16.42 ± 9.06 | |
| Change | 0.036 ± 0.317 | 0.067 ± 0.294 | 0.58 |
| Within-Group [3] | 0.71 | 0.36 | |
| HOMA-IR | | | |
| Baseline | 3.58 ± 2.13 | 4.10 ± 2.50 | |
| 28 Days | 3.63 ± 2.22 | 4.19 ± 2.94 | |
| Change | 0.055 ± 0.322 | 0.058 ± 0.337 | 0.94 |
| Within-Group [3] | 0.99 | 0.99 | |
| AST (U/L) | | | |
| Baseline | 23.48 ± 7.83 | 23.42 ± 9.93 | |
| 28 Days | 22.90 ± 7.45 | 24.29 ± 7.29 | |
| Change | −0.010 ± 0.141 | 0.088 ± 0.241 | 0.11 |
| Within-Group [3] | 0.99 | 0.05 | |
| ALT (U/L) | | | |
| Baseline | 30.35 ± 15.74 | 36.68 ± 23.74 | |
| 28 Days | 29.93 ± 15.16 | 34.93 ± 18.50 | |
| Change | −0.001 ± 0.138 | 0.008 ± 0.317 | 0.45 |
| Within-Group [3] | 0.42 | 0.28 | |
| GGT (U/L) | | | |
| Baseline | 29.71 ± 10.78 | 40.48 ± 23.01 | |
| 28 Days | 28.29 ± 10.31 | 34.22 ± 21.68 | |
| Change | −0.041 ± 0.113 | −0.160 ± 0.206 | 0.005 |
| Within-Group [3] | 0.12 | 0.0001 | |
| Alkaline Phosphatase (U/L) | | | |
| Baseline | 69.77 ± 21.00 | 67.64 ± 19.99 | |
| 28 Days | 71.58 ± 21.42 | 68.74 ± 19.88 | |
| Change | 0.029 ± 0.067 | 0.019 ± 0.069 | 0.66 |
| Within-Group [3] | 0.56 | 0.58 | |
| hsCRP (mg/dL) | | | |
| Baseline | 0.29 ± 0.23 | 0.34 ± 0.43 | |
| 28 Days | 0.30 ± 0.31 | 0.30 ± 0.41 | |
| Change | 0.201 ± 1.365 | 0.090 ± 0.740 | 0.79 |
| Within-Group [3] | 0.03 | 0.58 | |
| Ferritin (ng/mL) | | | |
| Baseline | 191.35 ± 95.77 | 241.05 ± 170.98 | |
| 28 Days | 188.07 ± 92.61 | 231.52 ± 163.94 | |
| Change | −0.001 ± 0.155 | −0.046 ± 0.206 | 0.32 |
| Within-Group [3] | 0.85 | 0.15 | |

[1] As mean and standard deviation for continuous variables and as frequency and percentage (%) for categorical. [2] Wilcoxon rank-sum test (Mann–Whitney); [3] Wilcoxon matched-pairs signed-rank test. Abbreviations: LDL, low-density lipoprotein; HDL, high-density lipoprotein; HOMA-IR, homeostatic model assessment for insulin resistance; AST, Aspartate Aminotransferase; ALT, Alanine Transaminase; GGT, Gamma-Glutamyl Transferase; hsCRP, high-sensitivity C-reactive protein.

### 3.3. *Orange Supplementation Reduces Liver Steatosis*

After four weeks of orange supplementation, we observed a reduction in liver steatosis as measured by CAP as a categorical variable (Figure 3B, 70.97% vs. 100.00%, $p < 0.004$), although this did not reach statistical significance in a continuous manner (Figure 3A).

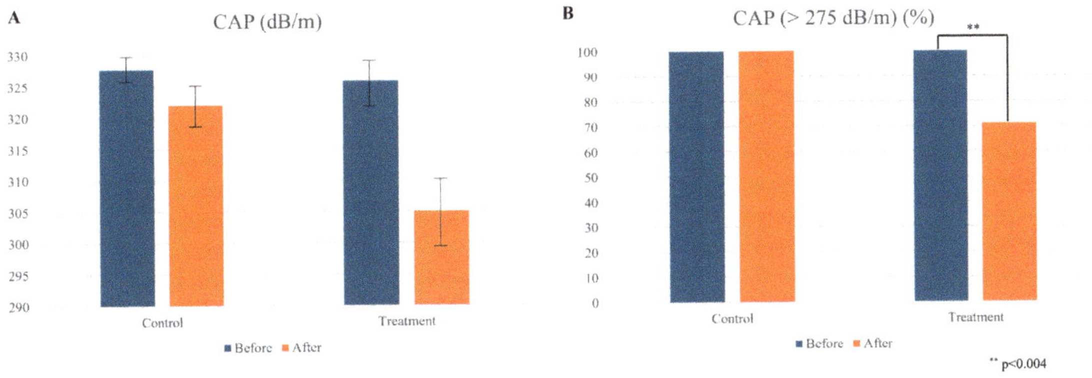


**Figure 3.** Impact of orange supplementation on liver steatosis. (**A**) Reduction in liver steatosis after four weeks of orange supplementation, as measured by controlled attenuation parameter (CAP = dB/m); (**B**) prevalence of liver steatosis based on CAP categorical analysis using a clinical cutoff of more than 275 dB/m [7]. Values are mean ± SEM.

When analyzing CAP as a categorical variable based on the clinical cutoff of 275 dB/m [7], we found a significant decrease in the prevalence of subjects in the treatment group (Figure 3, panel B), with 70.97% of participants showing liver steatosis compared to 100% in the control group ($p < 0.004$). This indicates a reduction in liver disease prevalence of approximately 30% attributable to orange supplementation. However, no statistically significant changes in fibrosis degree (kPa) were observed in either group after the four-week period. Plasma concentrations of AST, ALT, and alkaline phosphates remained unchanged after orange supplementation (Table 3). However, there was a significant reduction in plasma GGT levels (Table 3).

## 4. Discussion

In this randomized clinical trial, unlike others focusing on orange juice consumption [11], we investigated the effects of supplementation with whole oranges, including the albedo rich in polyphenols [18], on liver function and steatosis using transient elastography. Over a four-week period, we evaluated these outcomes alongside various liver and cardiometabolic markers in weight-stable overweight individuals with MASLD and a CAP score exceeding 275 dB/m. Our findings indicate that daily consumption of 400 g of whole oranges—approximately four oranges per day—for 28 days significantly reduced the prevalence of liver steatosis, independent of any changes in body weight.

Lifestyle-induced weight loss leads to a dose-dependent improvement in liver function and steatosis, with reductions exceeding 10% of body weight achieving a 90% resolution rate of steatohepatitis [19]. Our findings highlight the potential of specific foods rich in phytochemicals and antioxidant vitamins, such as whole fruits like oranges, to enhance liver function as an adjunct treatment for MASLD. The significant reduction in liver steatosis prevalence, independent of changes in body weight and adiposity, is consistent with preclinical research suggesting that the flavonoids, vitamin C, and riboflavin found in oranges may support liver function [12,13]. However, unlike preclinical studies, our data indicate that these compounds can promote liver health independently of weight loss or improvements in insulin sensitivity, inflammation, and glucose and lipid metabolism, which typically require a negative energy balance [20–22].

This effect may be achieved by activating lipolytic and lipid oxidation pathways, such as PPAR-α [23,24], while simultaneously inhibiting de novo lipogenesis through mechanisms involving Liver X receptor (LXR-α) [25,26] and the dimethylarginine dimethylaminohydrolase (DDAH)/asymmetric dimethylarginine (ADMA) pathway [13].

Numerous studies have shown that oranges are rich in flavonoids and anthocyanins, which can positively influence lipid metabolism [27–29]. Key components such as polymethoxyflavones, narirutin, naringenin, tangerine, and hesperidin have lipid-lowering and antioxidant properties, preventing liver lipid accumulation and subsequent portal inflammation [29,30]. Other polyphenol-rich fruits like pomegranate and lychee have also been shown to reduce hepatic steatosis and insulin resistance in rodents, likely due to alterations in gut microbiota [31–33]. Additionally, increased intake of antioxidant vitamin C and thiamine may further enhance liver health by reducing liver oxidative stress [34–36]. Riboflavin is also involved in mitochondrial energy production, reducing the risk of fat accumulation in the liver [37].

Therapeutical benefits of the fruit-derived components have been demonstrated in the onset and progression of NAFLD [38,39]. The preventive effect of orange and pomelo peel powder on NAFLD has been demonstrated in mice through the reduction in HFD-induced dyslipidemia with a positive effect on liver inflammation [40]. Pomegranate fruit pulp has recently been shown to reduce hepatic steatosis and insulin resistance in mice by the modulation of the gut microbiota [41].

In subjects with metabolic syndrome, a high content of polyunsaturated fatty acids, tocopherols, and phenolic compounds in the diet led to reduced insulin resistance and glucose levels, improving lipid parameters and modulating the leptin and adiponectin levels in the serum [42].

Consequently, dietary components can largely determine the success of nutritional interventions in patients with metabolic diseases [39]. For example, the Mediterranean diet is a gold benchmark to treat MAFLD for its ability to reduce body weight, BMI, hip circumference, fat mass, and hypertension [43].

In a recent study conducted on tissue-engineered fatty liver, naringenin, found in many citrus fruits such as oranges, demonstrated a potential NAFLD-ameliorative property by decreasing fatty acid absorption and de novo lipogenesis and enhancing fatty acid oxidation [44]. Recently, naringenin has been reported to inhibit the NOD-like receptor protein 3 (NLRP3)/ nuclear factor-kappaB (NF-κB) pathway in a methionine-choline deficient (MCD) model of mice as well as in hepatoma carcinoma (HepG2) cells, primary hepatocytes, and Kupffer cells (KCs) [45].

The study has some limitations, including a small sample size and the absence of liver biopsies for histopathological and mechanistic characterization. The major strengths of this study include the intention-to-treat randomized controlled trial design minimizing the potential for selection bias and the high retention rate of enrolled participants with excellent adherence to the study intervention. A notable distinction of this study compared to previous research is the selection criteria for participants. Unlike earlier studies, our subjects were specifically chosen as overweight individuals with CAP values greater than 256 dB/m. This criterion ensures that all participants had a quantifiable degree of liver steatosis, making the study's results more applicable to a clearly defined population of individuals with MASLD. This focused selection enhances the relevance and applicability of our findings to clinical practice for managing MASLD in overweight individuals.

## 5. Conclusions

Our findings underscore the potential effectiveness of whole fruit consumption, particularly citrus fruits, as a dietary strategy for reducing liver steatosis in overweight individuals with MASLD, independent of weight loss. This research adds to the growing evidence that fruits rich in vitamins, phytochemicals, and fiber can serve as adjunct therapy for preventing liver steatosis and MASLD. Future studies should explore the long-term effects of orange supplementation on fibrosis progression and overall metabolic health, as well as identify the specific bioactive compounds and microbial metabolites responsible for these benefits. Our study also suggests that daily consumption of whole oranges, including the albedo, as part of a balanced, moderately energy-restricted diet, combined with regular exercise, can be an effective preventive measure to reduce liver steatosis.

**Supplementary Materials:** The following supporting information can be downloaded at: https://www.mdpi.com/article/10.3390/nu16183191/s1, Table S1: List of foods rich in vitamin C.; Figure S1: Macronutrients and daily calorie consumption.

**Author Contributions:** Conceptualization, M.N.; methodology, V.D.N., V.T. and R.A.M.; software, V.D.N. and R.D; validation, L.F.; formal analysis, R.D.; investigation, A.M.C.; resources, G.G.; data curation, V.D.N.; writing—original draft preparation, M.N.; writing—review and editing, L.F.; visualization, V.G., M.Z. and M.C.; supervision, L.F. and G.G.; project administration, M.N.; funding acquisition, G.G. All authors have read and agreed to the published version of the manuscript.

**Funding:** This research was funded by the Italian Ministry of Health Ricerca Corrente 2024.

**Institutional Review Board Statement:** The study was approved by the Human Studies Committee of the IRCCS Oncological Hospital—Giovanni Paolo II, Bari, Italy (approval number #184 del 13 May 2022).

**Informed Consent Statement:** Informed consent was obtained from all subjects involved in the study.

**Data Availability Statement:** The original contributions presented in the study are included in the article. Further inquiries can be directed to the corresponding author.

**Acknowledgments:** We thank the biological farm Antonio Caruso for the kind donation of "Navelina" oranges.

**Conflicts of Interest:** The authors declare no conflicts of interest.

## References

1. Lippolis, T.; Cofano, M.; Caponio, G.R.; De Nunzio, V.; Notarnicola, M. Bioaccessibility and Bioavailability of Diet Polyphenols and Their Modulation of Gut Microbiota. *Int. J. Mol. Sci.* **2023**, *24*, 3813. [CrossRef] [PubMed]
2. Assini, J.M.; Mulvihill, E.E.; Huff, M.W. Citrus Flavonoids and Lipid Metabolism. *Curr. Opin. Lipidol.* **2013**, *24*, 34–40. [CrossRef] [PubMed]
3. Caponio, G.R.; Cofano, M.; Lippolis, T.; Gigante, I.; De Nunzio, V.; Difonzo, G.; Noviello, M.; Tarricone, L.; Gambacorta, G.; Giannelli, G.; et al. Anti-Proliferative and Pro-Apoptotic Effects of Digested Aglianico Grape Pomace Extract in Human Colorectal Cancer Cells. *Molecules* **2022**, *27*, 6791. [CrossRef] [PubMed]
4. Fiore, A.; La Fauci, L.; Cervellati, R.; Guerra, M.C.; Speroni, E.; Costa, S.; Galvano, G.; De Lorenzo, A.; Bacchelli, V.; Fogliano, V.; et al. Antioxidant Activity of Pasteurized and Sterilized Commercial Red Orange Juices. *Mol. Nutr. Food Res.* **2005**, *49*, 1129–1135. [CrossRef]
5. Grande, F.; Occhiuzzi, M.A.; Perri, M.R.; Ioele, G.; Rizzuti, B.; Statti, G.; Garofalo, A. Polyphenols from Citrus Tacle® Extract Endowed with HMGCR Inhibitory Activity: An Antihypercholesterolemia Natural Remedy. *Molecules* **2021**, *26*, 5718. [CrossRef]
6. Weisberg, S.P.; McCann, D.; Desai, M.; Rosenbaum, M.; Leibel, R.L.; Ferrante, A.W. Obesity Is Associated with Macrophage Accumulation in Adipose Tissue. *J. Clin. Investig.* **2003**, *112*, 1796–1808. [CrossRef]
7. Xu, H.; Barnes, G.T.; Yang, Q.; Tan, G.; Yang, D.; Chou, C.J.; Sole, J.; Nichols, A.; Ross, J.S.; Tartaglia, L.A.; et al. Chronic Inflammation in Fat Plays a Crucial Role in the Development of Obesity-Related Insulin Resistance. *J. Clin. Investig.* **2003**, *112*, 1821–1830. [CrossRef]
8. Subramanian, S.; Goodspeed, L.; Wang, S.; Kim, J.; Zeng, L.; Ioannou, G.N.; Haigh, W.G.; Yeh, M.M.; Kowdley, K.V.; O'Brien, K.D.; et al. Dietary Cholesterol Exacerbates Hepatic Steatosis and Inflammation in Obese LDL Receptor-Deficient Mice. *J. Lipid Res.* **2011**, *52*, 1626–1635. [CrossRef]
9. Subramanian, S.; Han, C.Y.; Chiba, T.; McMillen, T.S.; Wang, S.A.; Haw, A.; Kirk, E.A.; O'Brien, K.D.; Chait, A. Dietary Cholesterol Worsens Adipose Tissue Macrophage Accumulation and Atherosclerosis in Obese LDL Receptor–Deficient Mice. *Arter. Thromb. Vasc. Biol.* **2008**, *28*, 685–691. [CrossRef]
10. McNeill, K.; Fontana, L.; Ritter, J.; Russel-Jones, D.; Chowienczyk, P. Inhibitory Effects of Low-Density Lipoprotein on Endothelium-Dependent Relaxation Are Exaggerated in Men with NIDDM. *Diabetic. Med.* **1998**, *15*, S3–S4.
11. Dos Santos, K.G.; Yoshinaga, M.Y.; Glezer, I.; de Britto Chaves-Filho, A.; de Santana, A.A.; Kovacs, C.; Magnoni, C.D.; Lajolo, F.M.; Miyamoto, S.; Aymoto Hassimotto, N.M. Orange Juice Intake by Obese and Insulin-Resistant Subjects Lowers Specific Plasma Triglycerides: A Randomized Clinical Trial. *Clin. Nutr. ESPEN* **2022**, *51*, 336–344. [CrossRef] [PubMed]
12. Salamone, F. Moro Orange Juice Prevents Fatty Liver in Mice. *World J. Gastroenterol.* **2012**, *18*, 3862. [CrossRef] [PubMed]
13. Sorrenti, V.; Di Giacomo, C.; Acquaviva, R.; Cosenza, J.; Carota, G.; Galvano, F. Blond and Blood Juice Supplementation in High Fat Diet Fed Mice: Effect on Antioxidant Status and DDAH/ADMA Pathway. *RSC Adv.* **2019**, *9*, 11406–11412. [CrossRef] [PubMed]
14. Kaya, E.; Yilmaz, Y. Epidemiology, Natural History, and Diagnosis of Metabolic Dysfunction-Associated Fatty Liver Disease: A Comparative Review with Nonalcoholic Fatty Liver Disease. *Ther. Adv. Endocrinol. Metab.* **2022**, *13*, 204201882211396. [CrossRef] [PubMed]
15. Day, C.P.; James, O.F.W. Steatohepatitis: A Tale of Two "Hits"? *Gastroenterology* **1998**, *114*, 842–845. [CrossRef]

16. Eslam, M.; Newsome, P.N.; Sarin, S.K.; Anstee, Q.M.; Targher, G.; Romero-Gomez, M.; Zelber-Sagi, S.; Wai-Sun Wong, V.; Dufour, J.-F.; Schattenberg, J.M.; et al. A New Definition for Metabolic Dysfunction-Associated Fatty Liver Disease: An International Expert Consensus Statement. *J. Hepatol.* **2020**, *73*, 202–209. [CrossRef]
17. Boccatonda, A.; Andreetto, L.; D'Ardes, D.; Cocco, G.; Rossi, I.; Vicari, S.; Schiavone, C.; Cipollone, F.; Guagnano, M.T. From NAFLD to MAFLD: Definition, Pathophysiological Basis and Cardiovascular Implications. *Biomedicines* **2023**, *11*, 883. [CrossRef]
18. Smeriglio, A.; Cornara, L.; Denaro, M.; Barreca, D.; Burlando, B.; Xiao, J.; Trombetta, D. Antioxidant and Cytoprotective Activities of an Ancient Mediterranean Citrus (*Citrus Lumia Risso*) Albedo Extract: Microscopic Observations and Polyphenol Characterization. *Food Chem.* **2019**, *279*, 347–355. [CrossRef]
19. Vilar-Gomez, E.; Martinez-Perez, Y.; Calzadilla-Bertot, L.; Torres-Gonzalez, A.; Gra-Oramas, B.; Gonzalez-Fabian, L.; Friedman, S.L.; Diago, M.; Romero-Gomez, M. Weight Loss Through Lifestyle Modification Significantly Reduces Features of Nonalcoholic Steatohepatitis. *Gastroenterology* **2015**, *149*, 367–378e5. [CrossRef]
20. Kraus, W.; Bhapkar, M.; Huffman, K.M.; Pieper, C.F.; Das, S.K.; Redman, L.M.; Villareal, D.T.; Rochon, J.; Roberts, S.B.; Ravussin, E.; et al. 2 Years of Calorie Restriction and Cardiometabolic Risk (CALERIE): Exploratory Outcomes of a Multicentre, Phase 2, Randomised Controlled Trial. *Lancet Diabetes Endocrinol.* **2019**, *7*, 673–683. [CrossRef]
21. Green, C.L.; Lamming, D.W.; Fontana, L. Molecular Mechanisms of Dietary Restriction Promoting Health and Longevity. *Nat. Rev. Cell Biol.* **2022**, *23*, 56–73. [CrossRef] [PubMed]
22. Ruggenenti, P.; Abbate, M.; Ruggiero, B.; Rota, S.; Trillini, M.; Aparicio, C.; Parvanova, A.; Petrov Iliev, I.; Pisanu, G.; Perna, A.; et al. Renal and Systemic Effects of Calorie Restriction in Patients with Type 2 Diabetes with Abdominal Obesity: A Randomized Controlled Trial. *Diabetes* **2017**, *66*, 75–86. [CrossRef] [PubMed]
23. Hashimoto, T.; Cook, W.S.; Qi, C.; Yeldandi, A.V.; Reddy, J.K.; Rao, M.S. Defect in Peroxisome Proliferator-Activated Receptor α-Inducible Fatty Acid Oxidation Determines the Severity of Hepatic Steatosis in Response to Fasting. *J. Biol. Chem.* **2000**, *275*, 28918–28928. [CrossRef] [PubMed]
24. Seo, Y.S.; Kim, J.H.; Jo, N.Y.; Choi, K.M.; Baik, S.H.; Park, J.; Kim, J.S.; Byun, K.S.; Bak, Y.; Lee, C.H.; et al. PPAR Agonists Treatment Is Effective in a Nonalcoholic Fatty Liver Disease Animal Model by Modulating Fatty-acid Metabolic Enzymes. *J. Gastroenterol. Hepatol.* **2008**, *23*, 102–109. [CrossRef]
25. Kay, H.Y.; Kim, W.D.; Hwang, S.J.; Choi, H.-S.; Gilroy, R.K.; Wan, Y.-J.Y.; Kim, S.G. Nrf2 Inhibits LXRα-Dependent Hepatic Lipogenesis by Competing with FXR for Acetylase Binding. *Antioxid. Redox Signal* **2011**, *15*, 2135–2146. [CrossRef]
26. Kim, Y.W.; Kim, Y.M.; Yang, Y.M.; Kim, T.H.; Hwang, S.J.; Lee, J.R.; Kim, S.C.; Kim, S.G. Inhibition of SREBP-1c-Mediated Hepatic Steatosis and Oxidative Stress by Sauchinone, an AMPK-Activating Lignan in Saururus Chinensis. *Free Radic. Biol. Med.* **2010**, *48*, 567–578. [CrossRef]
27. Titta, L.; Trinei, M.; Stendardo, M.; Berniakovich, I.; Petroni, K.; Tonelli, C.; Riso, P.; Porrini, M.; Minucci, S.; Pelicci, P.G.; et al. Blood Orange Juice Inhibits Fat Accumulation in Mice. *Int. J. Obes.* **2010**, *34*, 578–588. [CrossRef]
28. FFujimori, A.S.; Ribeiro, A.P.; Pereira, A.G.; Dias-Audibert, F.L.; Tonon, C.R.; Dos Santos, P.P.; Dantas, D.; Zanati, S.G.; Catharino, R.R.; Zornoff, L.A.; et al. Effects of Pera Orange Juice and Moro Orange Juice in Healthy Rats: A Metabolomic Approach. *Metabolites* **2023**, *13*, 902. [CrossRef]
29. Pan, M.; Yang, G.; Li, S.; Li, M.; Tsai, M.; Wu, J.; Badmaev, V.; Ho, C.; Lai, C. Combination of Citrus Polymethoxyflavones, Green Tea Polyphenols, and Lychee Extracts Suppresses Obesity and Hepatic Steatosis in High-fat Diet Induced Obese Mice. *Mol. Nutr. Food Res.* **2017**, *61*, 1601104. [CrossRef]
30. Tsuda, T.; Horio, F.; Uchida, K.; Aoki, H.; Osawa, T. Dietary Cyanidin 3-O-β-D-Glucoside-Rich Purple Corn Color Prevents Obesity and Ameliorates Hyperglycemia in Mice. *J. Nutr.* **2003**, *133*, 2125–2130. [CrossRef]
31. Tangestani, H.; Jamshidi, A.; Farhadi, A.; Ghalandari, H.; Dehghani, P.; Moghaddas, N.; Safaei, Z.; Emamat, H. The Effects of Pomegranate (*Punica granatum*) on Nonalcoholic Fatty Liver Disease: A Systematic Review of in Vivo Interventional Studies. *Phytother. Res.* **2024**, *38*, 4189–4201. [CrossRef] [PubMed]
32. Sánchez-Terrón, G.; Martínez, R.; Morcuende, D.; Caballero, V.; Estévez, M. Pomegranate Supplementation Alleviates Dyslipidemia and the Onset of Non-Alcoholic Fatty Liver Disease in Wistar Rats by Shifting Microbiota and Producing Urolithin-like Microbial Metabolites. *Food Funct.* **2024**, *15*, 7348–7363. [CrossRef] [PubMed]
33. Jinato, T.; Chayanupatkul, M.; Dissayabutra, T.; Chutaputti, A.; Tangkijvanich, P.; Chuaypen, N. Litchi-Derived Polyphenol Alleviates Liver Steatosis and Gut Dysbiosis in Patients with Non-Alcoholic Fatty Liver Disease: A Randomized Double-Blinded, Placebo-Controlled Study. *Nutrients* **2022**, *14*, 2921. [CrossRef] [PubMed]
34. He, Z.; Li, X.; Yang, H.; Wu, P.; Wang, S.; Cao, D.; Guo, X.; Xu, Z.; Gao, J.; Zhang, W.; et al. Effects of Oral Vitamin C Supplementation on Liver Health and Associated Parameters in Patients with Non-Alcoholic Fatty Liver Disease: A Randomized Clinical Trial. *Front. Nutr.* **2021**, *8*, 5609. [CrossRef]
35. Lee, H.; Ahn, J.; Shin, S.S.; Yoon, M. Ascorbic Acid Inhibits Visceral Obesity and Nonalcoholic Fatty Liver Disease by Activating Peroxisome Proliferator-Activated Receptor α in High-Fat-Diet-Fed C57BL/6J Mice. *Int. J. Obes.* **2019**, *43*, 1620–1630. [CrossRef]
36. Kalyesubula, M.; Mopuri, R.; Asiku, J.; Rosov, A.; Yosefi, S.; Edery, N.; Bocobza, S.; Moallem, U.; Dvir, H. High-Dose Vitamin B1 Therapy Prevents the Development of Experimental Fatty Liver Driven by Overnutrition. *Dis. Model. Mech.* **2021**, *14*, dmm048355. [CrossRef]

37. Wang, Y.; Bian, X.; Wan, M.; Dong, W.; Gao, W.; Yao, Z.; Guo, C. Effects of Riboflavin Deficiency and High Dietary Fat on Hepatic Lipid Accumulation: A Synergetic Action in the Development of Non-Alcoholic Fatty Liver Disease. *Nutr. Metab.* **2024**, *21*, 1. [CrossRef]
38. Pathak, M.P.; Pathak, K.; Saikia, R.; Gogoi, U.; Patowary, P.; Chattopadhyay, P.; Das, A. Therapeutic Potential of Bioactive Phytoconstituents Found in Fruits in the Treatment of Non-Alcoholic Fatty Liver Disease: A Comprehensive Review. *Heliyon* **2023**, *9*, e15347. [CrossRef]
39. Beygi, M.; Ahi, S.; Zolghadri, S.; Stanek, A. Management of Metabolic-Associated Fatty Liver Disease/Metabolic Dysfunction-Associated Steatotic Liver Disease: From Medication Therapy to Nutritional Interventions. *Nutrients* **2024**, *16*, 2220. [CrossRef]
40. Hu, M.; Zhang, L.; Ruan, Z.; Han, P.; Yu, Y. The Regulatory Effects of Citrus Peel Powder on Liver Metabolites and Gut Flora in Mice with Non-Alcoholic Fatty Liver Disease (NAFLD). *Foods* **2021**, *10*, 3022. [CrossRef]
41. Song, H.; Shen, X.; Chu, Q.; Zheng, X. Pomegranate Fruit Pulp Polyphenols Reduce Diet-induced Obesity with Modulation of Gut Microbiota in Mice. *J. Sci. Food Agric.* **2022**, *102*, 1968–1977. [CrossRef] [PubMed]
42. Silva Figueiredo, P.; Carla Inada, A.; Marcelino, G.; Maiara Lopes Cardozo, C.; De Cássia Freitas, K.; De Cássia Avellaneda Guimarães, R.; Pereira de Castro, A.; Aragão do Nascimento, V.; Aiko Hiane, P. Fatty Acids Consumption: The Role Metabolic Aspects Involved in Obesity and Its Associated Disorders. *Nutrients* **2017**, *9*, 1158. [CrossRef] [PubMed]
43. Tsitsou, S.; Cholongitas, E.; Bali, T.; Neonaki, A.; Poulia, K.-A.; Papakonstantinou, E. Effects of Time-Restricted Hypocaloric Mediterranean Diet in Patients with Non-Alcoholic Fatty Liver Disease: Preliminary Data from the CHRONO-NAFLD Project. *Proceedings* **2024**, *91*, 359. [CrossRef]
44. Zhang, X.; Zhang, Y.; Gao, W.; Guo, Z.; Wang, K.; Liu, S.; Duan, Z.; Chen, Y. Naringin Improves Lipid Metabolism in a Tissue-Engineered Liver Model of NAFLD and the Underlying Mechanisms. *Life Sci.* **2021**, *277*, 119487. [CrossRef]
45. Wang, Q.; Ou, Y.; Hu, G.; Wen, C.; Yue, S.; Chen, C.; Xu, L.; Xie, J.; Dai, H.; Xiao, H.; et al. Naringenin Attenuates Non-alcoholic Fatty Liver Disease by Down-regulating the NLRP3/NF-κB Pathway in Mice. *Br. J. Pharmacol.* **2020**, *177*, 1806–1821. [CrossRef]

*nutrients*

MDPI

*Article*

# A Qualitative Study Supporting Optimal Nutrition in Advanced Liver Disease—Unlocking the Potential for Improvement

**Shaye Ludlow [1,2], Katherine Farragher [3], Kelly Squires [3], Susan Heaney [4], Jessica Orman [1,2], Sarah Pullen [1,2], John Attia [1,2,5] and Katie Wynne [1,2,5,*]**

1 John Hunter Hospital, Hunter New England Local Heath District, New Lambton Heights, NSW 2305, Australia; shaye.ludlow@health.nsw.gov.au (S.L.); jessica.orman@health.nsw.gov.au (J.O.); sarah.pullen@health.nsw.gov.au (S.P.); john.attia@newcastle.edu.au (J.A.)
2 Hunter Medical Research Institute, Equity in Health and Wellbeing, New Lambton Heights, NSW 2305, Australia
3 School of Health Sciences, University of Newcastle, Callaghan, NSW 2308, Australia; katherine.farragher@uon.edu.au (K.F.); kelly.squires@newcastle.edu.au (K.S.)
4 Department of Rural Health, University of Newcastle, Port Macquarie, NSW 2444, Australia; susan.heaney@newcastle.edu.au
5 School of Medicine and Public Health, The University of Newcastle, Callaghan, NSW 2308, Australia
* Correspondence: katiejane.wynne@health.nsw.gov.au

**Abstract:** Malnutrition rates in Advanced Liver Disease (ALD) are significantly higher than those in well-compensated liver disease. In addition to its physiological impact, malnutrition is detrimental for quality of life and social, emotional, and psychological well-being. Studies within oncology and renal supportive care have identified the influence of non-physiological factors on malnutrition risk. Integrating similar factors into malnutrition screening for ALD could improve identification of at-risk patients to optimize treatment planning. This qualitative study aimed to understand the holistic factors influencing nutritional status in the ALD population. Semi-structured interviews with 21 patients, carers, and clinicians explored the experiences of malnutrition in ALD. Thematic analysis revealed five key themes: (i) appropriateness of healthcare delivery; (ii) health- and food-related factors; (iii) high symptom burden, (iv) social support impacting well-being, and (v) physical and structural supports. Current screening methods do not adequately capture all potential drivers of malnutrition in the ALD population. Adopting a more supportive approach including both physiological and non-physiological factors in ALD malnutrition screening may promote more timely and comprehensive nutritional interventions that address the complex and holistic needs of patients living with ALD.

**Keywords:** liver disease; malnutrition; quality of life; social support; supportive care; palliative care; screening; assessment

## 1. Introduction

Malnutrition in Advanced Liver Disease (ALD) is common and contributes to high symptom burden, poorer health outcomes, increased hospital admissions, increased healthcare costs, decreased quality of life, and increased rates of mortality [1–6]. Studies have shown that 20% of people living with well-compensated liver disease suffer from malnutrition, with rates increasing to 60–85% in people in advanced stages of the disease [1–3,6]. Malnutrition directly impacts severe complications of liver cirrhosis, such as ascites, hepatic encephalopathy, and infections, worsening prognosis and reducing quality of life [6].

Early detection and diagnosis of malnutrition is essential in ALD. The European Society for Clinical Nutrition and Metabolism (ESPEN) guidelines recommend initial screening for malnutrition using a validated tool [1–3,6,7]. While most globally used validated screening tools seek to identify changes in dietary intake and weight, screening for malnutrition in ALD can be difficult. The fluid buildup from edema and ascites may mask weight changes, leading to inaccurate weight and body mass index calculations and thereby decreasing the accuracy of these tools and potentially underestimating malnutrition risk [6–8]. As a result, nutritional intervention is often delayed [6]. The Malnutrition Screening Tool (MST) is an example of a screening tool commonly used in clinical practice [3]. It is a popular tool as it is validated across multiple conditions, can be completed by any staff member, and can be easily applied in all settings [3]. However, it is less likely to be effective in this population as it only uses intake and weight as indicators of risk of malnutrition [3]. Some studies have shown that in patients with cirrhosis, the MST has poor diagnostic ability, with reduced sensitivity and lower prevalence of identified malnutrition risk when compared with other screening tools [2].

The Patient-Generated Subjective Global Assessment Short Form (PG-SGA Short Form) includes a wider range of nutritional symptoms such as nausea, taste change, and loss of appetite, with the option to include additional factors under the category of 'other' [9]. However, this 'other' information is reliant on a patient's health literacy or understanding of the condition to recognize key details to convey for effective identification and prioritization of need [9]. Alternatively, the Royal Free Hospital-Nutrition Prioritizing Tool (RFH-NPT) is recommended by the European Society for Enteral and Parenteral Nutrition (ESPEN) guidelines for malnutrition screening in patients with ALD as it is disease-specific and considers factors beyond intake and weight [1,3]. Included in the tool are disease-related complications such as ascites and general fluid overload, therefore improving its effectiveness for malnutrition risk detection in this population [6,10].

Non-physiological determinants such as personal, religious, and cultural values and psychological factors play a role in malnutrition etiology but are not routinely captured in current tools [3,6–8,11,12]. While there is limited evidence investigating the non-physiological determinants of malnutrition in ALD populations, studies in other patient groups with comparable high symptom burdens, such as oncology and renal supportive care, have shown that incorporating these additional factors leads to more timely nutritional intervention for those at risk of malnutrition [11,12]. This allows for better management of symptoms, improved physical function and independence, and improved quality of life [11,12].

Given the significant impact of malnutrition on ALD outcomes and emerging evidence regarding the benefit of incorporating non-physiological determinants of malnutrition in screening for ALD, a broader approach to malnutrition screening is required. The primary aim of this research is to identify these additional non-physiological factors for use in malnutrition screening for patients with ALD that could inform a patient-reported screening tool. Consumer engagement explored the lived experience of nutrition concerns in this patient group through qualitative methods. Such consumer involvement has been shown to increase the quality, impact, and reach of clinical research [13].

## 2. Materials and Methods

This qualitative study is reported in accordance with the 'Standards for Reporting Qualitative Research (SRQR): A Synthesis of Recommendations' [14]. Ethics approval was provided by Hunter New England Ethics Committee reference (2022/ETH02426) on 21 December 2022. Registration was granted by the Australian New Zealand Clinical Trials Registry (ANZCTR), ACTRN12624000472572.

### 2.1. Setting

This study was conducted within complex and supportive care liver clinics across one metropolitan and one regional Australian public health site.

### 2.2. Research Steering Committee

The research team comprised a ten-member steering committee consisting of researchers, doctors, nurses, and dieticians with experience in ALD. An early-career research dietician skilled in working with ALD patients and supportive care convened the research steering committee. The research dietician worked collaboratively under the guidance of the broader research steering committee, seeking feedback and direction on every aspect of the study design, implementation, and evaluation.

### 2.3. Consumer Input

For this study, it was vital to engage with a range of consumers to improve the researchers' understanding of the lived experience of malnutrition in ALD and to ensure the richness of the data. Consumers consisted of (i) patients and (ii) carers.

Patients were eligible if they were 18 years of age or older, attended one of the liver clinics in the research setting, were able to provide informed consent, and had Child–Pugh B or C liver disease. As a range of lived experience was sought, current malnutrition was not an inclusion criterion for the study; participants were invited if they had Child–Pugh B or C status as this group would be more likely to have a current or future risk of undernutrition and receive dietetic input. Carers of any patient meeting the eligibility criteria were invited to participate, with their participation dependent on receiving informed consent from the patient.

### 2.4. Clinician Input

Dieticians, nurses, social workers, and doctors who worked across either research site were eligible to participate. These health workers needed to be currently employed at one of the liver clinics in the setting, caring for patients who met the eligibility criteria and/or have experience working with the ALD population.

### 2.5. Recruitment

Recruitment occurred between January and March 2023. Eligible patients and carers were identified from those who attended a clinic within the research setting. In consultation with site leads for the Department of Nutrition and Dietetics, Gastroenterology and Supportive Care, the research dietician identified key staff members with experience in ALD who were purposefully sampled and invited to participate. Due to a limited number of dieticians available at the regional site, dieticians from an outlying health campus with expertise in ALD were nominated by department leads to provide a broader range of input and regional perspective. Clinicians who provided consent to participate were provided an information sheet prior to contact with the research dietician.

### 2.6. Data Collection

Semi-structured interviews were conducted with all consumers between January and March 2023. Interviews were facilitated by the research dietician (blinded for peer review) either in person, via phone, or virtually using Microsoft Teams. Interview guides were developed to promote consistency in the data collected (see Tables 1 and 2) based on the literature and the research team's knowledge and clinical experience. Thirteen clinicians were interviewed either individually or in small groups of two or three. All patients and carers were interviewed individually.

Adroit Transcription was used to transcribe a total of eleven interviews with thirteen participants, including two focus groups [15]. A glossary of terms was provided to transcribers to give context to the interviews for more accurate transcription (see Table S1). The remaining nine participant interviews were transcribed manually by the research team due to poor recording quality. Each transcript was then checked by two members of the research team (blinded for peer review) for accuracy.

**Table 1.** Interview Guide for Clinicians.

| **Welcome and Introductions.** |
|---|
| Experiences of nutrition care in complex liver clinics. |
| • What is your experience of using nutrition screening and assessment tools in standard practice?<br>• Can you explain the referral processes to the dietician currently used in standard care? Can you explain how these processes are effective or ineffective in identifying those patients requiring nutrition support?<br>• From your point of view, what are some of the factors influencing an ALD patient's nutrition?<br>• How do current nutrition screening tools account for these factors?<br>• Can you explain how non-physiological factors (for example, food security, culture, dentition, psychosocial and emotional well-being) influence nutrition for patients living with ALD? |
| Positive/negative comments. |
| • Can you explain the positive components of the nutrition screening tools currently used in standard practice? What works well?<br>• Can you explain the negative components of the nutrition screening tools currently used in standard practice? What doesn't work well? |
| Feedback and suggestions for screening tool development. |
| • What are your suggestions on how the screening of nutrition in ALD patients could be improved?<br>• How could the non-physiological determinants of nutrition be incorporated into a new nutrition screening tool for ALD patients?<br>• What are the main physiological and non-physiological components or considerations you think are important to include in the novel screening tool? |
| General suggestions. |
| • Do you have any general recommendations?<br>• Do you have any other comments? |

**Table 2.** Interview Guide for Patients and Carers.

| **Welcome and Introductions.** |
|---|
| We know that nutrition can affect more than just your physical health. It can also be important to people's connection with their family, quality of life, culture and social and emotional well-being. We'd like to ask you a few questions about nutrition, which will help us improve the way we plan and provide nutritional care |
| Experiences of care. |
| • Can you tell me how nutrition affects your daily life?<br>• Other than your physical health, can you explain how nutrition impacts other areas of your well-being? |
| Positive/negative comments. |
| • What are the things that make it hard for you to have good nutrition?<br>• What are the things that might help you have good nutrition? |
| Feedback. |
| • What things do you think are important for the healthcare team to consider when asking about your nutrition and how it affects your daily life? |
| General suggestions |
| • Do you have any general suggestions or comments? |

### 2.7. Data Analysis

Transcripts were de-identified and analyzed thematically using the Braun and Clarke method [16]. The initial coding was completed by two members of the research team (blinded for peer review) who spent time familiarizing themselves with the transcribed interviews by completing iterative readthroughs of each interview to gain maximum insight [16]. Codes were generated for as many topics as possible, ensuring that the code was not just a phrase but rather applied to a contextual segment of the interview. Two members of the research steering committee (the dietetic honors student and one senior research dietician) generated themes from the existing codes and sorted these into categories that best encompassed their meaning [16]. Themes were further refined during two consultations with the broader research steering committee for review, revisiting and reorganizing codes and subthemes until a consensus was obtained [16]. The sample size was deemed large enough to provide adequate information power due to the narrow focus of the study, specific sample population, and clinical expertise of the research team [17]. Supporting exemplars were then extracted from the text, aiding in the refining of the names of the themes, ensuring that they were conceptually parallel [16]. NVivo 12 software was used to assist in the organization and visualization of the data [18].

## 3. Results

There was a total of twenty-two participants included in this study: eleven clinicians, nine participants, and two carers. Five clinicians and two patients came from the regional sites. Six clinicians, seven patients, and two carers came from the metropolitan site (see Figure 1). Patient participants had a diagnosis of hepatitis B, hepatitis C, and/or alcoholic liver disease and had received dietician input into their care planning during standard care liver clinics in the six months prior to being recruited to the study. Two of these patient participants had been diagnosed with hepatocellular carcinoma, with one having received immunotherapy. There was a 100% participation rate with all patients, carers, and clinicians approached for the study agreeing to be interviewed. Interviews lasted between five and thirty minutes.

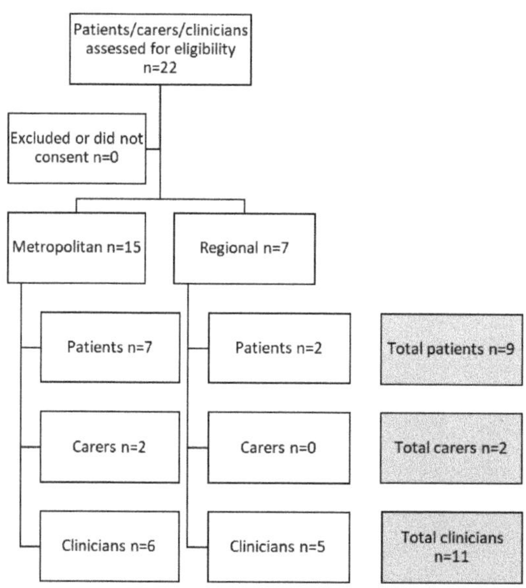


**Figure 1.** Flow chart for the recruitment of participants.

When exploring the factors influencing the nutritional status of the ALD population, five main themes were identified: (i) appropriateness of healthcare delivery; (ii) health- and food-related factors; (iii) high symptom burden, (iv) social support impacting well-being, and (v) physical and structural supports (see Table 3 for themes, sub-themes, and supporting quotes).

**Table 3.** Themes, sub-themes, and supporting quotes.

| Theme | Sub-Theme | Demonstrative Quotes—Patient or Carer | Demonstrative Quotes—Clinician |
| --- | --- | --- | --- |
| Appropriateness of Healthcare Delivery | Accurate Screening/Correct Referrals | "Yeah well didn't have the right people around her. I suppose it was month in, month off, every six weeks she'd end up in [de-identified] Hospital, um, she'd make little improvements, but there was no eating involved. Ah, she made little improvements then they'd send her home. Um, and you'd just wait five or six days and we're on the downhill slide again. Look, the only thing that changed (de-identified) life was meeting that lady in the waiting room that day and getting (de-identified) in the liver clinic, or my daughter would be dead." (carer) | "They might have already been in the hospital for say, five days, before we even know about them and I think that really is a reflection of the MST, not capturing the issues that the patient has." (clinician)<br>"If there was an effective screening tool, that would obviously create more referrals to a dietician, or more appropriate referrals, potentially. What I know across the hospital, is a malnutrition screening tool is, not sensitive enough to pick up the people who really need it or often results in multiple referrals for people who don't really need to see a dietician at all, so I think it really needs to be developed for the population that we are looking at, at the time, or using something more in depth than just a MST" (clinician)<br>"Very difficult with weight changes-increase in ascites [and] decrease in muscle mass." (clinician)<br>"it's just a bit of a hit and miss. . .it doesn't seem to be a real clear process. . . [of] who gets referred to the dietician". (clinician) |
| | Supportive Care Team | "If I needed to ring up and ask a question about if I could eat something or not, eat something which is great, like you guys jumped on. If you guys didn't know. I know you personally look up for me whether I should have it or how much I would like to have that." (patient)<br>"I was (de-identified) primary carer and the kids' primary carer, I had somebody. . .you blokes were ringing me up a couple of times per week, just to make sure how things were going and that. Do you know how much benefit that did for me? Do you know how much benefit that gave (de-identified)? Knowing somebody gave a s**t. . .but you blokes are liver specialists and dieticians and doctors and. . .mental health person, you know she was beautiful too. Having the right group around you, especially a group that sort of specialises in that stuff, if you like, when no-one else really took it very serious, so um, life changing, for both of us." (carer) | "entering a more. . .transient approach. . .being in the same room, or sharing notes, getting a bigger picture of what's happening in the world and bouncing off each other always seems to work really well." (clinician) |

**Table 3.** *Cont.*

| Theme | Sub-Theme | Demonstrative Quotes—Patient or Carer | Demonstrative Quotes—Clinician |
| --- | --- | --- | --- |
| Health- and Food-Related Factors | Dentition | "had to have a root canal the other week. So they've been pretty bad and there's more to be done there. . .I don't have the money, but I don't want to go around with no teeth either." (patient)<br>"they said if you don't. . .get that tooth fixed, you won't be able to eat on that side of your mouth." (patient)<br>"[food] gets stuck all over my dentures. . .I gotta keep going to the bathroom and cleaning my teeth out." (patient) | "We've had patients with dental issues that's impacted their nutrition" (clinician)<br>"issues with dentition" (clinician)<br>"changes to dentition of course changes what people can eat and what they can tolerate, that links in often with financial things, not being able to get their teeth fixed, or access the services that they need" (clinician) |
| | Food Literacy | "You know, last night I had a bit of cheese and flavoured milk and all that and that's always good, you know I'll drink flavoured milk rather than drink an apple juice, or something like that. yeah, yeah, so good education and meal suggestions [would help improve nutrition]" (patient)<br>"And the goodness [they're] getting from the food to make it worthwhile eating, hmm. Like common understanding of nutrition." (patient) | "I'd say, like cooking skills and food preparation skills are, on average, lower in this population". (clinician)<br>"the health literacy of a lot of the patients that come to clinic and I guess. . . it has to be balanced. . . a lot of patients would struggle or lose interest or not understand." (clinician)<br>"they've not had good, potentially, dietary or nutrition inputs until now and so those [negative] habits are formed." (clinician)<br>"I guess general knowledge about health because they probably, I know it's very stereo-typical but, um, they've not made positive, healthy, lifestyle choices, so it's hard to break that barrier as well, sometimes." (clinician) |
| | Alcohol Consumption | "I had wine and there was two and then there was three and then there was four long drinks. I'd drink right up until news was over at 7 o'clock, cook some dinner and have one bite and put it in the fridge, saying I'd have it tomorrow and it'd end up in the bin, so the alcohol was probably sustaining my hunger perhaps, I don't know, but it put me in the wrong frame of mind to get some tucker in to me and feeling healthy." (patient) | "There can often still be alcohol consumption, which can affect their nutrition." (clinician)<br>"a lot of people we do know still have a reliance on alcohol as well, which can impact their nutritional status, so I guess it's multi-factorial." (clinician) |

**Table 3.** *Cont.*

| Theme | Sub-Theme | Demonstrative Quotes—Patient or Carer | Demonstrative Quotes—Clinician |
| --- | --- | --- | --- |
| High Symptom Burden | Sickness | "Oh, um, well at the moment, 'cause being sick and all that, sort of affects [diet] probably different ways than what you'd probably expect." (patient)<br>"it's the absolute sickness." (patient)<br>"She spent more time with her head in a bucket, than she did with her head on a pillow" (carer) | "stage of disease [influences nutrition]." (clinician)<br>"the disease state is probably a big thing, in progression." (clinician) |
| | Unexpected Symptoms | "I was eating perfectly and then one day I just decided I didn't feel like eating anymore and yeah food just didn't interest me at all like nothing and it took a very long time to get that interest that I wanted to eat back that's for sure" (patient)<br>"I get full pretty quick." (patient) | "physiological things, ascites, nausea, vomiting, poor appetite, loss of taste," (clinician) |
| | Cascade | "And quite often when I eat I throw up. Just out of the blue. But with some nausea in the beginning or just randomly after eating... I ate and it makes it worse, because you're feeling so uncomfortable." (patient) | "a lot of people with liver disease, their ascites can cause nausea and... shortness of breath and things as their ascites can build up...and impact their diet in that way and changes to their bowels." (clinician) |
| | Loss of Interest in Food | "Yeah, that most people find it a really pleasurable thing whereas it's a bit of a chore for me [eating]." (patient)<br>"I do get a funny taste in my mouth...it's like a filter's been put over my tongue and my tastebuds. If I want to try and enjoy something and that filter's over there and I can't taste it, I think well what's the point?" (patient)<br>"I went to the butcher today and I bought all this stuff. I thought, well I'm really good at buying food, sometimes I'm good at preparing it, I'm just not good at eating it" (patient)<br>"No appetite, like I literally have to make myself eat" (patient)<br>"The ascites, I think, had a lot to do with it and having the NG tube made it harder to eat for me." (patient)<br>"He's gone off meat and everything like that, so it's hard to get him interested in food, to get him to eat." (carer) | "I think, a lot of the time I think there is loss of appetite." (clinician)<br>"The ascites is when they're really quite bloated, they find it difficult to eat." (clinician) |
| | Loss of Motivation | "It's just...it's just the energy level, I just can't be bothered making...I bought that Light and Easy, but I've gone off that, so...I really don't know what I'm going to do for...I just can't be bothered, type of thing." (patient)<br>"Sometimes it's day three of diarrhea and I feel rotten, so I can plan that sort of stuff but as far as a meal goes, food goes, I, plan it but...I won't go ahead with it." (patient)<br>"When I'm in a care situation and food's put in front of you...it's easier to do that. I need to get the motivation to cook for myself and enjoy that again." (patient) | "people may not have always had healthy eating habits and but it's also actually identifying do they actually see that as a problem, do they want help with that". (clinician)<br>"that motivation to cook and to...actually prepare the meals can be limited as well" |

**Table 3.** *Cont.*

| Theme | Sub-Theme | Demonstrative Quotes—Patient or Carer | Demonstrative Quotes—Clinician |
|---|---|---|---|
| | Confusion | "you're just too confused to even think about food." (patient) | "When they [are] confused, they just don't wanna eat. They get to the point where, yeah, they just don't wanna eat." (clinician) |
| | Loss of Energy | "Physically, I couldn't walk. I literally couldn't lift my three-month-old son up at the time, I barely could move off the lounge. I just slept all day. I had no energy whatsoever. . . I couldn't go to the shops, I couldn't carry any bags I couldn't take the kids to the park or out to the beach or anywhere like that because I physically couldn't walk more than 5 meters" (patient)<br>"My body's not absorbing protein so that makes me really tired and then you get tired and it's just like that wicked circle again, you get tired, you can't be bothered you just don't do and I'm just trying to step over that at the moment" (patient)<br>"she didn't have the strength, the energy, she didn't have um, the desire." (carer) | "One of the key symptoms that you see from the liver clinic which probably 90 per cent of people experience is lethargy and so preparing something that's nutritious and that doesn't come out of a packet somewhere or from a take-away store is. . .takes energy and that can steal something from their ability" (clinician)<br>"Their, energy levels, and you know, um, their desire to eat and prepare food." (clinician) |
| | Depression | "When I'm depressed I don't eat." (patient)<br>"Not having the nutrition that I needed to have, it depressed me a lot, it gave me depression I couldn't even take my daughter to school, I couldn't be there for her year 6 formal, yeah so my family missed out on a lot with their mum I guess as well like they suffered a lot for me being sick." (patient)<br>"If you're not eating and you're not getting that nutrition, you're not feeling like wanting to do anything. And then that affects your mental health, like it's a you know a horrid cycle." (patient) | "I think sometimes some of these people, like, you'd say 80 per cent of them are probably depressed. . .and that's got to have an impact on, on motivation." (clinician) |
| | Varices | | "Often may have swallowing difficulties or dysphagia related to varices" (clinician) |
| Social Support Impacting Well-being | Need for Support | "I do online shopping and I make it for a day and a time that I know that someone else is going to be here because they drop it to the door, which is great, but then I've got to get it from the door to the kitchen and I can't make it." (patient) | "I think it's important to know their level of support, at home, like carers. . .like meals on wheels, things like that, are they using any services, what services are there that can help." (clinician)<br>"Sometimes don't have good support networks so not only do they often forget or not hear the messages being given clearly during clinic they don't have that network to help keep them on the right path once at home and assist when needed/having a low health day." (clinician) |

**Table 3.** *Cont.*

| Theme | Sub-Theme | Demonstrative Quotes—Patient or Carer | Demonstrative Quotes—Clinician |
| --- | --- | --- | --- |
| | Loss of Independence/Challenges with Independence | "I was a very independent person, I did everything on my own, I never asked for help, I was very stubborn... Whereas now, I'm like, 'yes please, can you do this for me'. So that's kind of what's changed me a lot I suppose." (patient)<br>"My dad took care of me and my kids and did a lot of the grunt work for me cause I couldn't physically do it but he helped a lot and he helped a lot to get me to eat, he'd get me food that I thought I'd like to eat and not forcing me but re reassuring me that I had to eat pretty much that was the only way I was going to get better." (patient)<br>"I ended up moving me and my kids in with my dad to support me for a few months that I couldn't eat and couldn't function properly and so much. So you take my kids to school and run me to the doctor appointments and things like that because I couldn't drive because I was so malnutrition and I was so skinny." (patient)<br>"I was with the NG tube, I pretty much didn't eat at all. He tried to get me to have family meals with them guys, but I'd have a mouthful and that'd be enough. And gradually got to the point where I'd have lunch with them, and then I would have a family dinner. But I'll be little and then gradually got more and more. He'd buy me vanilla slices and things like that just to try and fatten me up a little bit and it worked and it definitely worked." (patient)<br>"If I didn't have his support too. I don't think I would have the energy or the will to even want to cook anything to eat or go to the shops to get anything that I'd like, which where he would do them things for me, which helped a lot." (patient)<br>"I try to always have a decent tea, you know, even if I've eaten nothing or, you know, rubbish, throughout the day, I will try to have like a normal tea, where we sit down, at the table, like a family, ah, if I'm not, ah, eating, I don't obviously, go to the table. You know, that takes away from that family sort of time." (patient)<br>"My daughter, she cooks meals every day and she will let me go maybe one or two days and then that's...she's like 'nah, that's it, you haven't had this for ages' and I'm like 'uh, but I don't feel like it' and she'll just dish me up something. And I will find, probably seven out of ten times, that I do eat it." (patient) | "somehow feeling responsible for what's happened to them and um, not worthy of some of the help that some people can easily access, is easily a barrier" (clinician)<br>"lack of social support...especially if they are living on their own and they're feeling so poorly." (clinician) |

**Table 3.** *Cont.*

| Theme | Sub-Theme | Demonstrative Quotes—Patient or Carer | Demonstrative Quotes—Clinician |
|---|---|---|---|
| | Social Isolation | "I didn't attend my grand-daughter's um, engagement party on Saturday, just because you know, I hadn't been eating and also too, because I am getting tired because also you don't eat so I'm 'I've got to sit down, I've got to sit down', you know I'd be forever feeling I was being that wet towel, always hanging around, so I just said I wasn't going to go and so I missed out on that." (patient) | "I mean there's a big difference in the patients who have a family or you know, have a partner and ah, patients who are single, and are on their own, yeah because I think you know, a lot of the older, single men, really struggle." (clinician) |
| Physical and Structural Supports | Socioeconomic Status | "my dad helped me financially." (patient) | "Being able to afford to eat the amount of protein or the amount of food, you know, or get all of those medical appointments in, travel back and forth to [regional hospital]. . .it's a huge impact, out here especially. (clinician)<br>"Patients can't afford to buy the appropriate foods, at times." (clinician)<br>"lower socioeconomic [status] as well, so financial barriers, transport barriers, things like that." (clinician)<br>"I think that food security is a bigger issue than we credit in a lot of different disease groups, that for a lot of people with um, liver disease, that could be an issue if they are no longer working, and they don't have a huge social network that can support them." (clinician) |
| | Affording Nutrition Treatment Options | "I'm on the DSP [Disability Support Pension] . . . I don't work at the moment, so I don't have that money to spend [on supplement drinks]" (patient)<br>"The dieticians that say "have those pro-biotic drinks" and this, that and the other, and they're not cheap, you know, like, I've got to provide for a family so I try and get stuff that we can all eat and so, yep, the finances would. . .would play a part in it. You know I buy different things for the family that I wouldn't have just for myself." (patient) | "They might be on a supplement here in hospital, but they simply can't afford that when they go home so we're often recommending things like up and go energisers, stuff like that, that they can easily pick up at the supermarket that might be a bit cheaper, so financial. . .those factors are, huge." (clinician)<br>"Socioeconomics is a big issue, you know, people being able to afford supplements." (clinician) |

### *3.1. Appropriateness of Healthcare Delivery*

Timely referrals and capturing and addressing what matters most to patients and their carers were highlighted by carers and clinicians as important factors in this study. Patients recognized the benefit of being able to "ring up and ask a question" and carers identified "having the right group around you, especially a group that sort of specializes in that stuff. . .when no-one else really took very serious, so um, life-changing, for both of us". Clinicians acknowledged that it was difficult to assess malnutrition risk with weight changes alone due to an "increase in ascites [and] decrease in muscle mass". This highlighted the need for a screening tool that could screen for more symptoms specific to the ALD population to allow for more appropriate referrals to dieticians. Clinicians identified that the current method of screening for malnutrition was "just a bit of a hit and miss" without "a real clear process of who gets referred to the dietician" and "not capturing the issues that the patient has".

### *3.2. Health- and Food-Related Factors*

One patient identified that having a "common understanding of nutrition" would help increase their intake as they would then be able to understand "the goodness [they're] getting from the food to make it worthwhile eating". For some patients, it was recognized by clinicians that "they've not had good, potentially, dietary or nutrition inputs until now and so those [negative] habits are formed", as well as "a lot of people we do know still have a reliance on alcohol as well" which can then make it "hard to break that barrier as well, sometimes." Clinicians noted that this impeded some patients' comprehension of the provided education regarding how food and nutrition may impact ALD.

It was identified by a clinician that there are "multi-factorial" components that can impact the nutrition of people with ALD. Clinicians reported the patients' "cooking skills and food preparation skills are, on average, lower in this population" and could adversely affect their nutritional status. Additionally, it was recognized that aspects such as "issues with dentition" could impact their nutritional status as it "changes what people can eat and what they can tolerate, that links in often with financial things, not being able to get their teeth fixed, or access the services that they need." This comment reflects difficulties patients have accessing public dental health services in Australia due to the associated costs, waiting times, limited transport options, and fewer dental practitioners in rural areas [19].

### *3.3. High Symptom Burden*

It was identified by patients, carers, and clinicians that the common physiological symptoms associated with ALD, such as ascites, nausea, vomiting, poor appetite, and loss of taste, could affect a patient's ability to maintain good nutrition. This was best described by one patient as the "absolute sickness" that would get in the way of their nutrition.

While for some patients the symptoms were unexpected without an apparent specific cause, for others, symptom burden was recognized as being complex and often interrelated, causing a cascade effect on intake: "I was eating perfectly, and then one day I just decided I didn't feel like eating anymore" and "Quite often when I eat, I throw up. Just out of the blue". As a result of these symptoms, there was a loss of interest in food, making eating more challenging and akin to an obligatory task. The motivation to eat could be quite transient and subject to frequent changes.

For some patients, despite best intentions, the experiences of symptoms impacted "that motivation to cook" and to "actually prepare the meals", as highlighted by one patient after frequent bouts of diarrhea impacted their ability to proceed with planned meals. Additionally, one clinician reported that "80 per cent of them [patients] are probably depressed," suggesting that low mood would further impact motivation and ability to look after one's nutrition. As a result of experiencing symptoms, patients' reduced energy levels were recognized as impacting their ability to prepare meals; this began even before the meal preparation stages, in being able to source food from the shops and get it home.

"Physically, I couldn't walk. I literally couldn't lift my three-month-old son up at the time, I barely could move off the lounge. I just slept all day".

### 3.4. Social Support Affecting Well-Being

Patients, carers, and clinicians identified the significance of social support for people living with ALD. Patients with ALD reported a loss of independence and the need for more support from family, friends, and carers, as exemplified by one patient's statement: "I was a very independent person, I did everything on my own, I never asked for help, I was very stubborn… Whereas now, I'm like, 'yes please, can you do this for me'. So that's kind of what's changed me a lot I suppose".

However, patients also recognized that their waning interest in food sometimes led them to decline social invitations for fear of bringing a negative atmosphere, resulting in missed opportunities for a supportive social dining experience. One patient responded that "I didn't attend my grand-daughter's um, engagement party on Saturday, just because you know, I hadn't been eating and also too, because I am getting tired because also you don't eat so I'm "I've got to sit down, I've got to sit down", you know I'd be forever feeling I was being that wet towel, always hanging around, so I just said I wasn't going to go and so I missed out on that."

Clinicians reported they noticed "a big difference in the patients who have a family, or you know, have a partner and patients who are single and are on their own". When patients had a "lack of social support…especially if they are living on their own and they're feeling so poorly", this would impact a patient's ability to maintain good nutrition due to difficulty shopping for food and preparing meals.

### 3.5. Physical and Structural Support

Financial concerns were raised by some patient participants, with one patient responding that "I'm on the DSP [Disability Support Pension] … I don't work at the moment, so I don't have that money to spend". It was identified by clinicians that a number of barriers could affect a patient's ability to maintain good nutrition; these were recognized as patients of "lower socioeconomic [status] as well, so financial barriers, transport barriers, things like that".

In the clinicians' experiences, finance had a big impact on "being able to afford to eat the amount of protein or the amount of food". This was reinforced by patients when they were required to purchase specialty items to manage their condition or when patients were required to access nutritional support to ensure they could meet their nutritional requirements. In some instances, clinicians stated that patients would respond "no" when asked if they could afford to purchase nutritional supplement drinks. As a result, the dieticians were altering recommendations to meet the financial needs of the patients.

## 4. Discussion

This novel study aimed to understand the non-traditional factors influencing the nutritional intake of the ALD population. Our findings highlight several barriers and non-physiological factors not included in standard malnutrition screening tools that influence the nutritional status of patients in this population.

Results from this study reinforce the impact of a high symptom burden in ALD on a patient's nutritional status. Symptoms such as ascites, nausea, vomiting, poor appetite, loss of taste, and low energy acted as barriers to maintaining adequate nutrition. Our study also highlighted the multifactorial nature of these symptoms in patients, which were often linked; for example, accumulation of ascites may cause nausea, resulting in changes to appetite and intake. This is consistent with the literature, which indicates that up to 50% of people with ALD will experience ascites and its consequent impact on nutrition, leading to heightened malnutrition rates of up to 85% in this population [1,20]. Despite these symptoms being commonly reported in our study population and consistently seen in the literature, only two of the seven validated malnutrition screening tools, the RFH-NPT and the PG-SGA Short Form, explore disease-related complications, such as ascites or general fluid overload [6,9,20,21]. In addition, the PG-SGA Short Form includes nutritional symptoms such as nausea, taste change, and low appetite, but doesn't capture fluid buildup from ascites or edema [9].

Evidence in the renal and oncology literature has identified that targeting non-physiological impacts can lead to better-managed symptoms and a greater quality of life [11,12]. In Australia, the PG-SGA Short Form is often preferred in renal and oncology settings. However, our study identified that patients in the ALD population have other complex needs not routinely picked up by current screening tools and experience non-physiological factors that impact their nutritional intake, such as financial status, level of social support, and food literacy levels.

It was highlighted by clinicians that the current screening tools used in this setting did not identify all factors that influenced the nutritional status of patients with ALD, which may impact timely and appropriate referrals for those at risk of malnutrition. As reported in the existing literature, the MST, commonly used in clinical settings, is found to have poor accuracy compared to tools such as the RFH-NPT [3,6]. Therefore, earlier detection and intervention for malnutrition, as recommended by the ESPEN guidelines, is essential to improve the quality of life and reduce the mortality rate of patients with ALD [1,6]. This study draws our attention to the importance of considering a patient-centered approach to improve outcomes and support optimal nutrition to meet the needs of patients with ALD.

To the authors' knowledge, this is the first exploration of malnutrition screening in ALD encompassing the important perspectives of patients, caregivers, and clinicians utilizing a collaborative and evidence-based approach with formal consumer engagement. As a result of their experiences, this study highlights the ineffectiveness of current screening methods and the need for more comprehensive malnutrition screening. Leveraging the consumer and clinician insights obtained in this study can inform clinical practice towards malnutrition screening that is consumer-focused and considers the unique lived experiences of this patient population. Designing effective patient-reported outcome measures could complement anthropometric or other measures to detect sarcopenia and biochemical methods of assessing nutritional status, for example, serum albumin level, total cholesterol level, and peripheral lymphocyte counts or the 'Controlling Nutritional Status' (CONUT) score [22]. It is important to acknowledge there was an unequal distribution of participants between the metropolitan and the regional sites. While it is not anticipated that this would have altered the themes identified in the study, it would be optimal for future research to further explore the experiences of regional and rural people with ALD in more depth due to the known health inequalities experienced by people in these regions [23]. This study did not include patient participants with Child–Pugh A status, and although it is anticipated that this would not have changed our themes, this could be another area of future study. Consideration of the health literacy of patients with ALD and the factors that may differentially influence meal frequency or meal quality may also benefit from future research. Additionally, while this study explored the experiences of patients, carers, and clinicians, there was an uneven distribution in the final numbers. As a result, there might be a lack of representation from specific groups, potentially impacting the comprehensiveness of the study [24]. Respondent validation of the findings could further support the data [24].

Future research in this area should focus on a supportive and holistic approach to nutritional management that considers economic, environmental, and psychosocial factors. The authors plan to develop a novel screening tool for ALD that will be evaluated in comparison to a comprehensive subjective global assessment. Furthermore, interdisciplinary care planning should be engaged to harness expertise in the management of both physiological and non-physiological determinants of malnutrition, which may improve not only the nutritional status of patients but also their quality of life.

## 5. Conclusions

Malnutrition rates in patients with ALD are higher when compared to patients with well-compensated liver disease. This study aimed to understand the non-traditional factors perceived to influence the nutritional status of patients with ALD which are not currently included in malnutrition screening tools. A wide range of physiological and non-physiological factors that can affect the nutrition status of patients with ALD were identified by the diverse group of stakeholders; these warrant consideration in the development and implementation of malnutrition screening tools for ALD. To our knowledge, no current published screening tools consider both the physiological and non-physiological factors of malnutrition in the ALD population. Therefore, we recommend the development of a novel screening tool that incorporates these aspects to screen for malnutrition in this population more accurately.

**Supplementary Materials:** The following supporting information can be downloaded at: https://www.mdpi.com/article/10.3390/nu16152403/s1, Table S1: Glossary of Terms.

**Author Contributions:** Conceptualization, S.P., J.A. and K.W.; methodology, S.L., S.P., J.A. and K.W.; software, S.L., K.F. and S.P.; validation, S.L., S.P., J.A. and K.W.; formal analysis, S.L., K.F., K.S. and S.H.; investigation, S.L. and J.O.; resources, S.L., S.P., J.A. and K.W.; data curation, S.L., K.F., K.S. and S.H.; writing—original draft preparation, S.L., K.F. and K.S.; writing—review and editing, S.L., K.F., K.S., S.H., J.O., S.P., J.A. and K.W.; visualization, S.L., K.F., K.S., S.H. and S.P.; supervision, K.S., S.H., S.P., J.A. and K.W.; project administration, S.L. and K.W.; funding acquisition, K.W. All authors have read and agreed to the published version of the manuscript.

**Funding:** This research was supported by seed funding from the Hunter Medical Research Institute (HMRI) Equity in Health and Wellbeing Research Program Seed Grant Scheme 2022 and the John Hunter Hospital Charitable Trust Grant Scheme 2022 Hunter New England Local Health District (HNELHD).

**Institutional Review Board Statement:** Ethics approval was granted by the Hunter New England Human Research Ethics Committee (2022/ETH02426, 21 December 2022). Governance site-specific approval was granted for Hunter New England (2022/STE04011, 18 January 2023; 2022/STE04012, 18 January 2023).

**Informed Consent Statement:** Informed consent was obtained from all subjects involved in the study.

**Data Availability Statement:** The original contributions presented in the study are included in the article/Supplementary Material; further inquiries can be directed to the corresponding author(s).

**Acknowledgments:** The authors thank Jane Kerr, Mary-Anne Dieckmann, Paulett Barnes, and all patients, carers, and clinicians for their involvement and insights.

**Conflicts of Interest:** The authors declare no conflicts of interest. The funders had no role in the design of the study; in the collection, analyses, or interpretation of data; in the writing of the manuscript; or in the decision to publish the results.

## References

1. Bischoff, S.C.; Bernal, W.; Dasarathy, S.; Merli, M.; Plank, L.D.; Schütz, T.; Plauth, M.; Peláez, R.B.; Irigoin, R.R. ESPEN practical guideline: Clinical nutrition in liver disease. *Nutr. Hosp.* **2022**, *39*, 434–472. [CrossRef] [PubMed]
2. Georgiou, A.; Papatheodoridis, G.V.; Alexopoulou, A.; Deutsch, M.; Vlachogiannakos, I.; Ioannidou, P.; Papageorgiou, M.-V.; Papadopoulos, N.; Tsibouris, P.; Prapa, A.; et al. Evaluation of the effectiveness of eight screening tools in detecting risk of malnutrition in cirrhotic patients: The KIRRHOS study. *Br. J. Nutr.* **2019**, *122*, 1368–1376. [CrossRef] [PubMed]
3. Tandon, P.; Raman, M.; Mourtzakis, M.; Merli, M.A. A practical approach to nutritional screening and assessment in cirrhosis. *Hepatology* **2017**, *65*, 1044–1057. [CrossRef] [PubMed]
4. Tsoris, A.; Marlar, C. *Use of the Child Pugh Score in Liver Disease*; StatPearls: Treasure Island, FL, USA, 2021.
5. UpToDate. Child-Pugh Classification of Severity of Cirrhosis. 2023. Available online: https://www.uptodate.com/contents/image?imageKey=GAST/78401 (accessed on 2 May 2023).
6. Wu, Y.; Zhu, Y.; Feng, Y.; Wang, R.; Yao, N.; Zhang, M.; Liu, X.; Liu, H.; Shi, L.; Zhu, L.; et al. Royal free hospital-nutritional prioritizing tool improves the prediction of malnutrition risk outcomes in liver cirrhosis patients compared with nutritional risk screening 2002. *Br. J. Nutr.* **2020**, *124*, 1293–1302. [CrossRef] [PubMed]
7. Reber, E.; Gomes, F.; Vasiloglou, M.F.; Schuetz, P.; Stanga, Z. Nutritional risk screening and assessment. *J. Clin. Med.* **2019**, *8*, 1065. [CrossRef] [PubMed]
8. Tandon, P.G.L. UpToDate: Evaluating Nutritional Status in Adults with Cirrhosis. 2023. Available online: https://www.uptodate.com/contents/nutritional-issues-in-adult-patients-with-cirrhosis (accessed on 22 May 2024).

9. Bauer, J.; Capra, S.; Ferguson, M. Use of the scored patient-generated subjective global assessment (PG-SGA) as a nutrition assessment tool in patients with cancer. *Eur. J. Clin. Nutr.* **2002**, *56*, 779–785. [CrossRef] [PubMed]
10. Borhofen, S.M.; Gerner, C.; Lehmann, J.; Fimmers, R.; Görtzen, J.; Hey, B.; Geiser, F.; Strassburg, C.P.; Trebicka, J. The royal free hospital-nutritional prioritizing tool is an independent predictor of deterioration of liver function and survival in cirrhosis. *Dig. Dis. Sci.* **2016**, *61*, 1735–1743. [CrossRef] [PubMed]
11. de van der Schueren, M.; Laviano, A.; Blanchard, H.; Jourdan, M.; Arends, J.; Baracos, V. Systematic review and meta-analysis of the evidence for oral nutritional intervention on nutritional and clinical outcomes during chemo (radio) therapy: Current evidence and guidance for design of future trials. *Ann. Oncol.* **2018**, *29*, 1141–1153. [CrossRef] [PubMed]
12. Stevenson, J.; Meade, A.; Randall, A.; Manley, K.; Notaras, S.; Heaney, S.; Chan, M.; Smyth, A.; Josland, E.; Brennan, F.P.; et al. Nutrition in renal supportive care: Patient-driven and flexible. *Nephrology* **2017**, *22*, 739–747. [CrossRef] [PubMed]
13. Hall, A.E.; Bryant, J.; Sanson-Fisher, R.W.; Fradgley, E.A.; Proietto, A.M.; Roos, I. Consumer input into health care: Time for a new active and comprehensive model of consumer involvement. *Health Expect.* **2018**, *21*, 707–713. [CrossRef] [PubMed]
14. O'Brien, B.C.; Harris, I.B.; Beckman, T.J.; Reed, D.A.; Cook, D.A. Standards for reporting qualitative research: A synthesis of recommendations. *Acad. Med.* **2014**, *89*, 1245–1251. [CrossRef] [PubMed]
15. *Androit Transcription Service*; Androit Research Pty Ltd.: Sunnybank, Australia; Available online: https://www.adroitresearch.com.au/services (accessed on 22 May 2024).
16. Braun, V.; Clarke, V. Using thematic analysis in psychology. *Qual. Res. Psychol.* **2006**, *3*, 77–101. [CrossRef]
17. Malterud, K.; Siersma, V.D.; Guassora, A.D. Sample size in qualitative interview studies: Guided by information power. *Qual. Health Res.* **2016**, *26*, 1753–1760. [CrossRef] [PubMed]
18. *NVivo Qualitative Data Analysis*, Version 12; QSR International Pty Ltd.: Doncaster, UK, 2018.
19. Australian Institute of Health and Welfare. Oral Health and Dental Care in Australia. 2023. Available online: https://www.aihw.gov.au/reports/dental-oral-health/oral-health-and-dental-care-in-australia (accessed on 18 June 2024).
20. Moore, K.P.; Aithal, G.P. Guidelines on the management of ascites in cirrhosis. *Gut* **2006**, *55* (Suppl. S6), vi1–vi12. [CrossRef] [PubMed]
21. Peng, J.-K.; Hepgul, N.; Higginson, I.J.; Gao, W. Symptom prevalence and quality of life of patients with end-stage liver disease: A systematic review and meta-analysis. *Palliat. Med.* **2019**, *33*, 24–36. [CrossRef] [PubMed]
22. González-Madroño, A.; Mancha, A.; Rodríguez, F.J.; Culebras, J.; I De Ulibarri, J. Confirming the validity of the CONUT system for early detection and monitoring of clinical undernutrition: Comparison with two logistic regression models developed using SGA as the gold standard. *Nutr. Hosp.* **2012**, *27*, 564–571. [PubMed]
23. Australian Institute of Health and Welfare. Rural and Remote Health. 2023. Available online: https://www.aihw.gov.au/reports/rural-remote-australians/rural-and-remote-health (accessed on 22 October 2023).
24. Tracy, S.J. Qualitative quality: Eight "big-tent" criteria for excellent qualitative research. *Qual. Inq.* **2010**, *16*, 837–851. [CrossRef]

nutrients

MDPI

*Review*

# Ultra-Processed Food and Its Impact on Bone Health and Joint Diseases: A Scoping Review

**Jacopo Ciaffi [1,2,*], Luana Mancarella [1], Claudio Ripamonti [1], Andrea D'Amuri [3], Veronica Brusi [1], Federica Pignatti [1], Lucia Lisi [1] and Francesco Ursini [1,2]**

1 Medicine & Rheumatology Unit, IRCCS Istituto Ortopedico Rizzoli, 40136 Bologna, Italy; luana.mancarella@ior.it (L.M.); claudio.ripamonti@ior.it (C.R.); veronica.brusi@ior.it (V.B.); federica.pignatti@ior.it (F.P.); lucia.lisi@ior.it (L.L.); francesco.ursini2@unibo.it (F.U.)

2 Department of Biomedical and Neuromotor Sciences (DIBINEM), Alma Mater Studiorum University of Bologna, 40123 Bologna, Italy

3 General Medicine Unit, Medical Department, ASST Mantova, Ospedale Carlo Poma, 46100 Mantova, Italy; dmrndr@unife.it

* Correspondence: jacopo.ciaffi@ior.it

**Abstract: Background/Objectives**: This scoping review explores the relationship between ultra-processed food (UPF), bone health, and joint diseases, focusing on its potential impact on bone mineral density (BMD), osteoporosis, osteoarthritis, and inflammatory arthritis, including rheumatoid arthritis (RA), gout, and spondyloarthritis. **Methods**: A search strategy was developed using key terms such as "ultra-processed food" and related terms like "fast food," alongside various definitions of bone health impairment, chronic degenerative joint diseases, and inflammatory arthritis. **Results**: A total of 19 studies were included: 12 on bone health, 3 on osteoarthritis, and 4 on inflammatory arthritis. Preclinical studies showed that UPF consumption negatively affects bone structure and strength. In studies on children and adults, four investigations (2013–2017) found no association between fast food intake and BMD. However, more recent large-scale cross-sectional studies linked higher UPF consumption to lower BMD, increased osteoporosis risk, and greater prevalence of osteopenia, particularly in postmenopausal women. UPF intake was associated with knee osteoarthritis risk, with evidence suggesting an interaction with cartilage thickness, though no association was found for hip osteoarthritis. In inflammatory arthritis, UK Biobank data indicated a higher risk of RA and gout in UPF consumers, while a Brazilian study reported worse metabolic profiles in RA patients. No significant differences in UPF intake were found in spondyloarthritis. **Conclusions**: This review highlights relevant considerations about the deleterious role of UPF on bone health and joint diseases, providing additional evidence to suggest healthier dietary patterns to patients and to the general population.

**Keywords:** ultra-processed; food; osteoporosis; bone; osteoarthritis; rheumatoid arthritis; gout

## 1. Introduction

According to the NOVA Food classification system, which categorizes foods based on the extent and purpose of their processing, ultra-processed foods (UPFs) are industrial formulations with little to no whole foods, containing additives, preservatives and artificial substances to enhance taste, texture, appearance and durability [1]. The most commonly consumed UPFs include soft and sweetened beverages, processed bread, refined breakfast



https://doi.org/10.3390/nu17071188

cereals, confectionery products, pre-packaged sauces, ready-to-heat meals and processed meat products [2].

UPFs are a highly relevant topic given the steadily increasing sales and consumption trends, not only in Western societies but also in low- and middle-income countries [3]. UPFs are widespread for several reasons: they are convenient, easy to consume on the go, require no preparation or utensils, are highly palatable, and are typically inexpensive [1]. These undesirable characteristics are further reinforced by aggressive and sophisticated marketing strategies that shape social norms, disproportionately affecting vulnerable groups, particularly children [4]. Nutritionally, UPFs are high in refined sugars, saturated fats, sodium and additives, yet lacking in essential nutrients such as fiber, protein, and key micronutrients including potassium, magnesium, vitamin C, vitamin D, zinc, phosphorus, vitamin B12, niacin and antioxidants [5,6].

These nutritional deficits are strongly linked to poor health outcomes. As energy-dense foods, UPFs contribute to excessive calorie intake and are associated with a 39% higher risk of obesity, a 79% increased risk of metabolic syndrome, and up to a 31% greater risk of diabetes [7,8]. Furthermore, diets rich in UPFs are linked to an elevated risk of coronary artery disease, stroke, cardiovascular mortality and all-cause mortality [9–11].

The health risks extend beyond metabolic disorders. UPF consumption has been associated with an increased risk of cancer, including an 11% higher risk of breast tumors, a 30% greater risk of colorectal tumors and a 49% increased risk of pancreatic cancer [12]. Moreover, as scientific research in this field advances, it continues to reveal further health implications. UPF consumption has been linked to cognitive decline, psychiatric disorders such as anxiety and depression, inflammatory bowel disease and demyelinating diseases such as multiple sclerosis [10,13–15].

Dietary patterns have long been recognized as key determinants of bone health and osteoporosis risk. Nutrient-rich diets, such as the Mediterranean diet, have been associated with higher bone mineral density (BMD) and lower fracture risk, likely due to their high content of calcium, vitamin D, polyphenols, and omega-3 fatty acids [16,17]. Conversely, Western dietary patterns, characterized by a high intake of refined carbohydrates, saturated fats, and processed foods, have been linked to lower BMD and an increased risk of osteoporosis [18,19]. Most research in this area has focused on specific nutrients, such as calcium, vitamin D, and protein, or on overall dietary patterns rather than on the role of UPF consumption as a distinct risk factor for bone fragility [20]. Given the rising global consumption of UPFs and their well-documented impact on metabolic and inflammatory pathways, investigating their effects on bone health, osteoporosis risk, and joint diseases is of increasing clinical importance [21].

## 2. Materials and Methods

This scoping review was conducted in accordance with the methodological guidelines of the Joanna Briggs Institute [22]. We used the Preferred Reporting Items for Systematic Reviews and Meta-Analysis extension for Scoping Reviews (PRISMA-ScR) checklist to guide the structured reporting of the review (Supplementary File) [23]. The protocol was registered in the Open Science Framework (OSF) Registries (https://doi.org/10.17605/OSF.IO/DEXGB) accessed on 14 February 2025. In line with scoping review's methodology, no critical appraisal or risk of bias assessment was performed in the included studies [22].

### 2.1. Eligibility Criteria and Study Selection

The Population, Concept, and Context (PCC) framework was used to formulate the research question and define the inclusion criteria. Studies were included if they met the following criteria:

- **Population:**
    - Preclinical studies: mice or rat models.
    - Human studies: children or adults.
- **Concept:**
    - Preclinical models: effects of UPF on bone health, bone growth, histomorphometric properties.
    - Clinical studies: impact of UPF on BMD, osteoporosis, osteoarthritis (OA) and inflammatory arthritis incidence; influence of UPF consumption on patients already diagnosed with chronic joint diseases, such as OA and inflammatory arthritis.
- **Context:**
    - Preclinical studies: animal models in which UPF-fed mice or rats underwent bone health assessments.
    - Bone health and disease risk: studies evaluating the association between UPF consumption and the risk of developing osteoporosis, low BMD, fractures, or inflammatory arthritis.
    - Impact on existing conditions: Studies investigating the effects of UPF intake on disease activity, progression, and related metabolic or inflammatory outcomes in patients with established chronic joint diseases.

We included randomized controlled trials (RCTs), quasi-RCTs, prospective and retrospective cohort studies, case–control studies, cross-sectional studies, and qualitative reports. Conference proceedings were also considered.

### 2.2. Search Strategy

After having registered the protocol on OSF, we conducted a comprehensive literature search in MedLine (via PubMed), Web of Science (WOS), and Embase, up to 14 February 2025. The search strategy included key terms related to UPF, bone health, and chronic joint diseases. Specifically, we used terms such as "ultra-processed food," "highly processed food," and "fast food" to identify dietary exposures. For the assessment of the outcomes, we included terms related to bone health (e.g., bone mineral density, osteoporosis, osteopenia, bone growth, bone health, bone diseases, fracture, bone loss) and chronic joint diseases (e.g., osteoarthritis, rheumatoid arthritis, psoriatic arthritis, spondyloarthritis, ankylosing spondylitis, gout). To ensure full transparency and reproducibility, the complete search strategy for each database is provided as a Supplementary File.

We also performed manual searches using relevant keywords and screened the references of included articles to find additional sources. The search strategy was developed and conducted by two independent authors (J.C. and L.M.) and supervised by a senior investigator (F.U.). No restrictions were applied on publication date.

### 2.3. Study Selection and Data Charting

After the removal of duplicate records, two reviewers (J.C. and L.M.) independently screened all titles and abstracts of the retrieved articles. Full-text assessment was performed for potentially eligible studies. Any discrepancies during the study selection process were resolved through discussion, and a senior investigator (F.U.) was consulted when consensus could not be reached.

For each included study, the following information was extracted: first author, year of publication, country, study design, sample size, study population (preclinical models or human participants), exposure assessment (UPF consumption), comparator groups (if applicable), outcomes assessed (e.g., bone mineral density, osteoporosis, fractures, osteoarthritis, inflammatory arthritis), and key findings related to UPF and musculoskeletal health.

### 2.4. Synthesis of Results

We conducted a narrative synthesis of the extracted data, structured into five main sections based on study populations and disease areas:

**Preclinical studies on bone health**

- This section summarizes findings from animal models assessing the impact of UPF consumption on bone health.
- Key outcomes include changes in bone biomechanical properties, histomorphometric parameters, bone growth, and mineralization in rodents fed with UPF diets.

**UPF and bone health in children and adolescents**

- This section compiles evidence from studies evaluating the relationship between UPF consumption and BMD or bone health markers in pediatric and adolescent populations.
- Findings include differences in BMD, bone turnover markers, and skeletal growth patterns in children with high UPF intake.

**UPF and bone health in adults**

- This section synthesizes clinical studies exploring the association between UPF intake and bone health in adults.
- Key outcomes include the impact of UPF on osteopenia, osteoporosis, fracture risk, and changes in BMD in different adult populations.

**UPF and osteoarthritis**

- This section summarizes studies investigating the link between UPF consumption and the risk or progression of OA.
- Outcomes include the prevalence and severity of OA, cartilage integrity, pain levels, and functional impairment in individuals with high UPF consumption.

**UPF and inflammatory arthritis**

- This section reviews evidence on UPF intake and the risk or progression of inflammatory arthritis, including rheumatoid arthritis (RA), spondyloarthritis (SpA), and gout.
- Findings cover the influence of UPF on disease incidence, inflammation markers, symptom severity, disease progression, and metabolic comorbidities in patients with inflammatory arthritis.

## 3. Results

The database search yielded a total of 119 studies (PubMed: 24, WOS: 50, Embase: 45). After removing 40 duplicates, 79 records remained for screening. Following title and abstract screening, 60 studies were excluded, leaving 19 full-text articles that met the inclusion criteria and were included in the qualitative synthesis (Table 1).

Of the 19 included studies, 12 focused on bone health, with 3 preclinical and 9 clinical studies, while 7 investigated chronic joint diseases. Additionally, four studies were conference proceedings. The studies were published between 2013 and 2025 and originated from the United States (5), China (4), Korea (3), Israel (2), Brazil (1), the United Kingdom (1), Portugal (1), Japan (1) and France (1).

A flowchart illustrating the study selection process is presented in Figure 1.

**Table 1.** Characteristics of the included studies.

| First Author | Year of Publication | Country of Affiliation of First Author | Publication Type | Study Design | Sample Size | Study Population | Exposure Assessment | Outcomes Assessed | Key Findings |
|---|---|---|---|---|---|---|---|---|---|
| Akkaya Z. [24] | 2024 | United States | Conference proceeding | Cross-sectional | 4330 | OA patients from the Osteoarthritis Initiative cohort | Self-reported UPF intake | Cartilage thickness in knee OA | Greater UPF intake was linked to thinner knee cartilage, particularly in women with OA. |
| Greatorex Brooks E.L. [25] | 2025 | United States | Full-text article | Cross-sectional | 5729 | adults from the NHANES cohort | UPF % of total energy intake | Osteoporosis prevalence and BMD | Higher UPF consumption was associated with increased osteoporosis prevalence and lower BMD in NHANES participants. |
| Lim H.S. [26] | 2018 | Korea | Full-text article | Cross-sectional | 161 | college students | Self-reported frequency of fast food consumption | Total body BMD and dietary influence | Frequent fast-food consumption was negatively associated with total body BMD in college students. |
| Mangano K.M. [27] | 2017 | United States | Full-text article | Prospective cohort | 2986 | adults | Dietary protein clusters, including "Fast food and full-fat dairy" | BMD and lean mass association | Higher protein intake, even from processed sources, was associated with greater lean mass but had no clear effect on BMD. |
| Monjardino T. [28] | 2015 | Portugal | Full-text article | Prospective cohort | 1007 | adolescents | Dietary patterns including "Fast food and sweets" cluster | BMD at the lumbar spine and femoral neck | Higher intake of fast food and sweets was associated with lower BMD at the lumbar spine and femoral neck in adolescents. |

**Table 1.** *Cont.*

| First Author | Year of Publication | Country of Affiliation of First Author | Publication Type | Study Design | Sample Size | Study Population | Exposure Assessment | Outcomes Assessed | Key Findings |
|---|---|---|---|---|---|---|---|---|---|
| Nguyen K. [29] | 2019 | France | Conference proceeding | Cross-sectional | 140 | SpA patients | Self-reported UPF consumption | Disease activity and quality of life | UPF intake was not significantly different between active and inactive SpA patients, but poor diet was associated with worse quality of life. |
| Noel S. [30] | 2023 | United States | Conference proceeding | Cross-sectional | 1254 | adults | Self-reported UPF intake frequency | Osteoporosis prevalence and BMD | Puerto Rican adults with high UPF intake had lower BMD and a higher prevalence of osteoporosis. |
| Saito M.K. [31] | 2024 | Japan | Full-text article | Prospective preclinical | 48 | rats | Cafeteria diet (highly processed) vs. standard chow | BMD, trabecular structure, and biomechanical properties | Rats fed a cafeteria diet exhibited lower BMD, reduced trabecular bone structure, and weaker biomechanical properties compared to controls. |
| Shin S. [32] | 2015 | Korea | Full-text article | Cross-sectional | 3573 | adults | Dietary patterns categorized, including "Fast food and soda" group | Association between dietary patterns and BMD | A "fast food and soda" dietary pattern was associated with lower BMD in adults. |
| Shin S. [33] | 2013 | Korea | Full-text article | Cross-sectional | 196 | adolescents | Dietary patterns categorized as "Fast food" vs. "Milk and Cereal" | BMD at the lumbar spine, femur, and total body | A diet rich in fast food was linked to lower BMD at multiple skeletal sites in adolescents. |

**Table 1.** *Cont.*

| First Author | Year of Publication | Country of Affiliation of First Author | Publication Type | Study Design | Sample Size | Study Population | Exposure Assessment | Outcomes Assessed | Key Findings |
|---|---|---|---|---|---|---|---|---|---|
| Sims W. [34] | 2024 | United States | Conference proceeding | Cross-sectional | 4796 | OA patients from the Osteoarthritis Initiative cohort | UPF % of total energy intake | OA-related pain, physical function, and disability | Higher UPF consumption was associated with worse OA-related pain and poorer physical function. |
| Smaira F.I. [35] | 2020 | Brasil | Full-text article | Cross-sectional | 56 | RA patients | Self-reported UPF intake frequency | Cardiovascular risk factors and metabolic health | RA patients consuming more UPF had worse metabolic profiles and higher cardiovascular risk. |
| Travinsky-Shmul T. [36] | 2021 | Israel | Full-text article | Prospective preclinical | 36 | mice | UPF diet with food additives vs. control diet | Bone strength, mechanical properties, and histological changes | Mice consuming a UPF-based diet had significantly reduced bone strength, altered mechanical properties, and increased histological abnormalities. |
| Vogel C. [37] | 2016 | United Kingdom | Full-text article | Ecological | 1107 | children | Number of fast food outlets near residence | Association between fast food exposure and BMD | Children living in areas with greater fast food availability had lower BMD, suggesting an environmental impact on bone health. |
| Wang S. [38] | 2024 | China | Full-text article | Cross-sectional | 4912 | adults from the NHANES cohort | UPF % of daily caloric intake | BMD at femoral neck and osteoporosis risk | Adults with high UPF intake had lower femoral neck BMD and a significantly greater risk of osteoporosis. |

**Table 1.** *Cont.*

| First Author | Year of Publication | Country of Affiliation of First Author | Publication Type | Study Design | Sample Size | Study Population | Exposure Assessment | Outcomes Assessed | Key Findings |
|---|---|---|---|---|---|---|---|---|---|
| Wei Y. [39] | 2024 | China | Full-text article | Prospective cohort | 163,987 | adults | UPF % of total caloric intake | Risk of knee and hip osteoarthritis | High UPF consumption increased the risk of knee osteoarthritis but had no significant effect on hip OA. |
| Zaretsky J. [40] | 2021 | Israel | Full-text article | Prospective preclinical | 40 | rats | UPF-based diet vs. control diet | Bone microarchitecture and endochondral ossification defects | UPF consumption led to impaired bone microarchitecture and disrupted endochondral ossification in rats, suggesting negative effects on bone quality. |
| Zhang T. [41] | 2024 | China | Full-text article | Prospective cohort | 181,559 | adults from the UK biobank study | UPF intake categorized by quartiles | Risk of developing gout and genetic interactions | Higher UPF consumption was associated with an increased risk of gout, particularly in genetically predisposed individuals. |
| Zhao H. [42] | 2024 | China | Full-text article | Prospective cohort | 207,012 | adults from the UK biobank study | UPF % of total dietary intake | Risk of developing rheumatoid arthritis | Individuals with high UPF intake had a 17% increased risk of developing RA. |

BMD: bone mineral density; OA: osteoarthritis; RA: rheumatoid arthritis; SpA: spondyloarthritis; UK: United Kingdom; UPF: ultra-processed food.

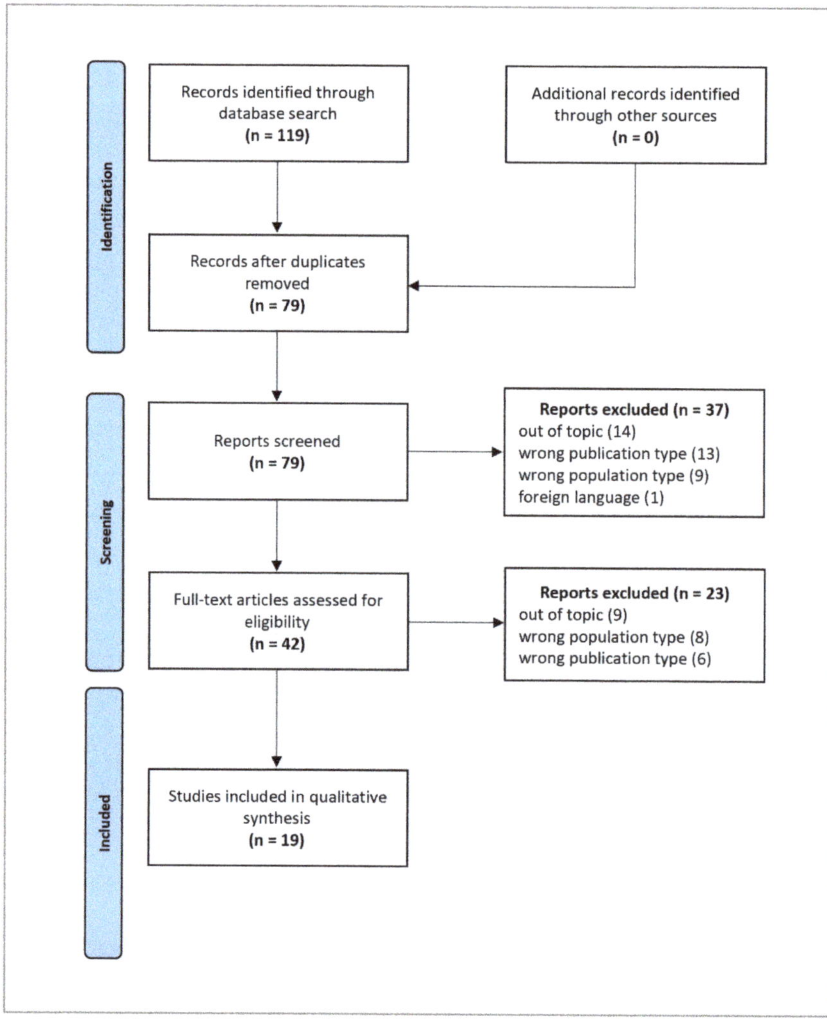


**Figure 1.** PRISMA 2020 flow diagram. Adapted From: Page MJ, McKenzie JE, Bossuyt PM, Boutron I, Hoffmann TC, Mulrow CD, et al. The PRISMA 2020 statement: an updated guideline for reporting systematic reviews [43].

### *3.1. Preclinical Studies on Bone Health*

Three preclinical studies have investigated the impact of UPF consumption on bone health, demonstrating detrimental effects on BMD, microarchitecture, and mechanical properties [31,36,40].

A study in young female mice found that UPF consumption resulted in a significant reduction in bone quality [40]. Micro-CT scans revealed impaired bone morphology and biomechanical testing showed inferior bone strength. Additionally, marrow adiposity was significantly increased, suggesting that UPF consumption alters bone remodeling processes and could predispose individuals to osteoporosis [40].

Similarly, in young rats, a high-fat, high-sugar UPF diet led to severe skeletal impairments, including growth retardation, lesions in the tibial growth plates, and a significant decrease in BMD [36]. Structural deterioration was observed in both trabecular and cortical bone. RNA sequencing revealed disruptions in extracellular matrix formation and mineralization processes. These findings suggest that UPF exposure during growth may lead to long-term skeletal fragility and increased fracture risk [36].

A third study examined the effects of a calorie-dense UPF "cafeteria" diet in male rats, investigating whether resistance exercise (ladder climbing) could counteract the diet's effects [31]. The results showed that UPF consumption led to a significant increase in adipose tissue, a reduction in BMD, and impaired biomechanical properties such as stiffness and maximum load capacity. Notably, exercise did not prevent the deterioration in bone quality, suggesting that dietary interventions are necessary to mitigate the negative skeletal effects of UPF consumption.

Collectively, these preclinical studies highlight the adverse effects of UPF on bone growth and integrity, demonstrating that UPF consumption negatively affects bone mass, structure, and strength, potentially leading to an increased risk of osteoporosis and fractures. Furthermore, exercise alone may not be sufficient to counteract these effects, and dietary modifications are needed to maintain bone health.

### 3.2. UPF and Bone Health in Children and Adolescents

We found four studies investigating the impact of UPF and fast food consumption on bone health in children and adolescents [26,28,33,37].

Lim et al. analysed the impact of fast food consumption on BMD in college students, finding a significant association between frequent fast food intake and lower BMD in both males and females [26]. The study also revealed nutrient imbalances, with excess sodium and protein intake coupled with deficiencies in vitamins A and C, suggesting that the poor micronutrient profile of UPFs may contribute to impaired bone metabolism. A UPF-rich diet may thus interfere with bone mineralization during young adulthood, a critical period for achieving peak bone mass [26].

The role of the food environment in childhood bone health was assessed by Vogel et al. in a study of young children from the Southampton Women's Survey [37]. Greater exposure to fast food outlets in residential areas was associated with lower BMD and bone mineral content at birth and during early childhood. Specifically, each additional fast food outlet near a child's home correlated with a 0.23 standard deviation decrease in BMD. In contrast, greater access to healthy food stores was associated with higher BMD at ages 4 and 6, suggesting that the availability of fast food influences long-term bone health outcomes from infancy onward [37].

In a longitudinal study of Portuguese adolescents, Monjardino et al. examined how dietary patterns affected bone accrual from ages 13 to 17 [28]. While no significant associations were found between the fast food dietary pattern and mean BMD at 13 years, girls who followed a diet characterized by lower food intake, including lower consumption of nutrient-dense foods, showed significantly lower BMD accrual over time (adjusted coefficient: $-0.451$ mg/cm$^2$/year). The findings suggest that nutrient-poor diets, which often include processed foods, may contribute to reduced bone mineralization during adolescence [28].

In a study of Korean adolescents, Shin et al. evaluated the impact of different dietary patterns on lumbar spine and femoral BMD [33]. No direct link was found between a fast-food-heavy diet and lower BMD, but the findings suggested a trend toward poorer bone health outcomes in those consuming higher amounts of UPF. Conversely, adolescents following a milk and cereal-rich dietary pattern had a 64% lower likelihood of low BMD, reinforcing the importance of whole, nutrient-rich foods in skeletal development [33].

These four studies highlight the potential risks of UPF consumption for bone health in children and adolescents. Frequent fast food intake and greater exposure to fast food outlets are associated with lower BMD, impaired bone accrual, and reduced bone strength.

### 3.3. UPF and Bone Health in Adults

Our search strategy identified five studies, including four full papers and one conference poster, that explored the association between UPF and bone health outcomes in adults, particularly in relation to BMD, osteoporosis, and fracture risk [25,27,30,32,38].

A large cross-sectional analysis by Greatorex Brooks et al. used NHANES data to examine UPF consumption in U.S. adults aged 50 and older [25]. The study found that higher UPF intake was significantly associated with an increased prevalence of osteopenia and osteoporosis, particularly in women. Individuals in the highest quintile of UPF consumption had a 52% greater likelihood of osteoporosis compared to those in the lowest quintile. Furthermore, each 1% increase in UPF intake correlated with a 1.9% increase in self-reported fractures among women, suggesting a direct link between UPF consumption and skeletal fragility [25].

Similarly, Wang et al. conducted a NHANES-based study and found that individuals whose diet consisted of more than 57.5% UPF had significantly lower BMD at the femoral neck and total femur, which are considered key sites for osteoporotic fractures [38]. High intake of UPF was associated with 78.9% increased odds of developing osteoporosis. The study also highlighted that physical activity could partially mitigate the negative impact of UPF on bone health, thus highlighting the role of lifestyle factors in influencing the skeletal deterioration related to UPF intake [38].

While these two studies demonstrated clear negative effects of UPF on bone health, Shin et al. examined dietary patterns in Korean adults and found no direct association between fast food intake and BMD [32]. However, the authors reported that a fruit, milk, and whole-grain-based dietary pattern was positively correlated with BMD, suggesting that a diet rich in essential nutrients may counteract bone loss. This highlights the complexity of dietary influences on bone health and suggests that the nutrient density of a diet may be more predictive of BMD than the presence of UPF alone [32].

Supporting the detrimental impact of UPF, a conference poster presented by Noel et al. investigated UPF consumption and osteoporosis in Puerto Rican adults aged 47–79 years [30]. The study found that higher UPF intake was significantly associated with increased odds of osteoporosis, particularly at the femoral neck and lumbar spine. Even after adjusting for key confounders like age, sex, BMI, and lifestyle habits, the association remained significant, reinforcing the idea that UPF consumption is an independent risk factor for osteoporosis [30].

Finally, Mangano et al. examined dietary protein sources and musculoskeletal health in the Framingham Third Generation cohort [27]. Among the different dietary patterns identified, one characterized by high fast food and full-fat dairy intake showed no significant association with BMD. However, higher total protein intake was linked to improved muscle mass and strength, indicating that protein consumption may help preserve musculoskeletal health, even in the presence of some UPF intake [27].

Taken together, these studies suggest a strong association between high UPF consumption and poor bone health outcomes in adults. Higher UPF intake is linked to lower BMD, increased osteoporosis risk, and greater fracture prevalence, particularly in older populations. However, some findings indicate that nutrient-dense dietary patterns and adequate protein intake may counteract these negative effects.

### 3.4. UPF and Osteoarthritis

We identified three studies, including two conference posters, that examined the relationship between UPF consumption and OA [24,34,39]. These studies focused on cartilage structure, pain severity, and OA risk in individuals with high UPF intake.

Wei et al. conducted a large prospective cohort study using data from the UK Biobank (n = 163,987 participants) to assess the impact of UPF consumption on hip and knee OA risk [39]. The study found that individuals in the highest quartile of UPF consumption had a 10% increased risk of developing knee OA compared to those in the lowest quartile, while no significant association was observed for hip OA. Additionally, replacing 20% of UPF intake with unprocessed or minimally processed food was linked to a 6% lower risk of knee OA, thus suggesting that dietary modifications could reduce the risk of developing OA [39].

A conference abstract by Akkaya et al. used Osteoarthritis Initiative (OAI) data to examine the association between UPF consumption and knee cartilage thickness in 4330 individuals [24]. The results showed a significant interaction between UPF intake, cartilage region, and sex. In women, higher UPF intake was associated with thinner cartilage in the medial tibia, medial femur, and lateral femur. In men, the association was weaker and mostly non-significant [24].

Another conference poster by Sims et al. analysed the relationship between UPF consumption and OA-related pain and functional outcomes in 4796 participants from the OAI cohort [34]. The study found that, after adjusting for potential confounders, including BMI, women consuming higher amounts of UPF experienced greater knee OA-related pain, worse activities of daily living, and lower physical performance compared to men [34].

These studies suggest that high UPF consumption could be linked to an increased risk of knee OA, reduced cartilage thickness, and worse pain outcomes, particularly in women. While no significant association was found for hip OA, findings from the UK Biobank and OAI cohorts indicate that reducing UPF intake could be a potential strategy for knee OA prevention and symptom management.

### 3.5. UPF and Inflammatory Arthritis

We identified four studies, including one conference abstract, that investigated the impact of UPF consumption on inflammatory arthritis, specifically RA, SpA, and gout [29,35,41,42]. These studies examined disease risk, symptom severity, and metabolic outcomes in individuals consuming high amounts of UPF.

A retrospective cohort study by Zhao et al. using the UK Biobank (n = 207,012 participants) evaluated the association between UPF consumption and RA incidence [42]. Participants in the highest quintile of UPF consumption had a 17% increased risk of developing RA compared to the lowest quintile. Mediation analyses suggested that inflammation, lipid profile changes, and liver enzyme alterations partially explained the link between UPF intake and RA risk, accounting for 3–15% of the association [42].

Another cross-sectional study by Smaira et al. examined the association between UPF consumption and cardiovascular risk in RA patients [35]. Among 56 individuals with RA, higher UPF intake was significantly associated with worsened metabolic and cardiovascular health, including an increased Framingham cardiovascular risk score and elevated glycated hemoglobin levels. Conversely, patients who consumed more unprocessed or minimally processed foods had a lower cardiovascular risk [35].

A prospective cohort study by Zhang et al. explored the relationship between UPF consumption, genetic predisposition, and gout risk in 181,559 participants from the UK Biobank [41]. The study found that higher UPF intake was associated with a 16% increased risk of developing gout. Additionally, individuals with both high genetic predisposition and high UPF intake had a nearly twofold increased risk of developing gout compared to those with low genetic predisposition and low UPF intake. The study also performed substitution analyses, showing that replacing 20% of daily UPF consumption with unprocessed or minimally processed foods reduced gout risk by 13% [41].

Finally, a conference abstract by Nguyen et al. investigated the dietary profiles of 140 patients with SpA and assessed their intake of UPF and its association with disease activity [29]. The study found no significant differences in UPF consumption between patients with active and inactive SpA [29].

Evidence from the four included studies on inflammatory arthritis suggests that higher UPF consumption is associated with increased risks of RA and gout, while its impact on SpA remains unclear. Moreover, among patients already diagnosed with RA, higher UPF intake was linked to worse metabolic health and increased cardiovascular risk.

## 4. Discussion

Our scoping review identified key insights into the relationship between UPF consumption, bone health, and chronic joint diseases. In the field of bone health and osteoporosis, there is a substantial body of evidence, encompassing both preclinical studies assessing bone microarchitecture and large-scale epidemiological studies evaluating osteoporosis and fracture risk. In contrast, research on UPF and chronic joint diseases remains limited, with only two large prospective cohort studies investigating the association between UPF intake and the risk of developing RA and gout.

This disparity was reflected in our review, as we identified 12 studies focusing on bone health, whereas only 7 studies addressed chronic joint diseases, of which only 4 were full-text articles, with the remaining being conference abstracts or posters. These findings highlight an important gap in the literature and the need for more robust, high-quality studies to explore the impact of UPF on musculoskeletal diseases, particularly in the context of inflammatory arthritis and OA progression.

Our findings were structured into five key research objectives. Preclinical studies consistently showed that UPF consumption deteriorates bone quality, leading to reduced BMD, altered trabecular structure, and impaired biomechanical properties [31,36,40]. These results suggest that early dietary exposure to UPF may have lasting negative effects on skeletal integrity, contributing to weakened bone strength and increased fracture risk. Further research is needed to clarify how inflammation and nutrient imbalances mediate these effects on bone remodeling.

We examined the association between UPF intake and bone health in children and adolescents. Studies linked higher UPF consumption to lower BMD at key skeletal sites, including the lumbar spine and femur [26,28]. Additionally, greater exposure to fast food environments correlated with reduced BMD in children, emphasizing the role of food accessibility in bone development [37]. Since early dietary habits shape peak bone mass and long-term skeletal health, these findings highlight the need for preventive strategies to limit UPF intake in youth and mitigate future skeletal risks [44,45].

In adults, large-scale observational studies found an association between increased UPF intake, lower BMD and increased osteoporosis risk, particularly in postmenopausal women and older individuals [25]. NHANES data confirmed this inverse relationship, raising concerns about UPF-driven skeletal aging [38]. Although the cross-sectional design of some studies limits causal inference, these findings align with evidence on the metabolic and inflammatory effects of UPFs, reinforcing the need for dietary modifications in osteoporosis prevention [46].

Furthermore, our review identified an association between high UPF intake and increased knee OA risk, though no significant effect was observed for hip OA [39]. UPF consumption was also correlated with worse pain, reduced physical function, and thinner knee cartilage, suggesting a role in disease progression via inflammatory and metabolic pathways [24,34]. However, the lack of significant findings for hip OA highlights inconsistencies, emphasizing the need for further research to clarify these associations [24,34].

Finally, we evaluated the impact of UPF consumption on inflammatory arthritis, including RA, SpA, and gout. Higher UPF intake was associated with a 17% increased risk of RA and a 16% increased risk of gout, according to large prospective studies [41,42]. However, findings on SpA were inconclusive, with no significant associations between UPF intake and disease activity. While existing cohort studies provide initial evidence linking UPFs to inflammatory arthritis, further research is needed to establish causality and mechanistic pathways, particularly regarding diet-induced inflammation. The evidence for SpA remains insufficient, underscoring the need for future studies on the role of UPF in disease onset and progression.

The findings of this review highlight the potential public health burden of UPF consumption on musculoskeletal health, reinforcing the need for dietary interventions and policy changes. The widespread availability, aggressive marketing, and affordability of UPFs have led to their increasing consumption across all age groups, including children, adolescents, and older adults, who are particularly vulnerable to bone fragility and joint diseases [47,48]. Given that UPFs are energy-dense but nutrient-poor, their high content of refined sugars, trans fats, sodium, and food additives, combined with their low levels of essential micronutrients such as calcium, vitamin D, magnesium, and antioxidants, may significantly contribute to bone loss, osteoporosis risk, and cartilage degeneration [7,49].

In addition, UPFs have been strongly linked to systemic inflammation, oxidative stress, metabolic syndrome, and obesity, all of which play a key role in osteoporosis, OA, and inflammatory arthritis [50,51]. The association between UPF consumption and an increased risk of RA and gout suggests that dietary modifications may be a potentially modifiable strategy for reducing the disease burden of inflammatory arthritis [52,53]. However, while the connection between UPFs and metabolic diseases such as obesity, diabetes, and cardiovascular disease is well established, their musculoskeletal effects remain underexplored, necessitating further research to determine causal pathways [5,8,54].

While our review highlights important associations between UPF consumption, bone health, and joint diseases, several limitations should be acknowledged. Most included studies were observational, preventing the establishment of causal relationships. Although some studies utilized prospective designs or genetic risk adjustment to strengthen causal inference, the possibility of reverse causation and residual confounding cannot be excluded [38,41]. The extent to which confounding factors were accounted for in the included studies is an important consideration. While 10 of the 16 clinical studies adjusted for confounders, the range and depth of adjustments varied considerably [25–28,32,33,38,39,41,42]. Most studies controlled for age, sex, BMI, and energy intake, but other key lifestyle and health factors, such as physical activity, smoking, alcohol consumption, socioeconomic status, corticosteroid use, and comorbid inflammatory conditions, were often not included in statistical models. Given the well-established influence of these factors on bone metabolism and joint health, their omission introduces the possibility of residual confounding, which may partially explain inconsistencies across studies.

To improve the quality and reliability of future research, greater efforts should be made to reduce methodological heterogeneity, particularly by incorporating more robust and standardized dietary assessment tools. Well-controlled longitudinal studies and Mendelian randomization approaches may help clarify causal pathways and minimize the risk of reverse causation and unmeasured confounding in this field [55].

Additionally, an important limitation of the included studies is the lack of consistency in how UPF exposure was assessed. There was substantial variability in the methods used to quantify UPF intake, which could contribute to heterogeneity in findings. Most studies relied on self-reported dietary data, often collected through food frequency questionnaires (FFQs) or 24 h dietary recalls, both of which are subject to recall bias and misclassification [56]. The classification of UPFs also varied across studies, with some using established food databases based on NOVA categorization, while others employed broader dietary pattern analyses, which may not fully capture UPF exposure. Moreover, some studies used indirect measures to assess UPF intake, such as fast-food outlet density in a given area, assuming that greater availability translates to higher individual consumption [37]. While such approaches provide valuable insights into environmental influences on diet, they do not directly measure personal dietary intake, making it difficult to draw precise conclusions about the relationship between UPF consumption and musculoskeletal health outcomes. This methodological variability may, at least in part, explain why the association between UPF intake, bone health, and joint diseases was not consistent across all studies. Differences in dietary assessment tools, classification criteria, and exposure measurement could have influenced the observed effect sizes and statistical significance, contributing to variability in findings. Standardizing UPF exposure assessment in future research could help improve comparability and reproducibility of results, ultimately providing stronger evidence on the role of UPFs in musculoskeletal health.

Notwithstanding the abovementioned limitations, from a public health perspective, the findings of our review support the need for nutritional education programs, clearer food labeling, and policies aimed at reducing UPF consumption, particularly among high-risk populations such as postmenopausal women, individuals with OA, and those predisposed to inflammatory arthritis. Strategies such as taxation of UPFs, restrictions on advertising to children, and incentives for healthier food choices could help curb the rising trend of UPF consumption and mitigate its long-term impact on bone and joint health [57]. Future studies should explore whether dietary interventions that reduce UPF intake can effectively slow disease progression and improve musculoskeletal outcomes, offering a cost-effective and accessible approach to musculoskeletal disease prevention.

## 5. Conclusions

The growing body of evidence on UPF consumption and adverse health outcomes highlights its detrimental impact not only on metabolic and cardiovascular diseases but also on bone health and chronic joint diseases. Our review suggests that high UPF intake is associated with reduced BMD, increased osteoporosis risk, and worse clinical outcomes in OA and inflammatory arthritis. However, most of the available evidence comes from observational studies, limiting the ability to draw causal conclusions. While some studies, such as those using prospective cohort designs or genetic risk adjustment, provide stronger evidence, methodological heterogeneity, including variability in dietary assessment methods and incomplete adjustment for confounders, remains a major limitation.

Despite accumulating evidence, research in this field is still in its early stages, particularly regarding the long-term impact of UPFs on musculoskeletal health. Given the global rise in UPF consumption, future studies should focus on well-controlled longitudinal research and intervention trials to determine whether reducing UPF intake could serve as a modifiable strategy to protect bone health and joint integrity. Additionally, standardized methods for UPF exposure assessment and more comprehensive adjustment for confounding factors will be essential for improving study comparability.

From a public health perspective, efforts should prioritize nutritional education and dietary interventions, promoting the consumption of whole, nutrient-dense foods to mitigate the growing burden of musculoskeletal diseases associated with UPFs.

**Supplementary Materials:** The following supporting information can be downloaded at: https://www.mdpi.com/article/10.3390/nu17071188/s1, PRISMA-ScR-checklist and search strategy.

**Author Contributions:** Conceptualization, J.C., L.M. and F.U.; methodology, J.C., L.M., C.R. and A.D.; software, V.B., F.P. and L.L.; validation, J.C. and F.U.; formal analysis, L.M., C.R., A.D. and F.P.; investigation, L.M., A.D., V.B., F.P. and L.L.; resources, C.R. and F.U.; data curation, J.C., A.D., F.P., L.L. and F.U.; writing—original draft preparation, J.C., L.M., C.R. and A.D.; writing—review and editing, J.C., L.M., C.R., A.D., V.B., F.P., L.L. and F.U.; visualization, J.C.; supervision, J.C. and F.U.; project administration, L.M., C.R. and V.B. All authors have read and agreed to the published version of the manuscript.

**Funding:** This research received no external funding.

**Data Availability Statement:** No new data were created or analyzed in this study. Data sharing is not applicable to this article.

**Conflicts of Interest:** The authors declare no conflicts of interest.

## References

1. Monteiro, C.A.; Cannon, G.; Levy, R.B.; Moubarac, J.-C.; Louzada, M.L.; Rauber, F.; Khandpur, N.; Cediel, G.; Neri, D.; Martinez-Steele, E.; et al. Ultra-Processed Foods: What They Are and How to Identify Them. *Public Health Nutr.* **2019**, *22*, 936–941. [CrossRef]
2. Wang, L.; Du, M.; Wang, K.; Khandpur, N.; Rossato, S.L.; Drouin-Chartier, J.-P.; Steele, E.M.; Giovannucci, E.; Song, M.; Zhang, F.F. Association of Ultra-Processed Food Consumption with Colorectal Cancer Risk among Men and Women: Results from Three Prospective US Cohort Studies. *BMJ* **2022**, *378*, e068921. [CrossRef]
3. Baker, P.; Machado, P.; Santos, T.; Sievert, K.; Backholer, K.; Hadjikakou, M.; Russell, C.; Huse, O.; Bell, C.; Scrinis, G.; et al. Ultra-Processed Foods and the Nutrition Transition: Global, Regional and National Trends, Food Systems Transformations and Political Economy Drivers. *Obes. Rev.* **2020**, *21*, e13126. [CrossRef] [PubMed]
4. Mallarino, C.; Gómez, L.F.; González-Zapata, L.; Cadena, Y.; Parra, D.C. Advertising of Ultra-Processed Foods and Beverages: Children as a Vulnerable Population. *Rev. Saude Publica* **2013**, *47*, 1006–1010. [CrossRef] [PubMed]
5. Juul, F.; Vaidean, G.; Parekh, N. Ultra-Processed Foods and Cardiovascular Diseases: Potential Mechanisms of Action. *Adv. Nutr.* **2021**, *12*, 1673–1680. [CrossRef] [PubMed]
6. Martini, D.; Godos, J.; Bonaccio, M.; Vitaglione, P.; Grosso, G. Ultra-Processed Foods and Nutritional Dietary Profile: A Meta-Analysis of Nationally Representative Samples. *Nutrients* **2021**, *13*, 3390. [CrossRef]
7. Pagliai, G.; Dinu, M.; Madarena, M.P.; Bonaccio, M.; Iacoviello, L.; Sofi, F. Consumption of Ultra-Processed Foods and Health Status: A Systematic Review and Meta-Analysis. *Br. J. Nutr.* **2021**, *125*, 308–318. [CrossRef]
8. Delpino, F.M.; Figueiredo, L.M.; Bielemann, R.M.; da Silva, B.G.C.; Dos Santos, F.S.; Mintem, G.C.; Flores, T.R.; Arcêncio, R.A.; Nunes, B.P. Ultra-Processed Food and Risk of Type 2 Diabetes: A Systematic Review and Meta-Analysis of Longitudinal Studies. *Int. J. Epidemiol.* **2022**, *51*, 1120–1141. [CrossRef]
9. Du, S.; Kim, H.; Rebholz, C.M. Higher Ultra-Processed Food Consumption Is Associated with Increased Risk of Incident Coronary Artery Disease in the Atherosclerosis Risk in Communities Study. *J. Nutr.* **2021**, *151*, 3746–3754. [CrossRef]
10. Bhave, V.M.; Oladele, C.R.; Ament, Z.; Kijpaisalratana, N.; Jones, A.C.; Couch, C.A.; Patki, A.; Garcia Guarniz, A.-L.; Bennett, A.; Crowe, M.; et al. Associations Between Ultra-Processed Food Consumption and Adverse Brain Health Outcomes. *Neurology* **2024**, *102*, e209432. [CrossRef]
11. Dai, S.; Wellens, J.; Yang, N.; Li, D.; Wang, J.; Wang, L.; Yuan, S.; He, Y.; Song, P.; Munger, R.; et al. Ultra-Processed Foods and Human Health: An Umbrella Review and Updated Meta-Analyses of Observational Evidence. *Clin. Nutr.* **2024**, *43*, 1386–1394. [CrossRef] [PubMed]
12. Isaksen, I.M.; Dankel, S.N. Ultra-Processed Food Consumption and Cancer Risk: A Systematic Review and Meta-Analysis. *Clin. Nutr.* **2023**, *42*, 919–928. [CrossRef] [PubMed]
13. Ejtahed, H.-S.; Mardi, P.; Hejrani, B.; Mahdavi, F.S.; Ghoreshi, B.; Gohari, K.; Heidari-Beni, M.; Qorbani, M. Association between Junk Food Consumption and Mental Health Problems in Adults: A Systematic Review and Meta-Analysis. *BMC Psychiatry* **2024**, *24*, 438. [CrossRef]
14. Narula, N.; Chang, N.H.; Mohammad, D.; Wong, E.C.L.; Ananthakrishnan, A.N.; Chan, S.S.M.; Carbonnel, F.; Meyer, A. Food Processing and Risk of Inflammatory Bowel Disease: A Systematic Review and Meta-Analysis. *Clin. Gastroenterol. Hepatol.* **2023**, *21*, 2483–2495.e1. [CrossRef]
15. Mannino, A.; Daly, A.; Dunlop, E.; Probst, Y.; Ponsonby, A.-L.; van der Mei, I.A.F.; Ausimmune Investigator Group; Black, L.J. Higher Consumption of Ultra-Processed Foods and Increased Likelihood of Central Nervous System Demyelination in a Case-Control Study of Australian Adults. *Eur. J. Clin. Nutr.* **2023**, *77*, 611–614. [CrossRef] [PubMed]

16. Rizzoli, R.; Biver, E.; Bonjour, J.-P.; Coxam, V.; Goltzman, D.; Kanis, J.A.; Lappe, J.; Rejnmark, L.; Sahni, S.; Weaver, C.; et al. Benefits and Safety of Dietary Protein for Bone Health—An Expert Consensus Paper Endorsed by the European Society for Clinical and Economical Aspects of Osteopororosis, Osteoarthritis, and Musculoskeletal Diseases and by the International Osteoporosis Foundation. *Osteoporos. Int.* **2018**, *29*, 1933–1948. [CrossRef]
17. Weaver, C. Nutrition and Bone Health. *Oral Dis.* **2017**, *23*, 412–415. [CrossRef]
18. Muñoz-Garach, A.; García-Fontana, B.; Muñoz-Torres, M. Nutrients and Dietary Patterns Related to Osteoporosis. *Nutrients* **2020**, *12*, 1986. [CrossRef]
19. Casey, C.; Kemp, B.J.; Cassidy, L.; Patterson, C.C.; Tully, M.A.; Hill, A.J.; McCance, D.R. The Influence of Diet and Physical Activity on Bone Density of Children Aged 5–7 Years: The Belfast HAPO Family Study. *Bone* **2023**, *172*, 116783. [CrossRef]
20. Ahmadieh, H.; Arabi, A. Vitamins and Bone Health: Beyond Calcium and Vitamin D. *Nutr. Rev.* **2011**, *69*, 584–598. [CrossRef]
21. Srour, B.; Kordahi, M.C.; Bonazzi, E.; Deschasaux-Tanguy, M.; Touvier, M.; Chassaing, B. Ultra-Processed Foods and Human Health: From Epidemiological Evidence to Mechanistic Insights. *Lancet Gastroenterol. Hepatol.* **2022**, *7*, 1128–1140. [CrossRef]
22. Peters, M.D.J.; Marnie, C.; Tricco, A.C.; Pollock, D.; Munn, Z.; Alexander, L.; McInerney, P.; Godfrey, C.M.; Khalil, H. Updated Methodological Guidance for the Conduct of Scoping Reviews. *JBI Evid. Implement.* **2021**, *19*, 3–10. [CrossRef] [PubMed]
23. Tricco, A.C.; Lillie, E.; Zarin, W.; O'Brien, K.K.; Colquhoun, H.; Levac, D.; Moher, D.; Peters, M.D.J.; Horsley, T.; Weeks, L.; et al. PRISMA Extension for Scoping Reviews (PRISMA-ScR): Checklist and Explanation. *Ann. Intern. Med.* **2018**, *169*, 467–473. [CrossRef] [PubMed]
24. Akkaya, Z.; Joseph, G.B.; Lynch, J.A.; McCulloch, C.; Gassert, F.; Pedoia, V.; Sims, W.; Lane, N.E.; Link, T.M. The Relationship Between Ultra-Processed Food Intake and Knee Cartilage Thickness in Men and Women:Data From Osteoarthritis Initiative. *Osteoarthr. Cartil.* **2024**, *32*, S357. [CrossRef]
25. Brooks, E.L.G.; Tangney, C.C.; Ritz, E.M. Ultra-Processed Food Intake and Prevalence of Osteoporosis in US Adults Aged 50 Years and Older: A Cross-Sectional Analysis. *Osteoporos. Int.* **2025**, *36*, 455–464. [CrossRef] [PubMed]
26. Lim, H.-S.; Ji, S.-I.; Hwang, H.; Kang, J.; Park, Y.-H.; Lee, H.-H.; Kim, T.-H. Relationship between Bone Density, Eating Habit, and Nutritional Intake in College Students. *J. Bone Metab.* **2018**, *25*, 181. [CrossRef]
27. Mangano, K.M.; Sahni, S.; Kiel, D.P.; Tucker, K.L.; Dufour, A.B.; Hannan, M.T. Dietary Protein Is Associated with Musculoskeletal Health Independently of Dietary Pattern: The Framingham Third Generation Study. *Am. J. Clin. Nutr.* **2017**, *105*, 714–722. [CrossRef]
28. Monjardino, T.; Lucas, R.; Ramos, E.; Lopes, C.; Gaio, R.; Barros, H. Associations between a Posteriori Defined Dietary Patterns and Bone Mineral Density in Adolescents. *Eur. J. Nutr.* **2015**, *54*, 273–282. [CrossRef]
29. Nguyen, K.; Vergne-Salle, P.; Fressinaud-Marie, A.-C.; Bertin, P. AB0709 Influence of Dietetary Intakes on Spondyloarthritis: An Observational Prospective Study. *Ann. Rheum. Dis.* **2019**, *78*, 1817. [CrossRef]
30. Noel, S.; Fouhy, L.; Flanagan, K.; Mangano, K.; Zhang, X.; Tucker, K. P23-058-23 Ultra-Processed Food Intake and Osteoporosis Among Puerto Rican Adults. *Curr. Dev. Nutr.* **2023**, *7*, 100168. [CrossRef]
31. Saito, M.; de Oliveira, B.; Macedo, A.; dos Santos, C.; Lopes, R.; Yamanaka, J.; Shimano, A. Cafeteria Diet Can Affect Bone Microarchitecture in Sedentary and Trained Male Rats. *J. Clin. Densitom.* **2024**, *27*, 101467. [CrossRef] [PubMed]
32. Shin, S.; Sung, J.; Joung, H. A Fruit, Milk and Whole Grain Dietary Pattern Is Positively Associated with Bone Mineral Density in Korean Healthy Adults. *Eur. J. Clin. Nutr.* **2015**, *69*, 442–448. [CrossRef] [PubMed]
33. Shin, S.; Hong, K.; Kang, S.W.; Joung, H. A Milk and Cereal Dietary Pattern Is Associated with a Reduced Likelihood of Having a Low Bone Mineral Density of the Lumbar Spine in Korean Adolescents. *Nutr. Res.* **2013**, *33*, 59–66. [CrossRef] [PubMed]
34. Sims, W.; Akkaya, Z.; Joseph, G.; Lynch, J.A.; Gassert, F.; McCulloch, C.; Lane, N.E.; Link, T.M. Association of Ultra-Processed Food Intake and Sex Differences in Osteoarthritis-Related Pain and Clinical Performance. *Osteoarthr. Cartil.* **2024**, *32*, S495. [CrossRef]
35. Smaira, F.I.; Mazzolani, B.C.; Peçanha, T.; Dos Santos, K.M.; Rezende, D.A.N.; Araujo, M.E.; Bonfiglioli, K.; Scagliusi, F.B.; Benatti, F.B.; De Sá Pinto, A.L.; et al. Ultra-Processed Food Consumption Associates with Higher Cardiovascular Risk in Rheumatoid Arthritis. *Clin. Rheumatol.* **2020**, *39*, 1423–1428. [CrossRef]
36. Travinsky-Shmul, T.; Beresh, O.; Zaretsky, J.; Griess-Fishheimer, S.; Rozner, R.; Kalev-Altman, R.; Penn, S.; Shahar, R.; Monsonego-Ornan, E. Ultra-Processed Food Impairs Bone Quality, Increases Marrow Adiposity and Alters Gut Microbiome in Mice. *Foods* **2021**, *10*, 3107. [CrossRef]
37. Vogel, C.; Parsons, C.; Godfrey, K.; Robinson, S.; Harvey, N.; Inskip, H.; Cooper, C.; Baird, J. Greater Access to Fast-Food Outlets Is Associated with Poorer Bone Health in Young Children. *Osteoporos. Int.* **2016**, *27*, 1011–1019. [CrossRef]
38. Wang, S.; Xie, J.; Zhai, D.; Wang, Z.; Qi, H.; Deng, M. Association between Ultra-Processed Food and Osteoporosis: A Cross-Sectional Study Based on the NHANES Database. *Nutr. Metab.* **2024**, *21*, 69. [CrossRef]
39. Wei, Y.; Zhang, T.; Liu, Y.; Liu, H.; Zhou, Y.; Su, J.; Chen, L.; Bai, L.; Xia, Y. Ultra-Processed Food Consumption, Genetic Susceptibility, and the Risk of Hip/Knee Osteoarthritis. *Clin. Nutr.* **2024**, *43*, 1363–1371. [CrossRef]

40. Zaretsky, J.; Griess-Fishheimer, S.; Carmi, A.; Travinsky Shmul, T.; Ofer, L.; Sinai, T.; Penn, S.; Shahar, R.; Monsonego-Ornan, E. Ultra-Processed Food Targets Bone Quality via Endochondral Ossification. *Bone Res.* **2021**, *9*, 14. [CrossRef]
41. Zhang, T.; Xu, X.; Chang, Q.; Lv, Y.; Zhao, Y.; Niu, K.; Chen, L.; Xia, Y. Ultraprocessed Food Consumption, Genetic Predisposition, and the Risk of Gout: The UK Biobank Study. *Rheumatology* **2024**, *63*, 165–173. [CrossRef]
42. Zhao, H.; Bai, Y.; Liu, Y.; Xing, Y.; Yan, Y.; Chen, G.; Chen, J.; Wang, X.; Chen, C.; Zhang, Z. Association of Ultraprocessed Food Consumption with Risk of Rheumatoid Arthritis: A Retrospective Cohort Study in the UK Biobank. *Am. J. Clin. Nutr.* **2024**, *120*, 927–935. [CrossRef] [PubMed]
43. Page, M.J.; McKenzie, J.E.; Bossuyt, P.M.; Boutron, I.; Hoffmann, T.C.; Mulrow, C.D.; Shamseer, L.; Tetzlaff, J.M.; Akl, E.A.; Brennan, S.E.; et al. The PRISMA 2020 Statement: An Updated Guideline for Reporting Systematic Reviews. *BMJ* **2021**, *372*, n71. [CrossRef] [PubMed]
44. Khoury, N.; Martínez, M.Á.; Garcidueñas-Fimbres, T.E.; Pastor-Villaescusa, B.; Leis, R.; De Las Heras-Delgado, S.; Miguel-Berges, M.L.; Navas-Carretero, S.; Portoles, O.; Pérez-Vega, K.A.; et al. Ultraprocessed Food Consumption and Cardiometabolic Risk Factors in Children. *JAMA Netw. Open* **2024**, *7*, e2411852. [CrossRef]
45. Suhett, L.G.; Filgueiras, M.D.S.; De Novaes, J.F.; Sukumar, D. Role of Diet Quality in Bone Health in Children and Adolescents: A Systematic Review. *Nutr. Rev.* **2023**, *82*, 47–59. [CrossRef]
46. Biver, E.; Herrou, J.; Larid, G.; Legrand, M.A.; Gonnelli, S.; Annweiler, C.; Chapurlat, R.; Coxam, V.; Fardellone, P.; Thomas, T.; et al. Dietary Recommendations in the Prevention and Treatment of Osteoporosis. *Jt. Bone Spine* **2023**, *90*, 105521. [CrossRef]
47. Calcaterra, V.; Cena, H.; Rossi, V.; Santero, S.; Bianchi, A.; Zuccotti, G. Ultra-Processed Food, Reward System and Childhood Obesity. *Children* **2023**, *10*, 804. [CrossRef] [PubMed]
48. Khandpur, N.; Neri, D.A.; Monteiro, C.; Mazur, A.; Frelut, M.-L.; Boyland, E.; Weghuber, D.; Thivel, D. Ultra-Processed Food Consumption among the Paediatric Population: An Overview and Call to Action from the European Childhood Obesity Group. *Ann. Nutr. Metab.* **2020**, *76*, 109–113. [CrossRef]
49. Luiten, C.M.; Steenhuis, I.H.; Eyles, H.; Ni Mhurchu, C.; Waterlander, W.E. Ultra-Processed Foods Have the Worst Nutrient Profile, yet They Are the Most Available Packaged Products in a Sample of New Zealand Supermarkets. *Public Health Nutr.* **2016**, *19*, 530–538. [CrossRef]
50. Martínez Leo, E.E.; Peñafiel, A.M.; Hernández Escalante, V.M.; Cabrera Araujo, Z.M. Ultra-Processed Diet, Systemic Oxidative Stress, and Breach of Immunologic Tolerance. *Nutrition* **2021**, *91–92*, 111419. [CrossRef]
51. Tristan Asensi, M.; Napoletano, A.; Sofi, F.; Dinu, M. Low-Grade Inflammation and Ultra-Processed Foods Consumption: A Review. *Nutrients* **2023**, *15*, 1546. [CrossRef] [PubMed]
52. Gioia, C.; Lucchino, B.; Tarsitano, M.G.; Iannuccelli, C.; Di Franco, M. Dietary Habits and Nutrition in Rheumatoid Arthritis: Can Diet Influence Disease Development and Clinical Manifestations? *Nutrients* **2020**, *12*, 1456. [CrossRef] [PubMed]
53. Zhang, Y.; Chen, S.; Yuan, M.; Xu, Y.; Xu, H. Gout and Diet: A Comprehensive Review of Mechanisms and Management. *Nutrients* **2022**, *14*, 3525. [CrossRef]
54. Qu, Y.; Hu, W.; Huang, J.; Tan, B.; Ma, F.; Xing, C.; Yuan, L. Ultra-Processed Food Consumption and Risk of Cardiovascular Events: A Systematic Review and Dose-Response Meta-Analysis. *eClinicalMedicine* **2024**, *69*, 102484. [CrossRef]
55. Qi, L. Mendelian Randomization in Nutritional Epidemiology. *Nutr. Rev.* **2009**, *67*, 439–450. [CrossRef] [PubMed]
56. Naska, A.; Lagiou, A.; Lagiou, P. Dietary Assessment Methods in Epidemiological Research: Current State of the Art and Future Prospects. *F1000Research* **2017**, *6*, 926. [CrossRef]
57. Popkin, B.M.; Barquera, S.; Corvalan, C.; Hofman, K.J.; Monteiro, C.; Ng, S.W.; Swart, E.C.; Taillie, L.S. Towards Unified and Impactful Policies to Reduce Ultra-Processed Food Consumption and Promote Healthier Eating. *Lancet Diabetes Endocrinol.* **2021**, *9*, 462–470. [CrossRef]

*nutrients*

MDPI

*Review*

# The Impact of Home Parenteral Nutrition on Survival and Quality of Life in Patients with Intestinal Failure and Advanced Cancer: A Comprehensive Review

**Miroslaw Perlinski [1,*] and Jacek Sobocki [2]**

[1] Fresenius Kabi Poland, Aleje Jerozolimskie 134, 02-305 Warsaw, Poland
[2] Department of General Surgery, and Clinical Nutrition, Medical Center of Postgraduate Education, Czerniakowska 231, 00-416 Warsaw, Poland; sobockij@gmail.com
* Correspondence: miroslaw.perlinski@gmail.com

**Abstract: Background and Aims:** Home parenteral nutrition (HPN) is essential in the management of chronic intestinal failure (CIF) and malignant bowel obstruction (MBO), particularly in cases where enteral feeding is not feasible. This review examines the evidence from 34 studies to evaluate the impact of HPN on survival and quality of life (QoL) in patients with MBO, CIF, and advanced cancer, as well as to identify clinical predictors of survival and address psychosocial challenges. **Methods:** A comprehensive review was conducted of 34 studies, focusing on the use of HPN in patients with MBO, CIF, and advanced cancer. Data were analyzed for survival outcomes, QoL metrics, and predictors of survival, including performance status, albumin levels, and the continuation of chemotherapy. The psychosocial aspects of HPN therapy were also assessed, particularly its influence on patient's daily lives and mental health. **Results:** Key predictors of improved survival included good performance status, higher albumin levels, and the ability to continue chemotherapy. While HPN extended survival in many cases, its impact on QoL varied significantly. Psychosocial challenges, including lifestyle disruption and mental health strain, were common among long-term HPN patients, underscoring the need for comprehensive patient support. **Conclusions:** HPN can be a life-sustaining therapy for patients with CIF, MBO, and advanced cancer, but its success depends on careful patient selection and management. Identifying predictors of survival helps optimize outcomes, while addressing psychosocial challenges is crucial to minimizing the negative impact on QoL. This review highlights the need for a balanced approach to maximize the benefits of HPN.

**Keywords:** home parenteral nutrition; chronic intestinal failure; quality of life; survival; oncology; malignant bowel obstruction; nutrition

## 1. Introduction

Home parenteral nutrition (HPN) is a critical, life-sustaining treatment for individuals with severe gastrointestinal (GI) disorders, particularly those with chronic intestinal failure (CIF) and malignant bowel obstruction (MBO) [1]. These conditions, often caused by complex diseases such as advanced cancers or severe bowel dysfunction, make normal enteral feeding insufficient or impossible, necessitating long-term intravenous nutrition. By delivering essential nutrients directly into the bloodstream, HPN supports metabolic functions and helps patients maintain body weight, muscle mass, and overall nutritional health when the digestive tract can no longer be relied upon.



https://doi.org/10.3390/nu17050905

The primary aim of HPN is to prolong survival and prevent malnutrition-related complications in patients who would otherwise face severe nutritional deficits. Research indicates that HPN significantly benefits survival rates for patients, especially when initiated early in the disease process and carefully monitored. Studies have shown that specific clinical indicators, including serum albumin levels, ECOG performance status, and hemoglobin levels, play a crucial role in determining patient outcomes, making patient selection and personalized HPN protocols essential for optimizing benefits [2,3].

However, while HPN can extend life, its long-term impact on patients' quality of life (QoL) is complex and multidimensional. Factors such as reduced mobility due to dependence on infusion equipment, increased social isolation, and the psychological burden of managing a chronic condition all contribute to QoL challenges. Patients and caregivers alike often face emotional and social difficulties, including anxiety, depression, and the need for intensive support networks. For this reason, the integration of psychosocial care and tailored patient education into HPN management has been suggested as essential to maximize quality of life [4–8].

This review synthesizes findings from 34 studies, offering a comprehensive evaluation of HPN's role in both survival and QoL outcomes. It identifies key clinical predictors that influence HPN outcomes and addresses the diverse physical, social, and psychological dimensions involved. By examining both the advantages and challenges of HPN, this review seeks to provide a balanced perspective on its application in advanced disease care and highlight strategies that may enhance patient and caregiver experiences with this complex, yet essential, therapy.

## 2. Methodology

A comprehensive literature search was conducted in the PubMed, Medline, and Cochrane databases, focusing on studies published from 2000 to 2024. Keywords included "home parenteral nutrition", "chronic intestinal failure", "quality of life", "survival", "oncology", "malignant bowel obstruction", "nutrition". The review included prospective and retrospective cohort studies, systematic reviews, and randomized controlled trials. All the studies meeting the above criteria have been included in this review. A total of 37 studies were analyzed, with a primary focus on survival, QoL, and clinical predictors.

## 3. Impact of HPN on Survival

HPN has been shown to significantly prolong survival in patients with MBO and CIF. Dzierżanowski and Sobocki found that patients receiving HPN for MBO had a median survival of 89 days. Survival was closely linked to the patient's performance status, with those scoring ECOG 0 or 1 having better outcomes. Serum albumin levels and the presence of water retention were also important prognostic factors [1].

Vashi et al. conducted a meta-analysis on patients with advanced cancer receiving HPN and found that the median survival was extended to 83 days, with the greatest benefit observed in patients who continued chemotherapy [2]. Similarly, Bozzetti et al. demonstrated that HPN in conjunction with chemotherapy significantly improved survival in cancer patients [3].

Naghibi et al. analyzed survival in patients with inoperable MBO and found that HPN prolonged survival by an average of 83 days. These findings were consistent across multiple studies, highlighting the role of HPN in stabilizing nutritional status and extending survival [1–3,9].

Several studies, including Cotogni and Fu, also emphasized the critical role of chemotherapy in improving survival. In their respective studies, patients receiving both chemotherapy and HPN experienced significantly longer survival compared to those who discontinued chemotherapy [10,11].

## 4. Impact of HPN on Quality of Life

While HPN is beneficial for survival, its effect on QoL varies greatly depending on several factors. Winkler et al. explored the QoL of patients on long-term HPN and found that patients often experience reduced physical and emotional functioning. Common issues include depression, dependence on caregivers, and disruption of social activities [4–6].

Sowerbutts et al. conducted a systematic review on the QoL of patients and caregivers receiving HPN. Their findings indicated that the frequency of infusions significantly impacted QoL, with fewer weekly infusions resulting in better physical and emotional outcomes [12]. This was also supported by Stanner et al. and Jones et al., who found that reducing infusion frequency improved overall well-being [7,13].

In pediatric populations, Tran et al. found that while HPN allowed children with intestinal failure to remain at home, it also introduced significant challenges, including dependency on caregivers and limitations in school attendance and social activities [14,15]. These findings were consistent across studies in both adult and pediatric populations, with the overall burden of HPN posing a significant challenge to QoL [4–7,12].

Other study led by French et al., explored the benefits of supportive interventions, such as telemedicine and psychological support, which helped improve patient satisfaction with HPN and mitigate some of the psychosocial challenges [16].

Patients on HPN face complex challenges that affect both their mental and physical well-being. Bond et al. emphasize that long-term HPN patients experience a high degree of dependence on caregivers, which can limit independence, mobility, and overall freedom. This reliance often results in social isolation and difficulties maintaining relationships and social activities, impacting emotional well-being [17].

Ablett et al. add that patients frequently report feelings of loneliness and limited daily life participation due to the rigid routines required by HPN. The structured nature of daily infusions and medical protocols restricts patients' ability to travel, work, or engage in social functions, which can lead to frustration and decreased life satisfaction [18].

Clement et al. extend this by noting that, while HPN improves clinical outcomes in some patients, it may exacerbate social challenges, as patients feel physically constrained by the need for regular infusions. For cancer patients, these limitations are often compounded by the mental toll of their illness, potentially leading to depression or anxiety [19].

The psychological burden of HPN, therefore, emphasizes the need for integrated psychosocial support, which can alleviate some emotional strain and improve coping skills. As studies show, providing access to social workers, psychologists, and supportive communities could positively influence the quality of life for HPN patients by fostering resilience and offering practical assistance.

The use of HPN for terminally ill patients raises ethical questions, particularly when treatment extends life without necessarily enhancing quality of life. Emanuel et al. discuss the importance of respecting patient autonomy and wishes in HPN decision making. Since HPN can be both a lifeline and a burden, it is crucial to assess whether treatment aligns with the patient's values and goals. In cases where HPN may prolong suffering, health professionals are encouraged to adopt a patient-centered approach, weighing the benefits against potential distress and preserving dignity. Additionally, ethical considerations include transparent communication with patients and families regarding the potential outcomes and limitations of HPN. Clinicians must carefully navigate the fine line between offering life-sustaining care and avoiding unnecessary interventions that might lead to a diminished quality of life [20].

Ma et al. contributes a vital perspective by showing that HPN can sustain the quality of life in patients with incurable gastric cancer undergoing salvage chemotherapy. In this study, HPN helped maintain body weight, stabilized nutritional parameters (e.g., protein, prealbumin, and cholesterol), and preserved global quality of life (QoL) scores comparable to those in the control group. These findings suggest that HPN, when introduced early, can support both nutritional health and QoL, even during aggressive treatments [21].

Bohnert et al. showed that while HPN contributes positively by stabilizing physical health and nutritional status, it often restricts daily activities, leading to limited mobility and dependence on structured routines. These limitations can contribute to feelings of social isolation and frustration, as patients are often unable to fully participate in previously enjoyed activities. This study highlights the dual effect of HPN, where physical benefits are tempered by significant social impacts [22].

Reber et al. further underscore the need for comprehensive psychosocial support in HPN care, showing that long-term HPN often leads to emotional distress and social isolation. According to their study, patients frequently report feelings of loneliness and emotional burden, indicating that HPN programs must incorporate access to social workers, counseling, and community resources to help patients cope. This psychosocial support could enhance resilience and provide a more balanced experience for individuals relying on HPN [23].

In conclusion, these studies [22,23] collectively underscore the importance of addressing not only the physical health but also the emotional and social needs of HPN patients. While HPN provides critical life-sustaining benefits, it is clear that a more integrated support system—including mental health resources and social support—can play a key role in improving overall quality of life for patients.

Kirk et al. examined the perspectives of healthcare providers in the UK regarding health-related quality of life (QoL) assessments for patients on HPN, highlighting both the importance and challenges of implementing QoL evaluations. The study revealed that although healthcare professionals recognize the value of assessing QoL to tailor care, routine implementation of these assessments is limited, with inconsistencies in both frequency and methodology across providers. This lack of standardized monitoring may lead to missed opportunities for early intervention in addressing patient needs. It was suggested that integrating regular, structured QoL assessments into HPN care would allow for a more personalized approach, helping providers identify and respond to social, emotional, and physical challenges faced by patients [24].

Hu et al. evaluated the quality of life (QoL) of adult patients on home parenteral nutrition (HPN) in North East England and Cumbria. The authors used the HPN-QOL (Home Parenteral Nutrition—Quality of Life) assessment tool, which measures various aspects of functioning and symptoms that may affect patients' quality of life on long-term HPN. Patients rated their ability to travel, physical functioning, employment, and sexual function as poor. Fatigue emerged as a primary limiting factor, having a significant impact on overall quality of life. The study also explored differences across age and gender. Male patients reported better scores for nutritional intake and support from healthcare teams but experienced more gastrointestinal symptoms. Patients over the age of 55 reported lower employment scores and more frequent gastrointestinal issues. The study suggests that QoL should be considered an integral part of clinical care for HPN patients, as many face challenges that affect their daily functioning and life satisfaction. Addressing these QoL factors may provide a more comprehensive and supportive approach to managing long-term HPN [8].

The study by Saqui et al. evaluated the impact of transitioning from stationary to portable infusion pumps on the QoL of HPN patients in Canada. It concludes that portable pumps offer significant QoL advantages over stationary models, particularly in reducing sleep disruption, increasing social flexibility, and enhancing overall satisfaction. The authors suggest that these QoL improvements justify the use of portable pumps for HPN patients, as they offer a meaningful enhancement to daily life and independence [25].

## 5. Clinical Predictors of HPN Outcomes

Several clinical and laboratory markers have been identified as critical predictors of HPN outcomes:

Performance status (ECOG): Numerous studies show that patients with an ECOG score of 0 or 1 are more likely to benefit from HPN, while those with higher scores have significantly shorter survival [1–3].

Serum albumin: Hypoalbuminemia (<2.5 g/dL) is consistently associated with poor outcomes, indicating severe malnutrition [1,2].

Hemoglobin: Anemia, even in mild forms, is linked to reduced survival, making it a key factor in determining patient eligibility for HPN [1,2].

Water retention: Patients with peripheral edema, ascites, or hydrothorax are less likely to benefit from HPN, with studies showing a significantly shorter survival in these populations [1].

Santarpia et al. examined predictive factors of survival in patients with MBO on HPN. Their findings indicated that low serum albumin levels and severe malnutrition were strongly associated with reduced survival. Patients with higher albumin levels and better overall nutritional status (e.g., absence of edema and other complications) demonstrated longer survival rates on HPN. This study emphasizes the importance of regular nutritional assessments, as maintaining higher albumin levels appears to be a critical factor for achieving better outcomes in patients on long-term HPN [26].

Ma et al. focused on identifying factors that predict survival in patients with incurable gastric cancer receiving HPN. This study highlighted that patients with a better Eastern Cooperative Oncology Group (ECOG) performance status (0–1), higher albumin levels, and improved nitrogen balance had significantly longer survival compared to those with poor ECOG scores and low albumin levels. The study underscores the importance of considering ECOG status and serum albumin as essential indicators in patient selection for HPN, as these parameters are closely associated with both survival and quality of life [21].

These findings contribute to a more comprehensive understanding of how specific clinical indicators—particularly serum albumin levels, ECOG performance status, and overall nutritional balance—impact the outcomes of patients on HPN. By closely monitoring these factors, healthcare providers can better assess which patients are likely to benefit from HPN and adjust treatment protocols to optimize results. Integrating such predictive markers into HPN management plans can significantly enhance patient outcomes, especially for those with advanced cancers and complex nutritional needs.

## 6. Clinical Outcomes of HPN

HPN has demonstrated substantial clinical benefits in stabilizing health, improving survival outcomes, and maintaining nutritional status in patients with severe intestinal failure and advanced cancer.

Pinto-Sanchez et al. focused on patients with short bowel syndrome (SBS) receiving HPN, a population at high risk of malnutrition due to limited absorptive capacity. Their study found that HPN significantly improved clinical outcomes, including stabilization of body weight, BMI, and vital nutritional parameters. HPN also helped prevent hospitalizations related to malnutrition, showcasing its role in maintaining health and reducing the need for acute medical interventions [27].

Senesse et al. explored HPN's benefits in patients with advanced cancer and intestinal failure. They observed that HPN not only improved nutritional status but also contributed to increased survival and reduced malnutrition-related complications. Cancer patients receiving HPN had greater tolerance to chemotherapy, suggesting that nutritional support through HPN may enhance treatment efficacy and improve overall clinical outcomes in oncology [28].

Cotogni et al. conducted a retrospective study on cancer patients receiving HPN, noting that it significantly stabilized their nutritional status and provided key support during cancer treatment. This study found that patients on HPN had fewer hospital admissions for complications related to malnutrition and were better able to withstand the side effects of intensive cancer therapies. These findings highlight HPN as an effective tool in enhancing the resilience of cancer patients and helping them manage the challenges of long-term treatment [10].

Bohnert et al. examined long-term clinical outcomes for patients on HPN, noting significant improvements in both survival and overall health status. The study underscored HPN's role in preventing deterioration in severely malnourished patients, particularly those with chronic or incurable conditions. By enabling patients to meet their nutritional needs at home, HPN reduced the frequency of hospitalizations, thus improving quality of life and allowing patients to remain in a more comfortable, familiar setting [22].

Reber et al. conducted a multicenter study that analyzed long-term HPN outcomes across various patient groups. Their findings indicated that HPN contributed to a sustained improvement in nutritional parameters, leading to better functional status and, in many cases, extended survival. The study emphasized the importance of personalized HPN protocols to address individual patient needs, optimizing both clinical outcomes and patient satisfaction [23].

Collectively, these studies underscore the essential role of HPN in supporting patients with complex nutritional requirements. For those with conditions such as SBS, advanced cancer, or other forms of intestinal failure, HPN provides a stable, sustainable source of nutrition, enhancing resilience, supporting treatment tolerability, and contributing to prolonged survival. Through effective HPN management, patients not only experience improved physical health but also gain greater independence and reduced reliance on hospital-based care, significantly enhancing their overall clinical outcomes.

A study by Van Gossum analyzed clinical outcomes for patients receiving HPN following bariatric surgery complications, such as anastomotic leaks, fistulas, severe protein deficiency (hypoalbuminemia), and vitamin deficiencies. The findings highlight that while HPN was effective in stabilizing nutritional status, it was primarily a temporary solution, often used as a "bridge" therapy until further surgical interventions could be performed.

Key Results:

- A high rate of rehospitalization (58%) was observed among patients on HPN, underscoring the complex needs and challenges faced by this population.
- Vascular complications, such as catheter-related issues, affected 41% of patients, indicating a significant risk associated with long-term HPN in these cases.

The study concludes that HPN provides critical support for patients with severe nutritional deficits due to postoperative complications; however, it is not without substantial risks. These findings suggest that HPN should be carefully managed, with attention to preventing complications and preparing for potential surgical solutions as patients stabilize. This research underscores the importance of assessing each patient's unique clinical factors, such as protein deficiency and post-surgical complications, to optimize HPN outcomes and anticipate possible rehospitalizations [29].

Lezo et al. [30], in their paper, provide valuable insights into long-term outcomes and the standard of care for pediatric patients on HPN due to CIF over a 28-year period in an Italian reference center. It was found that the survival rate was high among pediatric patients, with a notable percentage achieving enteral autonomy over time. For example, 74.5% of patients were weaned off HPN within two years, while dependence rates dropped significantly over time. The study also showed a decrease in catheter-related bloodstream infections (CRBSI) over the years, from 0.33 to 0.19 episodes per 1000 catheter days after implementing a taurolidine lock solution in 2011. Although QoL was not formally measured, data indicated that 90% of patients attended school, and 81% could go on holidays outside their region, with 48% participating in sports. Additionally, 67% of caregivers, mostly mothers, remained employed, suggesting a well-managed daily life despite HPN dependency. The study underscores the importance of standardized care protocols for pediatric HPN patients with CIF, which contribute to high survival rates, reduced complications, and improved quality of life. The data indicate that specialized HPN centers with multidisciplinary teams are essential in managing CIF effectively and enhancing both clinical and quality of life outcomes for pediatric patients.

Similar observations were made by Lowthian et al. and Meijerink et al. They postulate for a re-evaluation of HPN management to prioritize quality of life outcomes, suggesting that HPN care should go beyond merely sustaining life and instead focus on enhancing overall well-being. This includes better patient education, enhanced social support, and developing standardized outcome measures for quality of life to ensure that care aligns with the needs and values of patients [31,32].

## 7. Role of Chemotherapy and Other Interventions

The continuation of chemotherapy is a key factor in improving outcomes for patients on HPN. Dzierżanowski and Sobocki found that patients who continued chemotherapy while receiving HPN had significantly higher survival rates compared to those who discontinued chemotherapy [1]. Similarly, Cotogni and Dashti et al. emphasized the importance of integrating HPN with chemotherapy to maximize survival [10,33,34].

Additionally, psychological support, as highlighted by Senesse et al., were found to enhance QoL by providing additional resources for managing the challenges of HPN [28].

## 8. Limitations of Current Research and Future Directions

This review highlights the need for continued research on home parenteral nutrition (HPN) to enhance patient selection, quality of life (QoL), and treatment efficacy. Future studies should focus on:

1. Standardized QoL Assessment—develop and validate HPN-specific QoL tools (e.g., HPN-QoL, SBS-QoL) to improve cross-study comparisons and patient care.
2. Personalized Patient Selection—use predictive models to refine selection criteria, ensuring HPN benefits those most likely to improve.
3. Psychosocial Support—integrate telemedicine, support groups, and mental health interventions to mitigate the emotional burden of HPN.
4. Optimized Infusion Schedules—explore cyclic HPN and portable infusion technologies to enhance mobility and daily functioning.
5. Long-Term Outcomes and Cost-Effectiveness—assess the economic impact, hospitalizations, and alternatives like gut rehabilitation or intestinal transplantation.
6. Oncology and Palliative Care Integration—determine HPN's role in chemotherapy support, ethical considerations, and criteria for discontinuation.
7. Technological Advancements—develop AI-driven monitoring, smart infusion systems, and personalized nutrition formulations for better patient outcomes.

Future research should move beyond survival benefits, focusing on holistic patient care, improved QoL, and innovative treatment approaches to make HPN a more effective and sustainable therapy.

## 9. Conclusions

HPN is an indispensable intervention for patients with CIF and advanced cancers, particularly those who face significant challenges in achieving adequate nutrition through enteral feeding. This therapy provides critical nutritional support, helping to prevent malnutrition and extend survival for patients in both palliative and supportive care settings. Research consistently shows that HPN can stabilize or improve nutritional markers, such as albumin and hemoglobin levels, which are strongly associated with better clinical outcomes. For certain patients, especially those with favorable clinical indicators (e.g., ECOG performance scores of 0–1), HPN can sustain health and quality of life while enhancing the effectiveness of concurrent treatments like chemotherapy.

However, the impact of HPN on QoL remains multifaceted and often varies widely across individuals. QoL is influenced not only by the physical aspects of HPN, such as dependence on infusion devices and the risk of complications (e.g., catheter-related infections), but also by significant psychosocial and lifestyle factors. Studies, including those by Bohnert et al. [22] and Reber et al. [23] highlight challenges such as social isolation, decreased mobility, and emotional burdens. These findings underscore the need for a holistic approach to HPN, one that combines medical management with comprehensive psychosocial support systems, including mental health services, social networks, and educational resources for both patients and caregivers.

Key clinical predictors, including performance status, serum albumin levels, and the presence of water retention, have emerged as crucial factors for assessing the suitability and potential benefit of HPN. Patients who continue chemotherapy alongside HPN tend to have better survival outcomes, suggesting that HPN may help sustain their tolerance to aggressive cancer treatments.

Moving forward, a more personalized approach to HPN is essential, with ongoing research aimed at refining patient selection criteria to ensure that those who are most likely to benefit from HPN receive this support. Future studies should also explore the long-term psychosocial effects of HPN on both patients and caregivers, focusing on strategies to mitigate QoL challenges and improve patient satisfaction. Furthermore, advances in portable infusion technology and integrated care models, as indicated by Jones et al. and Hu et al. [8,13], have the potential to enhance patient autonomy and reduce the burden on daily life, thereby fostering a better overall experience with HPN.

Moving forward, HPN research must shift from a survival-focused approach to a patient-centered model that prioritizes personalized treatment, psychosocial well-being, and technological innovations. By integrating advanced predictive analytics, QoL-enhancing interventions, and ethical considerations, HPN can be optimized to not only sustain life but also improve the overall well-being of patients.

**Author Contributions:** M.P.: Conceptualization; Investigation; Methodology; Data curation; Validation; Visualization; Writing—original draft, Writing—review and editing. J.S.: Supervision; Validation; Investigation, Writing—review and editing. All authors have read and agreed to the published version of the manuscript.

**Funding:** This research did not receive any specific grant from funding agencies in the public, commercial, or not-for-profit sectors.

**Acknowledgments:** We would like to thank the authors and researchers of the 34 studies reviewed in this article for their invaluable contributions to the field of home parenteral nutrition and cancer care.

**Conflicts of Interest:** Author Miroslaw Perlinski was employed by the company Fresenius Kabi Poland. The remaining authors declare that the research was conducted in the absence of any commercial or financial relationships that could be construed as a potential conflict of interest.

## References


1. Dzierżanowski, T.; Sobocki, J. Survival of Patients with Multi-Level Malignant Bowel Obstruction on Total Parenteral Nutrition at Home. *Nutrients* **2021**, *13*, 889. [CrossRef] [PubMed]
2. Vashi, P.G.; Dahlk, S.; Popiel, B.; Lammersfeld, C.A.; Ireton-Jones, C.; Gupta, D. A longitudinal study investigating quality of life and nutritional outcomes in advanced cancer patients receiving home parenteral nutrition. *BMC Cancer* **2014**, *14*, 593. [CrossRef]
3. Bozzetti, F.; Cotogni, P.; Lo Vullo, S.; Pironi, L.; Giardiello, D.; Mariani, L. Development and validation of a nomogram to predict survival in incurable cachectic cancer patients on home parenteral nutrition. *Ann. Oncol.* **2015**, *26*, 2335–2340. [CrossRef] [PubMed]
4. Winkler, M.F. Quality of life in adult home parenteral nutrition patients. *JPEN J. Parenter. Enteral Nutr.* **2005**, *29*, 162–170. [CrossRef]
5. Winkler, M.F.; Hagan, E.; Wetle, T.; Smith, C.; Maillet, J.O.; Touger-Decker, R. An exploration of quality of life and the experience of living with home parenteral nutrition. *JPEN J. Parenter. Enteral Nutr.* **2010**, *34*, 395–407. [CrossRef] [PubMed]
6. Winkler, M.; Tappenden, K. Epidemiology, survival, costs, and quality of life in adults with short bowel syndrome. *Nutr. Clin. Pract.* **2023**, *38* (Suppl. 1), S17–S26. [CrossRef]
7. Stanner, H.; Zelig, R.; Rigassio Radler, D. Impact of infusion frequency on quality of life in patients receiving home parenteral nutrition. *JPEN J. Parenter. Enteral Nutr.* **2022**, *46*, 757–770. [CrossRef]
8. Hu, M.; Gemmal, L.; Leyland, H.; Leeds, J.; Mansour, D.; Thompson, N.; Mountford, C. Evaluating the quality of life of adult patients on home parenteral nutrition in North East England and Cumbria. *Clin. Nutr. ESPEN* **2017**, *22*, 116–147. [CrossRef]
9. Naghibi, M.; Smith, T.R.; Elia, M. A systematic review with meta-analysis of survival, quality of life and cost-effectiveness of home parenteral nutrition in patients with inoperable malignant bowel obstruction. *Clin. Nutr.* **2015**, *34*, 825–837. [CrossRef]
10. Cotogni, P.; Stragliotto, S.; Ossola, M.; Collo, A.; Riso, S.; On Behalf of the Intersociety Italian Working Group for Nutritional Support in Cancer. The Role of Nutritional Support for Cancer Patients in Palliative Care. *Nutrients* **2021**, *13*, 306. [CrossRef]
11. Fu, M.; Shi, M.; Li, M.; He, G. The Experience and Needs of Living with Home Parenteral Nutrition in Adult Patients: A Meta-Synthesis of Qualitative Studies. *J. Clin. Nurs.* **2024**, *33*, 4468–4483. [CrossRef]
12. Sowerbutts, A.M.; Jones, D.; Lal, S.; Burden, S. Quality of life in patients and in family members of those receiving home parenteral support with intestinal failure: A systematic review. *Clin. Nutr.* **2021**, *40*, 3210–3220. [CrossRef] [PubMed]
13. Jones, D.; Lal, S.; French, C.; Sowerbutts, A.M.; Gittins, M.; Gabe, S.; Brundrett, D.; Culkin, A.; Calvert, C.; Thompson, B.; et al. Investigating the Relationship between Home Parenteral Support and Needs-Based Quality of Life in Patients with Chronic Intestinal Failure: A National Multi-Centre Longitudinal Cohort Study. *Nutrients* **2023**, *15*, 622. [CrossRef]
14. Tran, L.C.; Lazonby, G.; Morello, R.; Pham, D.; Ellis, D.; Goldthorpe, J.; Iglesias, N.; Steele, J.; Zamvar, V.; Puntis, J.W.L.; et al. How good is quality-of-life for children receiving home parenteral nutrition?—A pilot study. *Clin. Nutr. ESPEN* **2019**, *29*, 119–124. [CrossRef] [PubMed]
15. Ross, V.M.; Smith, C.E. Longitudinal trends in quality of life after starting home parenteral nutrition: A randomized controlled study of telemedicine. *Clin. Nutr.* **2008**, *27*, 314–316. [CrossRef] [PubMed]
16. French, C.; Lal, S.; Jones, D.; Sowerbutts, A.M.; Brundrett, D.; Burch, N.; Calvert, C.; Cooper, S.C.; Donnellan, C.; Forbes, A.; et al. Impact of home parenteral nutrition on family members: A national multi-centre cross-sectional study. *Clin. Nutr.* **2022**, *41*, 500–507. [CrossRef]
17. Bond, A.; Soop, M.; Taylor, M.; Purssell, H.; Abraham, A.; Teubner, A.; Carlson, G.; Lal, S. Home parenteral nutrition and the older adult: Experience from a national intestinal failure unit. *Clin. Nutr.* **2020**, *39*, 1418–1422. [CrossRef]
18. Ablett, J.; Vasant, D.H.; Taylor, M.; Cawley, C.; Lal, S. Poor Social Support and Unemployment Are Associated with Negative Affect in Home Parenteral Nutrition-Dependent Patients With Chronic Intestinal Failure. *JPEN J. Parenter. Enteral Nutr.* **2019**, *43*, 534–539. [CrossRef]
19. Clement, D.S.; Brown, S.E.; Naghibi, M.; Cooper, S.C.; Tesselaar, M.E.; van Leerdam, M.E.; Ramage, J.K.; Srirajaskanthan, R. Feasibility of Home Parenteral Nutrition in Patients with Intestinal Failure Due to Neuroendocrine Tumours: A Systematic Review. *Nutrients* **2023**, *15*, 3787. [CrossRef]
20. Emanuel, A.; Rosenberger, F.; Krampitz, J.; Decker-Baumann, C.; Märten, A.; Jäger, D.; Rötzer, I. Effects of parenteral nutrition + best supportive nutritional care vs. best supportive nutritional care alone on quality of life in patients with pancreatic cancer-a secondary analysis of PANUSCO. *Support. Care Cancer* **2024**, *32*, 466. [CrossRef]
21. Ma, C.J.; Huang, C.W.; Yeh, Y.S.; Tsai, H.L.; Su, W.C.; Chang, T.K.; Sun, L.C.; Shih, Y.L.; Yu, F.J.; Wu, D.C.; et al. Supplemental home parenteral nutrition improved nutrition status with comparable quality of life in malnourished unresectable/metastatic gastric cancer receiving salvage chemotherapy. *Support. Care Cancer* **2021**, *29*, 1977–1988. [CrossRef]

22. Bohnert, H.; Maurer, M.; Calder, P.C.; Pratschke, J.; Thul, P.; Müller, V. Efficacy of a long-term home parenteral nutrition regimen containing fish oil-derived n-3 polyunsaturated fatty acids: A single-centre, randomized, double blind study. *Nutr. J.* **2018**, *17*, 113. [CrossRef]
23. Reber, E.; Staub, K.; Schönenberger, K.A.; Stanga, A.; Leuenberger, M.; Pichard, C.; Schuetz, P.; Mühlebach, S.; Stanga, Z. Management of Home Parenteral Nutrition: Complications and Survival. *Ann. Nutr. Metab.* **2021**, *77*, 46–55. [CrossRef] [PubMed]
24. Kirk, C.; Pearce, M.S.; Mathers, J.C.; Thompson, N.P.; Gemmell, L.; Jones, D.E. Quality of life and home parenteral nutrition: A survey of UK healthcare professionals' knowledge, practice and opinions. *J. Hum. Nutr. Diet.* **2023**, *36*, 687–696. [CrossRef]
25. Saqui, O.; Fernandes, G.; Allard, J.P. Quality of life analysis during transition from stationary to portable infusion pump in home parenteral nutrition patients: A Canadian experience. *Nutr. Clin. Pract.* **2014**, *29*, 131–141. [CrossRef]
26. Santarpia, L.; Orefice, R.; Alfonsi, L.; Marra, M.; Contaldo, F.; Pasanisi, F. The Anxiety Burden in Patients with Chronic Intestinal Failure on Long-Term Parenteral Nutrition and in Their Caregivers. *Nutrients* **2024**, *16*, 1168. [CrossRef] [PubMed]
27. Pinto-Sanchez, M.I.; Gadowsky, S.; McKenzie, S.; Raphael, M.J.; Childs, A.; Thabane, M.; Hansen, S.; Marshall, J.K.; Armstrong, D. Anxiety, Depression and Quality of Life Improve After One Month and Three Months of Home Parenteral Nutrition: A Pilot Study in a Canadian Population. *J. Can. Assoc. Gastroenterol.* **2019**, *2*, 178–185. [CrossRef]
28. Senesse, P.; Tadmouri, A.; Culine, S.; Dufour, P.R.; Seys, P.; Radji, A.; Rotarski, M.; Balian, A.; Chambrier, C. A prospective observational study assessing home parenteral nutrition in patients with gastrointestinal cancer: Benefits for quality of life. *J. Pain Symptom Manag.* **2015**, *49*, 183–191.e2. [CrossRef] [PubMed]
29. Van Gossum, A.; Pironi, L.; Chambrier, C.; Dreesen, M.; Brandt, C.F.; Santarpia, L.; Joly, F. Home parenteral nutrition (HPN) in patients with post-bariatric surgery complications. *Clin. Nutr.* **2017**, *36*, 1345–1348. [CrossRef]
30. Lezo, A.; D'Eusebio, C.; Riboldi, L.; Baldini, L.; Spada, M. HPN Standard of Care and Long-Term Outcomes of CIF Pediatric Patients: Twenty-Eight Years' Experience in a Reference Center. *Front. Nutr.* **2022**, *9*, 868273. [CrossRef]
31. Lowthian, T.J. Why are we settling? Improving home parenteral nutrition quality of life outcomes. *JPEN J. Parenter. Enteral Nutr.* **2023**, *47*, 827–829. [CrossRef] [PubMed]
32. Beurskens-Meijerink, J.; Huisman-de Waal, G.; Wanten, G. Evaluation of quality of life and caregiver burden in home parenteral nutrition patients: A cross sectional study. *Clin. Nutr. ESPEN* **2020**, *37*, 50–57. [CrossRef] [PubMed]
33. Dashti, H.S.; Rhyner, J.J.; Mogensen, K.M.; Godbole, M.; Saxena, R.; Compher, C.; Winkler, M.F. Infusion timing and sleep habits of adults receiving home parenteral and enteral nutrition: A patient-oriented survey study. *JPEN J. Parenter. Enteral Nutr.* **2023**, *47*, 130–139. [CrossRef] [PubMed]
34. Cotogni, P.; De Carli, L.; Passera, R.; Amerio, M.L.; Agnello, E.; Fadda, M.; Ossola, M.; Monge, T.; De Francesco, A.; Bozzetti, F. Longitudinal study of quality of life in advanced cancer patients on home parenteral nutrition. *Cancer Med.* **2017**, *6*, 1799–1806. [CrossRef]

MDPI AG
Grosspeteranlage 5
4052 Basel
Switzerland
Tel.: +41 61 683 77 34

*Nutrients* Editorial Office
E-mail: nutrients@mdpi.com
www.mdpi.com/journal/nutrients

www.ingramcontent.com/pod-product-compliance
Lightning Source LLC
Chambersburg PA
CBHW062031220926
51850CB00010B/2511